Updates in Clinical Dermatology

Series Editors

John Berth-Jones
Chee Leok Goh
Howard I. Maibach

More information about this series at http://www.springer.com/series/13203

Becky S. Li • Howard I. Maibach

Editors

Ethnic Skin and Hair and Other Cultural Considerations

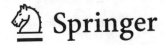 Springer

Editors
Becky S. Li
Department of Dermatology
Howard University Hospital
Washington, DC
USA

Howard I. Maibach
Department of Dermatology
University of California San Francisco
San Francisco, CA
USA

ISSN 2523-8884   ISSN 2523-8892   (electronic)
Updates in Clinical Dermatology
ISBN 978-3-030-64832-9   ISBN 978-3-030-64830-5   (eBook)
https://doi.org/10.1007/978-3-030-64830-5

This Springer imprint is published by the registered company Springer Nature Switzerland AG
The registered company address is: Gewerbestrasse 11, 6330 Cham, Switzerland

To my family, friends, and mentors –
Without you, I would not be who I am
and where I am today.

Preface

The United States of America is becoming increasingly diverse. According to projections by the Bureau of the Census, by 2044, there will be no clear racial or ethnic majority in the USA. Soon, ethnic and racial minorities will comprise over half of the population. With this demographic shift and the resultant increase in people of color seeking dermatological care, physicians must become adept at recognizing and treating dermatologic disease processes in patients of color. Inherent in effectively treating these cutaneous diseases is sufficient understanding of skin pigmentation, differences in skin structure and function in different populations, and common cutaneous manifestations in persons of color. It is also important to consider how historical, socioeconomic, and cultural factors can hinder the delivery of care, leading to health disparities for these populations. The aim of this text is to help educate dermatologists and general physicians of the challenges involved in treating skin of color in culturally appropriate ways.

Distinctly broken up into three parts for ease of use, the reader enters the text through a series of chapters meant to introduce the physician to the anatomical structure and makeup of patient with skin of color as well as the evolution of basic concepts for understanding and treatment. The second and longest part looks at diseases and cosmetic concerns covering some of the most common issues for patients of color. The last part offers cultural considerations to treatment and care. *Ethnic Skin and Hair* is complete with color photos alongside real patient case studies. Written by some of the leading names in dermatological treatment of skin of color, this text will prove to be a concise and thorough tool for dermatologists at every stage in their career.

We hope this text can be an addition to the repertoire available for skin of color, as well as inspire others to continue to investigate and educate us all. We sincerely thank all the committed contributing authors to skin of color.

Washington, DC, USA
San Francisco, CA, USA

Becky S. Li
Howard I. Maibach

Contents

Contributors

Oma N. Agbai, MD University of California, Davis, Department of Dermatology, Sacramento, CA, USA

Aya J. Alame, MD University of Texas Southwestern Medical Center, Department of Dermatology, Dallas, TX, USA

Andrew F. Alexis, MD, MPH Mount Sinai Morningside and Mount Sinai West, Department of Dermatology, Mount Sinai Doctors, New York, NY, USA

Umer Ansari, MD University of Maryland Medical Systems, Baltimore, MD, USA

Katherine Omueti Ayoade, MD, PhD University of Texas Southwestern Medical Center, Department of Dermatology, Dallas, TX, USA

Enzo Berardesca, MD San Gallicano Dermatological Institute, Rome, Italy

Micah Christine Brown, MS Howard University College of Medicine, Washington, DC, USA

Valerie D. Callender, MD Howard University College of Medicine, Department of Dermatology, Washington, DC, USA
Callender Dermatology & Cosmetic Center, Glenn Dale, MD, USA

Norma Cameli, MD San Gallicano Dermatological Institute, Department of Dermatology, Rome, Italy

Jessica Dawson, BS University of Washington School of Medicine, Seattle, WA, USA

Nada Elbuluk, MD, MSc Department of Dermatology, University of Southern California, Keck School of Medicine, Los Angeles, CA, USA

Steven R. Feldman, MD, PhD Wake Forest School of Medicine, Department of Dermatology, Winston-Salem, NC, USA

Donald A. Glass II, MD, PhD University of Texas Southwestern Medical Center, Department of Dermatology, Dallas, TX, USA

Valerie M. Harvey, MD, MPH Hampton Roads Center for Dermatology, The Hampton University Skin of Color Research Institute, Hampton University, Hampton, VA, USA

William W. Huang, MD Wake Forest School of Medicine, Department of Dermatology, Winston-Salem, NC, USA

Chesahna Kindred, MD, MBA, FAAD Kindred Hair and Skin Center, Columbia, MD, USA

Department of Dermatology, Howard University Hospital, Washington, DC, USA

Loren Krueger, MD The Ronald O. Perelman Department of Dermatology, New York University, New York, NY, USA

Porcia B. Love, MD River Region Dermatology and Laser, Montgomery, AL, USA

University of Alabama School of Medicine, River Region Dermatology and Laser, Montgomery, AL, USA

Howard I. Maibach, MD University of California, San Francisco, School of Medicine, Department of Dermatology, San Francisco, CA, USA

Karra K. Manier, BA, MA Howard University College of Medicine, Washington, DC, USA

Amy J. McMichael, MD Wake Forest School of Medicine, Department of Dermatology, Winston-Salem, NC, USA

Callie R. Mitchell, BS River Region Dermatology and Laser, Montgomery, AL, USA

Aldo Morrone, MD San Gallicano Dermatological Institute IRCCS, Rome, Italy

Andrea T. Murina, MD Tulane Medical Center, Tulane University, Department of Dermatology, New Orleans, LA, USA

Kamaria Nelson, MD, MHS George Washington University, Medical Faculty Associates, Department of Dermatology, Washington, DC, USA

Amanda A. Onalaja, MD Loyola University Medical Center, Maywood, IL, USA

Lauren C. Payne, MD, MS, FAAD Veteran Affairs Medical Center, Howard University Hospital, George Washington University, Department of Dermatology, Washington, DC, USA

Jodie Raffi, BA UC Irvine School of Medicine, Department of Dermatology, Beverly Hills, CA, USA

Cynthia O. Robinson, MD Dermatology Associates of Uptown, Cedar Hill, TX, USA

Edward W. Seger, MS Wake Forest School of Medicine, Department of Dermatology, Winston-Salem, NC, USA

Titilola Sode, MD U.S. Dermatology Partners Dallas Hillcrest, Dallas, TX, USA

U.S. Dermatology Partner Dallas Presbyterian, Dallas, TX, USA

Whitney A. Talbott, MD, BSc Icahn School of Medicine at Mount Sinai, Department of Dermatology, New York, NY, USA

Susan C. Taylor, MD Department of Dermatology, Perelman School of Medicine at the University of Pennsylvania, Philadelphia, PA, USA

Part I

Introduction/Overview

Defining Skin of Color

Amanda A. Onalaja and Susan C. Taylor

Abbreviations

AD	Atopic dermatitis
AGA	Androgenetic alopecia
AKN	Acne keloidalis nuchae
CAM	Complementary and alternative medicine
CCCA	Central centrifugal cicatricial alopecia
DLE	Discoid lupus erythematosus
EDP	Erythema dyschromicum perstans
LP	Lichen planus
PFB	Pseudofolliculitis barbae
PIH	Postinflammatory hyperpigmentation
PR	Pityriasis rosea
SLE	Systemic lupus erythematosus

A. A. Onalaja
Loyola University Medical Center,
Maywood, IL, USA
e-mail: Amanda_Onalaja@URMC.Rochester.edu

S. C. Taylor (✉)
Department of Dermatology, Perelman School of
Medicine at the University of Pennsylvania,
Philadelphia, PA, USA
e-mail: Susan.Taylor@pennmedicine.upenn.edu

Introduction

Skin of color is generally used to identify individuals of South and East Asian, African, Native American, and Pacific Island descent. This population is rapidly growing worldwide [1]. The United States Census Bureau currently estimates that more than half of the country's population will identify as a race other than non-Hispanic white by the year 2044 [2]. The implication for dermatologists as this population increases is that there will be an increased demand for healthcare by individuals with skin of color. The ability to recognize the vast clinical presentations of skin and hair disorders in these patients will be critical. One barrier to understanding cutaneous diversity is in the nuances in the terminology found in the literature. The term "ethnic skin" has historically been used in dermatology and has come under recent controversy. The descriptor has been critiqued as being a reductive catch-all term used to refer to non-Caucasian individuals [3, 4]. The gold standard for classifying skin types is the well-known Fitzpatrick scale. With this scale, individuals are classified based on their skin's response to UV radiation [5]. Individuals with skin of color are often regarded as having IV, V, and VI Fitzpatrick phototype. However, this scale has been called into question as being too Eurocentric since the propensity to "suntan" and "sunburn" do not usually relate to members of the black community [6]. Others have developed

© Springer Nature Switzerland AG 2021
B. S. Li, H. I. Maibach (eds.), *Ethnic Skin and Hair and Other Cultural Considerations*, Updates in
Clinical Dermatology, https://doi.org/10.1007/978-3-030-64830-5_1

skin classification systems that may be more clinically relevant to skin of color [7–10].

Despite the limitations of the words and categories used to classify humans as members of social groups, cutaneous diseases may have a genetic component that causes them to manifest differently in certain populations [11]. If population-based differences in skin disorders do in fact exist, it is reasonable to assume that defining and understanding those differences will lead to better care and better treatment outcomes. This chapter will provide an overview on the current literature addressing differences in skin of color including special considerations on the dermatological implications of cultural practices by individuals with skin of color, variations in normal pigmentation, variations in the clinical presentation of skin disorders in skin of color and non-skin of color, and prevalent skin disorders in patients with skin of color.

Cultural Practices and the Dermatological Implications: An Overview

According to the United States Office of Management and Budget, the individuals with skin of color in the United States are African American/Black, Alaskan Native, American Indian, Asian American, Hispanic/Latino, Native Hawaiian, or other Pacific Islander [12]. Currently about 40% of the US population are people of color, with this percentage expected to exceed over 50% by the year 2044. The resultant increase in individuals with skin of color seeking dermatological care requires an understanding of how these individuals interact with the healthcare system. It is also important to know how their cultural practices affect healthcare delivery. It has been documented in numerous studies that even when accounting for a lack of healthcare access, patients of color generally receive poorer quality of care when receiving healthcare [13, 14]. When compared to patients of European descent, Hispanics and African Americans experience more discrimination on the part of healthcare

providers [15]. Unfortunately, this often leads to poorer health outcomes [16]. Cultural competency can be partially defined as an understanding of "the importance of social and cultural influences on patients' health beliefs and behaviors" [17]. Therefore, dermatologists may be able to ameliorate the disparities in healthcare for patients of color by improving their communication on disease and treatments with their patients. This requires dermatologists to be receptive to diverse cultural health beliefs on hair and skin in order to better understand how to tailor care to patients of color.

Hispanic Cultural Practices and the Dermatological Implications

The United States Census Bureau uses the term "Hispanic or Latino" in reference to a person of Cuban, Mexican, Puerto Rican, South and Central American, or other Spanish culture or origin, regardless of race [18]. Between 2000 and 2010, the Hispanic population in the United States grew to 50.5 million (roughly 16%) with about three-quarters of this population reported as Mexican, Puerto Rican, or Cuban descent. Additionally, in 2000 and in 2010, the "Some Other Race" population was reportedly the third largest racial group primarily due to reporting by Hispanics who did not identify with any of the other US Office of Management and Budget race categories [19]. Clearly, Hispanics in the United States are not racially or ethnically homogenous, and their socioeconomic status and views on healthcare and health risks vary significantly depending on country of origin [20]. However, they may share similar values and beliefs about healthcare with Hispanics born outside the United States.

For Hispanics, the concept known as *familismo* encompasses loyalty to the family and is more important than the needs of the individual. However, studies indicate that this prioritization of family over the individual may lessen with acculturation [21]. Patients may feel the need to include their loved ones in decisions about treatment options and/or lifestyle modifications. In addition, traditional gender roles tend to apply to Hispanic families. Women may be considered the primary caretakers, but men will often speak to their wives about health concerns [22]. *Machismo*, meaning the set of identities and attitudes associated with the Hispanic concept of masculinity, may also have an impact on healthcare. If men believe that they are expected to behave in ways that are considered fearless, they may suffer from illnesses for as long as necessary before seeking medical care. On the other hand, due to the cultural expectation that Hispanic men must provide for their households, illnesses that affect an ability to fulfill these expectations may paradoxically increase patient adherence to medical care [22].

Other cultural views that can influence health behavior in Hispanics are *personalismo* and *fatalismo*. The term *fatalismo* refers to the belief that God's will directs each individual and that the fate of disease processes cannot be altered because it is part of destiny [23]. *Personalismo* refers to the expectation that a Hispanic patient will garner a kinship with the healthcare provider. Thus, *fatalismo* and a lack of *personalismo* may result in Hispanic patients being less likely to adhere to their recommended treatment plan. Many Hispanic health beliefs take origin from a variety of sources. Interestingly, there are some health beliefs in the form of folk medicine that have withstood the ethnic, racial, and geographical divide of Hispanic populations. *Curanderos* are healers who use herbs and plants to treat sicknesses. *Santeros* are healer that use *santería*, a religion that petitions the assistance of the spirits, to treat individuals. These naturalist healers are sought to aid in social, physical, and psychological matters. In one survey, 17% of Hispanics sought care from a folk healer, 32% from a healthcare professional, and the remainder self-treated [24]. Folk medicine has a long-standing place in Hispanic-American culture. It is in the best interest of dermatologists to be able to understand these cultural practices and respect the patient's identity.

African American Cultural Practices and the Dermatological Implications

It is well known that the origins of humanity have been traced back to the continent of Africa. In a literal sense then, all human beings despite racial identification are "of African descent." However, this phrase is more often connoted for individuals that racially identify as black and African American. This can be confusing as race and ethnicity are not clear-cut categories and are not always readily apparent. Nevertheless, black people make up an impressive percentage of the global population. While the exact numbers are difficult to obtain, there were an estimated 970 million individuals that occupied sub-Saharan Africa in 2015 [25]. Coupled with the estimated more than 140 million individuals that make up the African diaspora [26], it can be estimated that blacks make up almost 16% of the world's 7 billion people. In 2010, over 42 million blacks were counted by the Unites States Census Bureau [27]. Surveys on the top dermatological concerns for black Americans have revealed that acne, pigmentary disorders, alopecia, acne keloidalis nuchae, scalp folliculitis, and keloids appear frequently [28]. Even when taking geographical location into account, variations in the diagnoses reported in the black population are seemingly small [28, 29]. This section serves as a brief dermatological guide on the cultural practices of African Americans and will empower physicians to have informed conversations with their patients regarding them.

Skin care in the African American community tends to center on achieving skin that is adequately moisturized and maintaining an even complexion. Skin moisturizers come in the form of oils, creams, lotions, and ointments that are applied and often reapplied over the course of a day. Xerosis can cause the skin to itch, crack, and bleed. It can also cause an undesirable appearance that patients may refer to as "ashy." Patients who continue to complain of xerosis despite use of ointments and creams may have an underlying diagnosis of atopic dermatitis and may require a prescription treatment.

African Americans encompass a spectrum of darker skin tones, and pigmentary disorders occur frequently in this population. An even skin complexion is highly desired by this population, and the use of skin lightening agents for hyperpigmentation is common. It is important to acknowledge the negative psychological impact pigmentary disorders may have on patients with skin of color. While many Africans and African Americans love the natural hue of their skin, skin bleaching is not an uncommon practice for some segments of the population since having lighter skin often affords certain social benefits [30, 31]. Despite the racial implications the practice of skin bleaching may have, it is important for dermatologists to discourage patients from seeking skin bleaching products, particularly those that contain corticosteroids, heavy metals, and high levels of hydroquinone.

The culture of hair and hair styling for African American men and women reflects their history. Hairstyles could indicate tribal and other social status in early African civilizations [32]. The ravaging of Africa due to the transatlantic slave trade displaced over 12.5 million Africans [33]. Those that made it to the New World and were enslaved were forced to denounce their former hair care practices. Despite slavery being abolished in most of the world during the nineteenth century, the shadow of white supremacy continued to mount a social pressure for black people in the United States. Many African Americans sought to blend in and change their hair accordingly by chemically straightening (also called relaxers or perms) it well into the 1950s and 1960s. The black hair industry grew to meet the needs of thousands of new consumers. Black entrepreneurs at the time such as Madame C.J. Walker, the first female self-made millionaire in the United States, made their money selling hair products.

A change emerged in the 1960s with the afro during the Civil Rights Movement to protest against racial segregation and oppression. The black power fist comb or afro pick was designed in the 1970s as a response to the buzzing racial politics at that time. In the 1980s and 1990s, the

use of chemical straightening was widespread. With the turn of the century, braids, hair twists, hair extensions, and straightened hair styles reigned supreme. The hairstyling culture for African American women today and for the last decade has continued to diversify and encompasses all of the above as well as the utilization of fashion wigs.

Currently, the two predominant hair style categories for women of African descent are natural and chemically treated. "Natural hair" connotes hair that has not been permanently straightened with relaxers. The clinical impact of long-term chemical straightening or straightening with heat has not yet been determined; however, there are reports in the literature of scarring alopecia, hair color change, and chemical burns following the application of relaxers [34]. Twists, braids, and hair extensions are popular styles for those with natural hair. These styles are often used to camouflage existing areas of alopecia. They are also seen as "protective styles" for some in the African diaspora and can be worn for a period of a couple days to a couple of months. The seemingly protective nature of these styles is that they allow the wearer to cease manipulation of their hair and reduce "weathering" of the hair during the duration of the style. However, traction alopecia can be a complication of these styles if the braids or twists are pulled too tightly or if the adhesive to secure the wig or hair extensions are improperly removed.

Asian Cultural Practices and the Dermatological Implications

Asia is the world's largest continent boasting a population of over 4 billion people. In 2010 in the United States, Asians made up almost 5% of the total population. Among this population, the majority identified as Chinese (except Taiwanese), Asian Indian, and Filipino as the third largest group [35]. Suffice to say, Asians come from numerous cultural backgrounds and encompass a range of skin phototypes from skin type II to VI [28]. Additionally, there are certain skin disorders that have different manifestations, prevalence, and social significance among Asian patients. For example, vitiligo can negatively impact quality of life among South Asians [36]. These patients are often considered to be outcasts. East Asian women consider porcelain-white facial skin to be the ultimate mark of beauty and therefore tanning is highly avoided. With widespread immigration, the sharing of certain Asian traditions has led to a diversity of cultural practices seen here in the United States. Traditional approaches to treatments of the body and the skin have become popular in their own right (i.e., herbal medicine and acupuncture) or claimed to be within the realm of complementary and alternative medicine (CAM). With the increasing prevalence of Asian cultural traditions being practiced outside of Asia, dermatologists should be aware of the diverse approaches for treating skin conditions that their patients might integrate into their own care.

Herbal medicine is widely used in Asia and the United States [37]. It is the use of plants and other herbs for therapeutic purposes. The plant material can be used fresh or dry and be prepared into powders, topical agents, tablets, or capsules. There are claims in the literature that herbal medicine can be used to treat a variety of skin conditions including psoriasis, atopic dermatitis, and cutaneous fungal infections; however, evidence-based studies to show its benefit are scant [38–41]. The potential harm with herbal medicine is in the unregulated preparation. Reports have described an assortment of adverse effects from herbal medicine [42, 43]. It is difficult to know whether contamination of herbal medicines with other herbs, pathogens, pesticides, heavy metals, or drugs could account for these reactions [44].

Acupuncture is considered a subset of traditional Chinese medicine and involves using a combination of needles, heat, and pressure to stimulate specific points on the body, known as acupoints [45]. This healing process is intended to balance *Qi*, the body's energy. The National Health Interview Survey of 2002 revealed that 1.1% (approximately two million) of adults in the United States had used acupuncture within the past 12 months [46]. Dermatologically, acu-puncture has been documented as a treatment for several disorders and cosmetic concerns such as atopic dermatitis, urticaria, herpes zoster, psoriasis, acne, melasma, rhytides, and hyperhidrosis [47, 48]. Acupuncture is regarded as a safe procedure when it is practiced by a well-trained, qualified practitioner [49].

Cupping therapy is an ancient therapeutic procedure practiced throughout various civilizations. It was described in the early Han dynasty that with "acupuncture and cupping, more than half of the ills [are] cured" [50]. The most common variations of cupping are characterized as dry cupping or wet cupping. Dry cupping involves applying a heated cup directly on the skin of the back, abdomen, chest, or buttock. Negative pressure suctions the skin into the cup and patients are often left with circular erythematous patches due to traumatized superficial blood vessels. Wet cupping is different from dry cupping in that it involves puncturing the skin and bloodletting [50]. Cupping has been used to treat pain, cardiovascular diseases, immune system diseases and metabolic diseases, herpes zoster, Behçet disease, secondary amenorrhea, depression and anxiety, fatigue, metabolic syndrome, and acne vulgaris [51]. There are limited quality studies on the dermatological application of cupping; therefore, the clinical evidence for cupping is low.

Moxibustion is a traditional technique that, like acupuncture, stimulates the body's vital energy. Moxibustion involves the burning of the herb *Artemesia vulgaris* L. close to the skin, usually near acupuncture points. A systematic review of moxibustion for pain found moxibustion reduced pain associated with osteoarthritis and may reduce pain in scleroma and herpes zoster [52]. Acupuncture and moxibustion are recommended in Chinese medicine clinical practice guidelines for treating the acute symptoms of herpes zoster [53], and are frequently used in combination in clinical practice. A literature review showed overall insufficient evidence from high quality studies reporting positive outcomes of this practice [54].

Ayurveda, Yoga and naturopathy, Unani, Siddha, and Homeopathy comprise the AYUSH system. The AYUSH system is popular in India because of its accessibility, low cost, and perceived lack of side effects [55]. Other countries including Russia, Germany, Italy, the United Kingdom, and the United States have also taken an interest in Ayurveda [56–58]. Ayurveda employs techniques such as removal of toxins, herbal and dietary regimens, and behavioral advice into the treatment of various diseases. The three main constitutional types, *vaata*, *pitta*, and *kapha* are understood to present as differing skin pathologies and require different Ayurvedic prescriptions [59]. Unfortunately, toxic amounts of heavy metals such as arsenic, lead, cadmium, and mercury have been shown to be included in certain Ayurvedic preparations [37].

Coining is a form of dermabrasion therapy still widely practiced in China and South East Asia, especially Vietnam. This ancient method of treatment is employed to rid the body of negative energies. This technique is done by lubricating the skin with oil or an ointment and using a coin to firmly and repetitively rub the skin. There is one case of a 45-year-old female that sustained serious injury from a severe burn due to receiving coining treatment [60].

Normal Variations in Individuals with Skin of Color

Skin pigmentation is generally believed to be an adaptive response of humans to the environment, namely ultraviolet rays [61]. Skin pigmentation can vary among members of the same ethnic background and even on a single individual. For example, some darkly pigmented areas are regarded as normal, such as the extensor joints and the knuckles. Knowledge about normal variations in skin color is needed to understand abnormal skin discolorations.

Pigmentary Demarcation Lines

Pigmentary demarcation lines are the physiological abrupt transition between light and dark skin. They were first documented in 1913 in the Japanese population as lines spreading over the upper and lower extremities [62]. Various cross-sectional reports, surveys, and case reports have expanded the characteristics of pigmentary demarcation lines, and there are currently eight documented types in the literature [63] (Table 1.1). One study reported that about 79% percent of black women have at least one type of pigmentary demarcation line as opposed to about 15% of white women [64]. These lesions are benign and require no clinical intervention. However, pigmentary demarcation lines must be distinguished from other varied patterns of pigmentation in the skin such as pigmentary mosaicism as this may warrant additional workup. There are several variations in pigmentation that typically follow lines of Blaschko and can be associated with systemic pathology including linear and whorled nevoid hypermelanosis and hypomelanosis of Ito [65]. Therefore, patients with large areas of cutaneous involvement should be considered for pathologic workup.

Longitudinal Melanonychia

Longitudinal melanonychia are longitudinal brown-black pigmented nail bands commonly found in individuals with skin of color including those of African and Asian descent [66]. The number of affected nails and the degree of pigmentation tends to increase with age [67, 68].

Table 1.1 Pigmentary demarcation lines

Type	Location
Type A	Lateral area of upper anterior arm, extending across to pectoral region
Type B	Posterior medial leg
Type C	Vertical hypopigmented patches in pre- and para-sternal skin
Type D	Skin surrounding posterior medial spine
Type E	Lateral chest, extending from mid-third of clavicle to periareolar area
Type F	V-shaped hyperpigmented patch extending from malar prominence to temple
Type G	W-shaped hyperpigmented patch extending from malar prominence to temple
Type H	Hyperpigmented patches extending from angle of mouth to lateral chin

The main goal for the clinician regarding longitudinal melanonychia is to exclude subungual melanoma. Suggestive features of malignant melanoma of the nail include the presence of longitudinal melanonychia confined to only one finger or toe, the sudden appearance in adulthood, irregular shape or color variation of the band, and the extension of pigmentation to adjacent nail folds and cuticle, also referred to as Hutchinson's sign [69]. Comprehension of the various causes of nail hyperpigmentation when evaluating clinical cases can aid in preventing a potentially fatal misdiagnosis.

Oral Mucous Membrane Pigmentation

Oral mucous membrane pigmentation represents various clinical patterns that can range from pathologic manifestations of systemic diseases to normal variations [70]. Oral pigmentation is more common in individuals with darker skin and is frequently not one uniform color throughout. This is due to increased activity of melanocytes rather than an increase in melanocyte number [71]. Intraoral pigmentation is most frequently found on the gingivae, but also occurs on the buccal mucosa, hard palate, and tongue [72]. The differential diagnosis includes drug-induced hyperpigmentation, smoker's melanosis, oral mucosal melanoma, postinflammatory changes, and melanocytic nevi.

Monogolian Spots

Mongolian spots are a form of congenital dermal melanocytosis characterized as irregular, non-blanching dark blue-gray macules present in some infants [73]. The lesions are estimated to occur in 98% of African American infants, 90% of Native American infants, 81% of Asian American infants, 40–70% of Hispanic infants, and 10% of Caucasian infants [74]. These blue-grayish hyperpigmented variants are due to incomplete melanocytic migration through the embryonic dermis, also referred to as the Tyndall effect [75]. Most cases resolve over time, however, nonresolving congenital blue-gray skin pigmentation can be the result of blue nevi, nevus of Ota, or nevus of Ito. Mongolian spots can also be mistaken for bruises and have been incorrectly implicated in child abuse [76].

Diagnosing Lesions in Skin of Color

It is important that dermatologists and other clinicians are familiar with the variations not only in disease incidence and treatment, but also in clinical appearance in patients with skin of color. There are intrinsic differences in skin of color that contribute to these variations. For example, although the increased melanin content in skin of color provides some level of inherent protection against sun damage, it is also responsible for variants in the appearance of several cutaneous disorders.

Discoid Lupus Erythematosus

Discoid lupus erythematosus (DLE) is a chronic inflammatory disorder that occurs more often in women. Ethnic heritage is thought to be a major risk factor for developing DLE as its predilection for some populations is almost as strong as that of gender. A cohort study of over 2000 people with systemic lupus erythematosus (SLE) reported that DLE was more common in African Americans (28.6%), followed by Caucasians (12.6%), Puerto Rican Hispanics (10.9%), and Texan Hispanics (6.2%) [77]. The lesion associated with DLE begins as localized, edematous erythematous plaques, which spread outward on sun-exposed skin. Patients with skin of color can have scattered depigmented and erythematous patches with rims of hyperpigmentation surrounding these patches (Fig. 1.1).

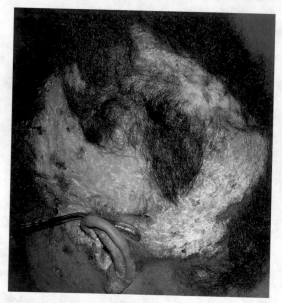

Fig. 1.1 Discoid lupus erythematosus affecting the head

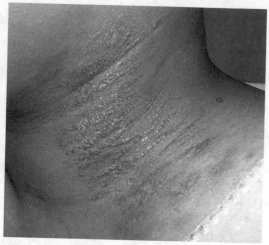

Fig. 1.2 Lichen planus on the neck

Lichen Planus

Lichen planus (LP) is a papulosquamous disease of unknown etiology. A typical LP lesion is described as polygonal, flat-topped, and violaceous. However, in darker skin tones, the hue of these lesions may appear brown, gray-brown, or slate-gray (Fig. 1.2). Patients with skin of color who have LP may develop postinflammatory hyperpigmentation that persists after their LP has resolved. Common anatomic sites that are affected include wrists, ankles, penis, and lumbar area; however, the oropharynx can be involved.

Pityriasis Rosea

Pityriasis rosea (PR) is another common papulosquamous disease of unknown etiology. Patients will develop an initial round lesion, the herald patch, and then days to weeks later have involvement of the trunk and proximal extremities. These lesions may appear salmon-colored with dark, erythematous edges; however, in patients with dark skin tones, the characteristic

lesions PR of may appear gray with a fine scale. Additionally, some studies of PR in African American children reported a variant characterized by lesions with thicker scale and diminished erythema, more facial involvement, and significantly worse pruritus in comparison to PR in white children [78].

Sarcoidosis

Sarcoidosis is a systemic granulomatous disorder of unknown etiology with skin involvement in 20–35% [79]. The cutaneous changes include an eruption of papules, plaques, and ulcerations that can appear over several months. There is a considerable racial difference in disease predominance and presentation. African Americans have a higher annual incidence and lifetime risk than whites [80]. Facial involvement and the angiolupoid variant appear more common among Taiwanese than in individuals from western countries [81]. The typical "apple jelly" hue of sarcoidosis seen in pale skin is rarely present in darkly pigmented skin [82]. The papules may instead display a hypochromic appearance that can help to distinguish them; however, they also may look flesh-colored, pink, purple, or less often hyperpigmented (Fig. 1.3).

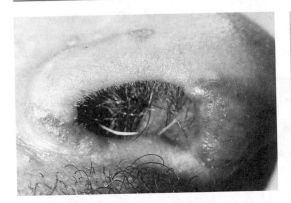

Fig. 1.3 Sarcoidosis papule on the nose

Tinea Versicolor

Tinea versicolor is a superficial fungal infection by *Malassezia furfur*. The lesions can manifest as hypopigmented or hyperpigmented, ivory to gray, slightly scaly macules and patches (Fig. 1.4). The lesions can be seen on the trunk, arms, neck, and face. Hypopigmented lesions may appear more prominent in skin of color given the contrast with the normal brown skin. The hypopigmentation induced by *Malassezia furfur* can be explained on the basis of its production of azelaic acid [83, 84]. Azelaic acid is a competitive inhibitor of tyrosinase, an enzyme involved in the production of melanin, and is used as a topical cream for hyperpigmentation. It is also thought that *Malassezia furfur* has direct cytotoxic effect on hyperactive melanocytes [84]. The pathogenesis of hyperpigmentation tinea versicolor is also not fully understood.

Atopic Dermatitis

Atopic dermatitis (AD) is a dermatitis related to atopy characterized by cycles of exacerbations and periods of remissions. AD is common on the face and flexural areas of extremities. While many dermatologists feel comfortable identifying AD, the transient erythema associated with inflammatory conditions may be difficult to see in skin of color or may appear violaceous in patients with AD. Therefore, it is important to note variations in skin types presenting with AD. Other clinical

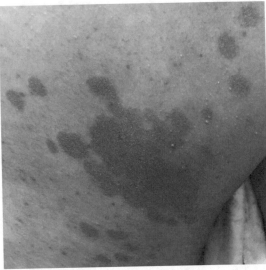

Fig. 1.4 Tinea versicolor on the back

features of AD that can present in skin of color include lichenification, postinflammatory hyper- or hypopigmentation, and follicular accentuation. Eczematous variants such as nummular, xerotic, and dyshidrotic eczema are also seen with increased frequency in patients with skin of color. These conditions may also result with postinflammatory hyperpigmentation.

Skin Disorders More Common in Skin of Color Patients

Physicians must address a host of cutaneous diseases that commonly occur in individuals with skin of color. The importance of epidemiologic studies of dermatologic diseases is clear; however, there is a scarcity of data in populations with skin of color [85, 86]. This section will provide a brief overview of some of the most frequently encountered pigmentary, scarring, and hair disorders in those with skin of color.

Disorders of Pigmentation

Disorders of pigmentation commonly occur in individuals with skin of color. The genetic code determines an individual's constitutive levels of pheomelanin and eumelanin [87]. Eumelanin is alleged to be more important in determining an individual's degree of pigmentation than pheomelanin [88]. In one study by Wakamatsu and colleagues, whites reportedly had the least amount of eumelanin, Asian Indians had more, and African Americans had the highest amount [88]. Additionally, melanosomes in patients with darker skin are larger, more active in producing melanin, and are packaged, distributed, and broken down differently than in white skin [87]. The increased amount of eumelanin content in the skin of people of color and the reactivity of this pigment likely account for the increased prevalence of pigmentary disorders in this population.

Melasma

Melasma is a common acquired relapsing skin disorder estimated to affect more than five million people in the United States [89]. This hypermelanosis is characterized by irregular brown, gray, or blue-tinted macules and patches on sun-exposed areas of the face. Melasma is primarily a disease of women and predominately affects women of Latino, Asian, African, and Native American descent [28]. A US study of Hispanic women in Dallas, Texas, reported that 8.8% had melasma and 4% had reported having it in the past [90]. Additionally, a population-based study conducted in Nepal reported that melasma was the fourth most frequent diagnosis and the most commonly reported pigmentary disorder [91]. The exact etiology of melasma remains unknown; however, a correlation between ultraviolet and visible light exposure, genetics, certain medication use, and hormonal influences have been reported [92].

Postinflammatory Hyperpigmentation

Postinflammatory hyperpigmentation (PIH) is an acquired, transient disorder. It is characterized by an excess of melanin following skin injury or inflammation, such as with acne vulgaris. Acne prevalence and the sequela of PIH predominately affect individuals with darker skin types; with over one third of African American women being afflicted [93]. PIH was also reported to cause higher levels of psychosocial distress in darker skinned patients than their white counterparts [94]. Numerous other diseases are associated with PIH including, but not limited to, atopic dermatitis, impetigo, contact dermatitis, papulosquamous diseases such as psoriasis or lichen planus, vesiculobullous diseases, and drug reactions. The pathophysiology of PIH remains largely unelucidated. It is thought that melanocyte stimulation by inflammatory mediators cause increased melanin synthesis [95]. The hyperpigmentation negatively affects quality of life for these patients and can take months to years to fade.

Erythema Dyschromicum Perstans

Erythema dyschromicum perstans (EDP), also known as ashy dermatosis, is a chronic pigmentary disorder in which brown-blue-gray macules and patches are located on the trunk, upper extremities, neck, and face [96, 97]. EDP occurs most frequently in Central and South America and the South Central US [98], although cases have been described from different parts of the world such as Korea and Japan [99, 100]. The exact etiology is unknown; however, this disease can be induced by drug and toxin ingestion, infections, and allergic contact allergy.

Keloidal and Hypertrophic Scarring

Keloidal and hypertrophic scarring are sequelae of wound healing characterized by excessive fibrous connective tissue deposition in the dermis. The two terms are often interchangeably used in the literature but are not synonymous. The excess connective tissue deposited in the keloid tends to be persistent and extends beyond the area of the original wound. In contrast, the excess tissue deposited in hypertrophic scarring is restricted to the area within the original wound and usually resolves over time [101]. Keloid formation is seen in individuals of all races, but dark-skinned individuals have been found to be 15 times more susceptible to keloid formation [102]. A retrospective study of cleft lip repairs reported that the presence of hypertrophic scarring at 1 year postoperatively was significantly higher in Hispanic patients (32.2%) and Asian patients (36.3%) and lowest in Caucasian patients (11.8%) [103]. Another study of postoperative patients in Hong Kong reported a higher incidence of hypertrophic scaring among the Chinese population when compared to whites [104]. Keloid and hypertrophic scarring can be disfiguring and significantly diminishing on a patient's quality of life [105].

Disorders of the Hair and Hair Follicle

Disorders of hair and hair follicles in individuals of color can range from susceptibility to acneiform diseases triggered by depilation to traction-induced hair loss from improper grooming practices. Variation in human hair morphology has been implicated in these hair disorders. In people of Asian descent, hair fibers are typically straight and round in cross section [106]. Those of European descent generally have straight, wavy, or curly hair fibers that are round or oval shaped in cross section [106]. For people of African descent, hair fibers are typically helical, coiled, or spiraled and flattened in cross section [106]. Additionally, the curvature of the hair follicles in people of African ancestry is related to a greater prevalence of pseudofolliculitis barbae [107]. This section will provide an overview on disorders of hair that typically affect individuals with skin of color.

Pseudofolliculitis Barbae and Acne Keloidalis Nuchae

Pseudofolliculitis barbae (PFB) and acne keloidalis nuchae (AKN) are inflammatory hair disorders that affect individuals with skin of color with tightly coiled hair. They are conditions that predominately affect men of African descent [108, 109]. PFB presents as papules or plaques most commonly in the beard on the neck, whereas the occipital scalp and posterior neck are afflicted in AKN. Both are sometimes referred to as "razor bumps." The etiology of AKN is poorly understood, but androgens, ingrowing hairs, genetics, trauma, and inflammation have been proposed as contributory factors [110]. PFB is thought to be due to curled shaved hairs penetrating inwards and inciting an inflammatory response, but genetics have also been implicated [107, 111, 112]. The consequences of these hair disorders often result in scarring and postinflammatory hyperpigmentation. Other complications include pain, pruritus, subcutaneous abscesses with draining sinuses, and scarring alopecia in the involved areas [109, 113]. Avoidance of close cutting or shaving through the use of laser hair removal, chemical depilatories, and increased beard length may be helpful. There are also topical or procedural options that patients can seek. While these lesions are for the most part benign, they are often a cosmetic as well as medical concern and can affect quality of life for these individuals.

Central Centrifugal Cicatricial Alopecia

Central centrifugal cicatricial alopecia (CCCA) is a chronic and progressive form of scarring hair loss. CCCA is responsible for more cases of scarring alopecia than all other forms in women of African descent [114]. Hair loss is centered on the crown or vertex of the scalp and will expand symmetrically to the frontal, parietal, and occipital scalp. Patients may complain of pruritus, tenderness, or soreness, but many patients are asymptomatic adding to the insidious nature of this disease. The exact pathogenesis of CCCA is still unknown; however, there are reports that previously held notions of the use of chemical hair straightening treatments, hot combs, and other hair styling methods are not etiologic factors [115]. Instead, a genetic predisposition is likely and has been reported by Dlova and colleagues [116].

Traction Alopecia

Traction alopecia is a gradual, patchy hair loss produced by chronic tension primarily at the frontal hairline. It is primarily seen in black patients and is the result of tightly pulled hairstyles and chemical and thermal straightening. Prevention of permanent traction alopecia in adulthood should begin in childhood; therefore, dermatologists should discourage tight braiding and excessive chemical hair processing in children and adolescents.

Androgenetic Alopecia

Androgenetic alopecia (AGA) is a type of hair loss due to changes in androgen levels as well as to genetic inheritance. AGA is sometimes referred to as patterned hair loss as men and women experience a difference in alopecia patterns. Men experience thinning at the temples and vertex with loss of the frontal hairline. Women tend to experience thinning at the vertex and less temporal and frontal hairline involvement than men. The age of onset is usually the third and fourth decades, but the hair loss can progress after puberty. There are racial as well as age-related differences in the incidence and severity of hair loss in AGA. Androgenetic alopecia (AGA) is the most common type of hair loss in Asian men [117]. Takashima and colleagues reported that AGA in Japanese patients was minimal before age 40 and that, although the incidence increased with age, it remained lower than whites [118]. Furthermore, the prevalence and severity of AGA were reported to be lower in Asian and black men than in whites [117]. AGA has various psychosocial impacts on the affected individual and can cause emotional distress [119].

Conclusion

For dermatologists and other clinicians, the current population shift in the United States will mean an increase in individuals with skin of color seeking care. Among certain populations of color, there is a growing sense of frustration at healthcare providers in the United States who do not understand the particular needs of their distinctive skin types and heritages. Particularly, most African American patients believe their providers do not know how to diagnose and care for patients with darker skin [120]. To provide culturally competent care will require the study of texts to develop the skills and understanding needed to manage skin of color. An emphasis on the distinct clinical patterns of cutaneous disorders that affect this population and the unique cultural practices that may implicate those disorders are greatly needed now more than ever.

References

1. United Nations, Department of Economic and Social Affairs, Population Division. World Population Prospects: the 2017 Revision, Key Findings and Advance Tables [Internet]. New York: United Nations; 2017 [cited 2018 Aug 23]. Available from: https://esa.un.org/unpd/wpp/publications/Files/WPP2017_KeyFindings.pdf.
2. Colby SL, Ortman JM. U.S. Census Bureau. Projections of the size and composition of the U.S. population: 2014 to 2060 [Internet]. 2015 [cited 2018 Aug 23]. Available from: https://www.census.gov/library/publications/2015/demo/p25-1143.html.
3. Adamson AS. Should we refer to skin as "ethnic?". J Am Acad Dermatol. 2017;76:1224–5.
4. Torres V, Herane MI, Costa A, Martin JP, Troielli P. Refining the ideas of "ethnic" skin. An Bras Dermatol. 2017;92(2):221–5.
5. Fitzpatrick TB. The validity and practicality of sun-reactive skin types I through VI. Arch Dermatol. 1988;124(6):869–71.
6. Pichon LC, Landrine H, Corral I, Hao Y, Mayer JA, Hoerster KD. Measuring skin cancer risk in African Americans: is the Fitzpatrick skin type classification scale culturally sensitive? Ethn Dis. 2010;20(2):174–9.
7. Taylor SC, Westerhof W, Im S, Lim J. Noninvasive techniques for the evaluation of skin color. J Am Acad Dermatol. 2006;54(5 Suppl 2):S282–90.
8. Kawada A. UVB-induced erythema, delayed tanning, and UVA-induced immediate tanning in Japanese skin. Photo-Dermatology. 1986;3:327–33.
9. Willis I, Earles MR. A new classification system relevant to people of African descent. J Cosmet Dermatol. 2005;18(3):209–16.
10. Roberts WE. The Roberts skin type classification system. J Drugs Dermatol. 2008;7(5):452–6.

11. DeStefano GM, Christiano AM. The genetics of human skin disease. Cold Spring Harb Perspect Med. 2014;4(10):a015172.

12. The White House Office of Management and Budget. Revisions to the standards for the classification of federal data on race and ethnicity [Internet]. 1997 [cited 2018 Aug 26]. Available from: www.whitehouse.gov/wp-content/uploads/2017/11/Revisions-to-the-Standards-for-the-Classification-of-Federal-Data-on-Race-and-Ethnicity-October30-1997.pdf.

13. Sue S, Dhindsa MK. Ethnic and racial health disparities research: issues and problems. Health Educ Behav. 2006;33(4):459–69.

14. Landrine H, Corral I. Advancing research on racial-ethnic health disparities: improving measurement equivalence in studies with diverse samples. Front Public Health. 2014;2:282.

15. Sorkin DH, Ngo-Metzger Q, De Alba I. Racial/ethnic discrimination in health care: impact on perceived quality of care. J Gen Intern Med. 2010;25(5):390–6.

16. Mays VM, Cochran SD, Barnes NW. Race, race-based discrimination, and health outcomes among African Americans. Annu Rev Psychol. 2007;58:201–25.

17. Betancourt JR, Green AR, Carrillo JE, Ananeh-Firempong O. Defining cultural competence: a practical framework for addressing racial/ethnic disparities in health and health care. Public Health Rep. 2003;118(4):293–302.

18. Ennis SR, Rios-Vargas M, Albert NG. The Hispanic population: 2010 [Internet]. 2011 [cited 2018 August 26]. Available from: www.census.gov/prod/cen2010/briefs/c2010br-04.pdf.

19. The United States Census Bureau. Research to improve data on race and ethnicity [Internet]. 2017 [cited 2018 Aug 26]. Available from: https://www.census.gov/about/our-research/race-ethnicity.html.

20. Morales LS, Lara M, Kington RS, Valdez RO, Escarce JJ. Socioeconomic, cultural, and behavioral factors affecting Hispanic health outcomes. J Health Care Poor Underserved. 2002;13(4):477–503.

21. Sabogal F, Marín G, Otero-Sabogal R, Marín BV, Perez-Stable EJ. Hispanic familism and acculturation: what changes and what doesn't? Hisp J Behav Sci. 1987;9(4):397–412.

22. Caballero AE. Understanding the Hispanic/Latino patient. Am J Med. 2011;124(10 Suppl):S10–5.

23. Caban A, Walker EA. A systematic review of research on culturally relevant issues for Hispanics with diabetes. Diabetes Educ. 2006;32:584–95.

24. World Health Organization. Legal status of traditional medicine and complementary/alternative medicine: a worldwide review. Geneva, Switzerland: World Health Organization; 2002. p.43–8.

25. United Nations, Department of Economic and Social Affairs, Population Division. World Population Prospects: the 2017 revision (custom data acquired via website) [Internet]. New York: United Nations; 2017 [cited 2018 Aug 27]. Available from: https://esa.un.org/unpd/wpp/DataQuery.

26. Bodomo A. African diaspora remittances are better than foreign aid funds: diaspora driven development in the 21st Century [Internet]. 2013 [cited 2018 Aug 27]. Available from: https://www.researchgate.net/publication/258338566_African_diaspora_remittances_are_better_than_foreign_aid_funds_diaspora-driven_development_in_the_21st_Century.

27. Rastogi S, Johnson TD, Hoeffel EM, Drewery, MP Jr. The Black population: 2010 [Internet]. 2011 [cited 2018 Aug 27]. Available from: www.census.gov/prod/cen2010/briefs/c2010br-06.pdf.

28. Taylor SC. Epidemiology of skin diseases in ethnic populations. Dermatol Clin. 2003;21(4):601–7.

29. Dunwell P, Rose A. Study of the skin disease spectrum occurring in an Afro-Caribbean population. Int J Dermatol. 2003;42(4):287–9.

30. Hunter ML. Buying racial capital: skin-bleaching and cosmetic surgery in a globalized world. J Pan Afr Stud. 2011;4(4):142–64.

31. Hunter ML. "If You're Light You're Alright": light skin color as social capital for women of color. Gend Soc. 2002;16:175–93.

32. Thompson C. Black women and identity: what's hair got to do with it? [thesis]. Ann Arbor: MPublishing, University of Michigan; 2009. Available from: http://hdl.handle.net/2027/spo.ark5583.0022.105

33. The Trans-Atlantic Slave Trade Database [homepage on Internet]. [cited 2018 Aug 28]. Available from: http://www.slavevoyages.org/.

34. Barbosa VH. Impact of traditional African American cultures on healthcare practices. In: Taylor SC, Kelly AP, Lim HW, Anido Serrano AM, editors. Taylor and Kelly's dermatology for skin of color. 2nd ed. New York: McGraw-Hill; 2016. p. 31–9.

35. Hoeffel EM, Rastogi S, Kim MO, Shahid H. The Asian population: 2010 [Internet]. 2012 [cited 2018 Aug 27]. Available from: www.census.gov/prod/cen2010/briefs/c2010br-11.pdf.

36. Nouveau S, Agrawal D, Kohli M, Bernerd F, Misra N, Nayak CS. Skin hyperpigmentation in Indian population: insights and best practice. Indian J Dermatol. 2016;61(5):487–95.

37. Lilly E, Kundu RV. Dermatoses secondary to Asian cultural practices. Int J Dermatol. 2012;51(4):372–9.

38. Damevska K, França K, Lotti T, Nikolovska S, Pollozhani N. Complementary and integrative therapies for psoriasis: looking forward. Dermatol Ther. 2018;31(5):e12627.

39. Gu S, Yang AW, Li CG, Lu C, Xue CC. Topical application of Chinese herbal medicine for atopic eczema: a systematic review with a meta-analysis. Dermatology. 2014;228(4):294–302.

40. Hughes R, Ward D, Tobin AM, Keegan K, Kirby B. The use of alternative medicine in pediatric patients with atopic dermatitis. Pediatr Dermatol. 2007;24(2):118–20.

41. Lewith G, Robinson N. Complementary and alternative medicine: what the public want and how it may be delivered safely and effectively. J R Soc Med. 2009;102(10):411–4.

42. Lim YL, Thirumoorthy T. Serious cutaneous adverse reactions to traditional Chinese medicines. Singap Med J. 2005;46(12):714–7.

43. Teschke R, Zhang L, Long H, Schwarzenboeck A, Schmidt-Taenzer W, Genthner A, et al. Traditional Chinese medicine and herbal hepatotoxicity: a tabular compilation of reported cases. Ann Hepatol. 2015;14(1):7–19.

44. Shenefelt PD. Herbal treatment for dermatologic disorders. In: Benzie IFF, Wachtel-Galor S, editors. Herbal medicine: biomolecular and clinical aspects. 2nd ed. Boca Raton: CRC Press/Taylor & Francis; 2011. Available from: https://www.ncbi.nlm.nih.gov/books/NBK92761/.

45. Vashi NA, Patzelt N, Wirya S, Maymone MBC, Kundu RV. Dermatoses caused by cultural practices: cosmetic cultural practices. J Am Acad Dermatol. 2018;79(1):19–30.

46. Barnes PM, Powell-Griner E, McFann K, Nahin RL. Complementary and alternative medicine use among adults: United States, 2002. Adv Data. 2004;343:1–19.

47. Yun Y, Choi I. Effect of thread embedding acupuncture for facial wrinkles and laxity: a single-arm, prospective, open-label study. Integr Med Res. 2017;6(4):418–26.

48. van den Berg-Wolf M, Burgoon T. Acupuncture and cutaneous medicine: is it effective? Med Acupunct. 2017;29(5):269–75.

49. Kim TH, Kang JW, Park WS. The reporting quality of acupuncture-related infections in Korean literature: a systematic review of case studies. Evid Based Complement Alternat Med. 2015;2015:273409.

50. Soliman Y, Hamed N, Khachemoune A. Cupping in dermatology: a critical review and update. Acta Dermatovenerol Alp Pannonica Adriat. 2018;27(2):103–7.

51. Chen B, Li MY, Liu PD, Guo Y, Chen ZL. Alternative medicine: an update on cupping therapy. QJM. 2015;108(7):523–5.

52. Lee MS, Choi TY, Kang JW, Lee BJ, Ernst E. Moxibustion for treating pain: a systematic review. Am J Chin Med. 2010;38(5):829–38.

53. Liu ZS, Peng WN, Liu BY, Wang J, Wang Y, Mao M, et al. Clinical practice guideline of acupuncture for herpes zoster. Chin J Integr Med. 2013;19(1):58–67.

54. Coyle ME, Liang H, Wang K, Zhang AL, Guo X, Lu C, et al. Acupuncture plus moxibustion for herpes zoster: a systematic review and meta-analysis of randomized controlled trials. Dermatol Ther. 2017;30(4):1–8.

55. Gupta D, Thappa DM. Dermatoses due to Indian cultural practices. Indian J Dermatol. 2015;60(1):3–12.

56. Ragozin BV. The history of the development of Ayurvedic medicine in Russia. Anc Sci Life. 2016;35(3):143–9.

57. Warrier M. Seekership, spirituality and self-discovery: ayurveda trainees in Britain. Asian Med (Leiden). 2009;4(2):423–51.

58. Morandi A. The first international research seminar on Ayurveda (2014), Birstein, Germany. Anc Sci Life. 2015;34(4):238–44.

59. Narahari SR, Prasanna KS, Sushma KV. Evidence-based integrative dermatology. Indian J Dermatol. 2013;58:127–31.

60. Amshel CE, Caruso DM. Vietnamese "coining": a burn case report and literature review. J Burn Care Rehabil. 2000;21(2):112–4.

61. Osborne DL, Hames R. A life history perspective on skin cancer and the evolution of skin pigmentation. Am J Phys Anthropol. 2014;153(1):1–8.

62. Selmanowitz VJ, Krivo JM. Pigmentary demarcation lines. Comparison of negroes with Japanese. Br J Dermatol. 1975;93(4):371–7.

63. Zhang R, Zhu W. Coexistence of pigmentary demarcation lines types C and E in one subject. Int J Dermatol. 2011;50(7):863–5.

64. James WD, Carter JM, Rodman OG. Pigmentary demarcation lines: a population survey. J Am Acad Dermatol. 1987;16(3 Pt 1):584–90.

65. Kromann AB, Ousager LB, Ali IKM, Aydemir N, Bygum A. Pigmentary mosaicism: a review of original literature and recommendations for future handling. Orphanet J Rare Dis. 2018;13(1):39.

66. Bilemjian AP, Piñeiro-Maceira J, Barcaui CB, Pereira FB. Melanonychia: the importance of dermatoscopic examination and of nail matrix / bed observation. An Bras Dermatol. 2009;84(2):185–9.

67. André J, Lateur N. Pigmented nail disorders. Dermatol Clin. 2006;24(3):329–39.

68. Baran R, Kechijian P. Longitudinal melanonychia (melanonychia striata): diagnosis and management. J Am Acad Dermatol. 1989;21(6):1165–75.

69. Kamyab K, Abdollahi M, Nezam-Eslami E, Nikoo A, Balighi K, Naraghi ZS, et al. Longitudinal melanonychia in an Iranian population: a study of 96 patients. Int J Womens Dermatol. 2016;2(2):49–52.

70. Sreeja C, Ramakrishnan K, Vijayalakshmi D, Devi M, Aesha I, Vijayabanu B. Oral pigmentation: a review. J Pharm Bioallied Sci. 2015;7(Suppl 2):S403–8.

71. Feller L, Masilana A, Khammissa RA, Altini M, Jadwat Y, Lemmer J. Melanin: the biophysiology of oral melanocytes and physiological oral pigmentation. Head Face Med. 2014;10:8.

72. Kauzman A, Pavone M, Blanas N, Bradley G. Pigmented lesions of the oral cavity: review, differential diagnosis, and case presentations. J Can Dent Assoc. 2004;70(10):682–3.

73. Cordova A. The Mongolian spot: a study of ethnic differences and a literature review. Clin Pediatr (Phila). 1981;20(11):714–9.

74. Kelly AP, Heidelberg KA. Nuances in skin of color. In: Taylor SC, Kelly AP, Lim HW, Anido Serrano AM, editors. Taylor and Kelly's dermatology for skin of color. 2nd ed. New York: McGraw-Hill; 2016. p. 123–30.

75. Richey PM, Norton SA. John Tyndall's effect on dermatology. JAMA Dermatol. 2017;153(3):308.

76. Gupta D. Mongolian spots: how important are they? World J Clin Cases. 2013;1(8):230.

77. Santiago-Casas Y, Vilá LM, McGwin G Jr, Cantor RS, Petri M, Ramsey-Goldman R, et al. Association of discoid lupus erythematosus with clinical manifestations and damage accrual in a multiethnic lupus cohort. Arthritis Care Res (Hoboken). 2012;64(5):704–12.

78. Amer A, Fischer H, Li X. The natural history of pityriasis rosea in black American children: how correct is the "classic" description? Arch Pediatr Adolesc Med. 2007;161(5):503–6.

79. Fernandez-Faith E, McDonnell J. Cutaneous sarcoidosis: differential diagnosis. Clin Dermatol. 2007;25:276–87.

80. Dubrey S, Shah S, Hardman T, Sharma R. Sarcoidosis: the links between epidemiology and aetiology. Postgrad Med J. 2014;90:582–9.

81. Wu MC, Lee JY. Cutaneous sarcoidosis in southern Taiwan: clinicopathologic study of a series with high proportions of lesions confined to the face and angiolupoid variant. J Eur Acad Dermatol Venereol. 2013;27:499–505.

82. Petit A, Dadzie OE. Multisystemic diseases and ethnicity: a focus on lupus erythematosus, systemic sclerosis, sarcoidosis and Behcet disease. Br J Dermatol. 2013;169(Suppl 3):1–10.

83. Ashbee HR, Evans EGV. Immunology of diseases associated with Malassezia species. Clin Microbiol Rev. 2002;15(1):21–57.

84. Shah A, Koticha A, Ubale M, Wanjare S, Mehta P, Khopkar U. Identification and speciation of Malassezia in patients clinically suspected of having pityriasis versicolor. Indian J Dermatol. 2013;58(3):239.

85. Davis SA, Narahari S, Feldman SR, Huang W, Pichardo-Geisinger RO, McMichael AJ. Top dermatologic conditions in patients of color: an analysis of nationally representative data. J Drugs Dermatol. 2012;11(4):466–73.

86. Alexis AF, Sergay AB, Taylor SC. Common dermatologic disorders in skin of color: a comparative practice survey. Cutis. 2007;80(5):387–94.

87. Taylor SC. Skin of color: biology, structure, function, and implications for dermatologic disease. J Am Acad Dermatol. 2002;46:S41–62.

88. Wakamatsu K, Kavanagh R, Kadekaro AL, Terzieva S, Sturm RA, Leachman S, et al. Diversity of pigmentation in cultured human melanocytes is due to differences in the type as well as quantity of melanin. Pigment Cell Res. 2006;19:154–62.

89. Grimes PE. Melasma. Etiologic and therapeutic considerations. Arch Dermatol. 1995;131(12):1453–7.

90. Werlinger KD, Guevara IL, González CM, Rincón ET, Caetano R, Haley RW, et al. Prevalence of self-diagnosed melasma among premenopausal Latino women in Dallas and Fort Worth. Tex Arch Dermatol. 2007;143(3):424–5.

91. Walker SL, Shah M, Hubbard VG, Pradhan HM, Ghimire M. Skin disease is common in rural Nepal: results of a point prevalence study. Br J Dermatol. 2008;158:334–8.

92. Ortonne JP, Arellano I, Berneburg M, Cestari T, Chan H, Grimes P, et al. A global survey of the role of ultraviolet radiation and hormonal influences in the development of melasma. J Eur Acad Dermatol Venereol. 2009;23(11):1254–62.

93. Perkins AC, Cheng CE, Hillebrand GG, Miyamoto K, Kimball AB. Comparison of the epidemiology of acne vulgaris among Caucasian, Asian, Continental Indian and African American women. J Eur Acad Dermatol Venereol. 2011;25(9):1054–60.

94. Callender VD, Alexis AF, Daniels SR, Kawata AK, Burk CT, Wilcox TK, et al. Racial differences in clinical characteristics, perceptions and behaviors, and psychosocial impact of adult female acne. J Clin Aesthet Dermatol. 2014;7(7):19–31.

95. Tomita Y, Maeda K, Tagami H. Melanocyte-stimulating properties of arachidonic acid metabolites: possible role in postinflammatory pigmentation. Pigment Cell Res. 1992;5(5 Pt 2):357–61.

96. Ramirez CO. Los cenescientos: problema clinic. In: Proceedings of the First Central American Congress of Dermatology. San Salvador, El Salvador; 1957. p. 122–30.

97. Tlougan BE, Gonzalez ME, Mandal RV, Kundu RV, Skopicki D. Erythema dyschromicum perstans. Dermatol Online J. 2010;16(11):17.

98. Silverberg NB, Herz J, Wagner AL, Paller AS. Erythema dyschromicum perstans in prepubertal children. Pediatr Dermatol. 2003;20:398–403.

99. Chang SE, Kim HW, Shin JM, Lee JH, Na JI, Roh MR, et al. Clinical and histological aspect of erythema dyschromicum perstans in Korea: a review of 68 cases. J Dermatol. 2015;42(11):1053–7.

100. Oiso N, Tsuruta D, Imanishi H, Kobayashi H, Kawada A. Erythema dyschromicum perstans in a Japanese child. Pediatr Dermatol. 2012;29(5):637–40.

101. Gauglitz GG, Korting HC, Pavicic T, Ruzicka T, Jeschke MG. Hypertrophic scarring and keloids: pathomechanisms and current and emerging treatment strategies. Mol Med. 2011;17(1–2):113–25.

102. Ogawa R. Keloid and hypertrophic scars are the result of chronic inflammation in the reticular dermis. Int J Mol Sci. 2017;18(3):606.

103. Soltani AM, Francis CS, Motamed A, Karatsonyi AL, Hammoudeh JA, Sanchez-Lara PA, et al. Hypertrophic scarring in cleft lip repair: a comparison of incidence among ethnic groups. Clin Epidemiol. 2012;4:187–91.

104. Li-Tsang CWP, Lau JCM, CCH C. Prevalence of hypertrophic scar formation and its characteristics among the Chinese population. Burns. 2005;31(5):610–6.

105. Bock O, Schmid-Ott G, Malewski P, Mrowietz U. Quality of life of patients with keloid and hypertrophic scarring. Arch Dermatol Res. 2006;297(10):433–8.

106. Imadojemu S, Seykora J. Biology of hair. In: Taylor SC, Kelly AP, Lim HW, Anido Serrano AM, editors.

Taylor and Kelly's dermatology for skin of color. 2nd ed. New York: McGraw-Hill; 2016. p. 87–90.

107. Winter H, Schissel D, Parry DA, Smith TA, Liovic M, Birgitte Lane E, et al. An unusual Ala12Thr polymorphism in the 1A alpha-helical segment of the companion layer-specific keratin K6hf: evidence for a risk factor in the etiology of the common hair disorder pseudofolliculitis barbae. J Invest Dermatol. 2004;122(3):652–7.

108. Alexander AM, Delph WI. Pseudofolliculitis barbae in the military. A medical, administrative and social problem. J Natl Med Assoc. 1974;66(6):459–64. 479

109. Awosika O, Burgess CM, Grimes PE. Considerations when treating cosmetic concerns in men of color. Dermatol Surg. 2017;43(Suppl 2):S140–50.

110. Ogunbiyi A. Acne keloidalis nuchae: prevalence, impact, and management challenges. Clin Cosmet Investig Dermatol. 2016;9:483–9.

111. Halder RM. Pseudofolliculitis barbae and related disorders. Dermatol Clin. 1988;6(3):407–12.

112. Taylor SC, Barbosa V, Burgess C, Heath C, McMichael AJ, Ogunleye T, et al. Hair and scalp disorders in adult and pediatric patients with skin of color. Cutis. 2017;100(1):31–5.

113. Kundu RV, Patterson S. Dermatologic conditions in skin of color: part II. Disorders occurring predominately in skin of color. Am Fam Physician. 2013;87(12):859–65.

114. Sperling LC, Sau P. The follicular degeneration syndrome in black patients. "Hot comb alopecia" revisited and revised. Arch Dermatol. 1992;128(1):68–74.

115. Gathers RC, Jankowski M, Eide M, Lim HW. Hair grooming practices and central centrifugal cicatricial alopecia. J Am Acad Dermatol. 2009;60(4):574–8.

116. Dlova NC, Jordaan FH, Sarig O, Sprecher E. Autosomal dominant inheritance of central centrifugal cicatricial alopecia in black South Africans. J Am Acad Dermatol. 2014;4:679–8.

117. Tanaka Y, Aso T, Ono J, Hosoi R, Kaneko T. Androgenetic alopecia treatment in Asian men. J Clin Aesthet Dermatol. 2018;11(7):32–5.

118. Takashima M, Iju K, Sudo M. Alopecia androgenica: its incidendce in Japanese and associated conditions. In: Orfanos CE, Montagna W, Stutgen G, editors. Hair research status and future aspects. Berlin: Springer-Verlag; 1981. p. 287–93.

119. Lee W-S, Lee H-J. Characteristics of androgenetic alopecia in Asian. Ann Dermatol. 2012;24(3):243–52.

120. Gathers RC, Mahan MG. African American women, hair care, and health barriers. J Clin Aesthet Dermatol. 2014;7(9):26–9.

Skin of Color: Biology, Physiology, Structure, and Function

Enzo Berardesca and Norma Cameli

Ethnic differences in skin physiology and reaction to environmental stimuli are more and more described [1], but notwithstanding the increasing number of studies, data are often conflicting. In fact, it is difficult to define and interpret the cutaneous pathophysiologic phenomena that are not only anatomical and functional characteristics of ethnic groups but also the result of socioeconomic, hygienic, and nutritional factors. Furthermore, skin status may be influenced by climate, circadian rhythms, and changes in circulating sex hormones or stress hormones. Indeed, even though it is well established that all humans belong to the same species, many physical differences exist among human population. Stratum corneum is equally thick in different races [2–5]. However, Weigand et al. demonstrated that the stratum corneum in Blacks contains more cell layers and requires more cellophane tape strips to be removed than the stratum corneum of Caucasians [6], while Kampaore and Tsuruta showed that Asian skin was significantly more sensitive to stripping than Black skin [7]. Weigand also found great variance in values obtained from Black subjects, whereas data from White subjects were more homogeneous. No correlation was found between the degree of pigmentation and the number of cell layers. These data could be explained due to the greater intercellular cohesion in Blacks, resulting in an increased number of cell layers and an increased resistance to stripping. This mechanism may involve lipids [8], because the lipid content of the stratum corneum ranges from 8.5 to 14 percent, with higher values in Blacks [5, 9]. This result was confirmed by Weigand et al. who showed that delipidized specimens of stratum corneum were equal in weight in the two races [6]. Johnson and Corah found that the mean electrical resistance of an adult Black skin is doubled in adult White skin, suggesting an increased cohesion of the stratum corneum [10]. In fact, La Ruche and Cesarini found that, in comparison with White skin, the Black skin stratum corneum is equal in thickness but more compact: about 20 cell layers are observed in Blacks versus 16 layers in Whites [5].

Corcuff et al. [11] investigated the corneocyte surface area and the spontaneous desquamation and found no differences among Black, White, and oriental skin. However, an increased desquamation (up to 2.5 times) was found in Blacks. They concluded that the differences may be related to a different composition of the intercellular lipids of the stratum corneum. Sugino et al. [12] found significant differences in the amount of ceramides in the stratum corneum, with the lowest levels in Blacks followed by Caucasian,

E. Berardesca (✉)
San Gallicano Dermatological Institute, Rome, Italy
e-mail: berardesca@berardesca.it

N. Cameli
San Gallicano Dermatological Institute, Department of Dermatology, Rome, Italy

© Springer Nature Switzerland AG 2021
B. S. Li, H. I. Maibach (eds.), *Ethnic Skin and Hair and Other Cultural Considerations*, Updates in Clinical Dermatology, https://doi.org/10.1007/978-3-030-64830-5_2

Hispanics, and Asians. In this experiment, ceramide levels were inversely correlated with TEWL and directly correlated with water content. Meguro et al. confirmed these correlations [13]. These data may partially explain the controversial findings in the literature on the mechanisms of skin sensitivity.

Changes in skin permeability and barrier function have been reported: Kompaore et al. [7, 14] evaluated TEWL and lag time after application of a vasoactive compound (methyl nicotinate) before and after removal of the stratum corneum by tape stripping. Before tape stripping, TEWL was 1.3 times greater in Blacks and Asians compared to Caucasians. No difference was found between Blacks and Asians, whereas after stripping they found a significantly higher TEWL in Blacks and Asians than in Whites. In particular, after stripping, Asians showed the highest TEWL (Asians 1.7 times greater than Caucasians). They conclude that, similar to previous studies [15, 16], skin permeability measured by TEWL is higher in Blacks than in Caucasians. They also concluded that Asian skin has the highest permeability among the groups studied. However, these findings have not yet been confirmed by other groups. In fact, Sugino et al. [12] also included Asians in their study but found that baseline TEWL was, in decreasing order, Blacks > Caucasians ≥ Hispanics ≥ Asians. Another study [17] about Asian skin has compared TEWL in Asians and Caucasians and found no statistically significant differences at baseline or after stripping; however, no vasoactive substance was applied.

Reed et al. [18] found differences in the recovery of the barrier between subjects with skin type II/III compared to skin type V/VI, but no differences between Caucasians in general and Asians. Darker skin recovered faster after barrier damage induced by tape stripping.

Clinical Effects of Changes in Skin Barrier

Conflicting findings have been reported on the incidence of allergic contact dermatitis in Blacks. Kenney reported a decreased rate (5% in Black

patients in his own private practice). Marshall and Heyl reported that the incidence of industrial contact dermatitis in South Africa is less in darkly pigmented Blacks [19]. Bantus showed a 7.4% prevalence [20]. Scott noted that contact dermatitis was less frequent in Bantus handling detergents, waxes, and fuels [21]. Despite a previous report describing an increased sensitization rate in Whites, Kligman and Epstein found no significant difference in the two races after testing many topical materials [22]. Fisher reported an approximately equal incidence of contact dermatitis in Blacks and Whites [23]. Paraphenylenediamine, nickel, and potassium bichromate appeared to be the most common allergens.

In Nigeria, nickel was the most frequent sensitizer, with an incidence of 12.3% [24] compared with 11% in North America. In Lagos, the female:male ratio is 1:1, whereas Fregert et al. recorded a ratio of 6:1 [25]. In North America, the ratio is 3:1 and in Stockholm, it is 7:3.

Clinically, acute contact dermatitis with exudation, vesiculation, or bullae is more common in Whites, whereas Blacks more commonly develop disorders of pigmentation and lichenification. Hypopigmentation has been described from contact with phenolic detergents [26], alkyphenols, and monobenzylether of hydroquinone [27]. Hyperpigmentation occurs more readily in Black patients after contact with mild irritants. Keratolytics and other chemicals used in acne therapy often cause hyperpigmentation in Blacks. The epidemiology studies are different to interpret for reasons related to exposure and the like.

Studies of transdermal clonidine permitted identification of certain racial and sex-related differences in sensitization. The occlusive transdermal patch is applied for 1 week. The sensitization rate was as follows: Caucasian women 34%, Caucasian men 18%, Black women 14%, and Black men 8%. These differences are large and presumably biologically significant (unpublished data).

A proneness of Blacks to "pomade acne" has been suggested. This eruption, consisting mainly of comedones on the forehead and temporal area, seems to be a peculiar response of Black skin to topical agents, because this reaction can be detected in Black children from 1 to 12 years of age [28]. Plewig et al. examined 735 Blacks and found that 70% of long-term users of pomades had a form of acne [29]. The more elaborate formulations induced pomade acne more frequently and more intensively than simpler preparations such as mineral oil and petroleum jelly. The distribution of the lesions corresponded to the area of contact. Comparable data for Whites are lacking.

Kaidbey and Kligman studied race-dependent cutaneous reactivity to topical coal [30]. There was a strikingly different response in the two groups: in Whites, the response was primarily inflammatory, with development of papules and papulopustules in about 2 or 3 weeks, whereas in Blacks the inflammatory response was largely absent and, after about 14 days, an eruption of small open comedones appeared. The follicles of White subjects responded early, with rupture of the wall and outpouring of follicular contents in the dermis, whereas in Blacks, the first response was proliferative with production and retention of horny cells. That is, in Blacks, the skin reacts to a comedogenic compound with hyperkeratoses rather than with disintegration of follicles, suggesting a greater resistance to irritants.

The postocclusive hyperemic reaction before and after a single 1-hour application of clobetasol 0.05% was determined by laser Doppler velocimetry to elucidate different racial responses [31]. In Black subjects, there were a decreased area under the curve response, decreased peak response, and a decreased decay slope after peak blood flow. These data are consistent with a different reactivity of blood vessels in Black skin and possibly not related to the transcutaneous penetration of the chemical compound.

References

1. Berardesca E, Maibach H. Racial differences in skin pathophysiology. J Am Acad Dermatol. 1996;34:667–72.
2. Freeman RG, Cockerell EG, Armstrong J, et al. Sunlight as a factor influencing the thickness of epidermis. J Invest Dermatol. 1962;39:295–7.
3. Thomson ML. Relative efficiency of pigment and horny layer thick-ness in protecting the skin of European and Africans against solar ultraviolet radiation. J Physiol Lond. 1955;127:236.
4. Lock-Andersen J, Therkildsen P, de Fine OF, et al. Epidermal thickness, skin pigmentation and constitutive photosensitivity. Photodermatol Photoimmunol Photomed. 1997;13(4):153–8.
5. La Ruche G, Cesarini JP. Histology and physiology of black skin. Ann Dermatol Venereol. 1992;119(8):567–74.
6. Weigand DA, Haygood C, Gaylor JR. Cell layers and density of Negro and Caucasians stratum corneum. J Invest Dermatol. 1974;62:563–5.
7. Kompaore F, Tsuruta H. In vivo differences between Asian, black and white in the stratum corneum barrier function. Int Arch Occup Environ Health. 1993;65(1 Suppl):S223–5.
8. Coderch L, Lopez O, de la Maza A, Parra JL. Ceramides and skin function. Am J Clin Dermatol. 2003;4(2):107–29.
9. Rienertson RP, Wheatley VR. Studies on the chemical composition of human epidermal lipids. J Invest Dermatol. 1959;32:49–51.
10. Johnson LC, Corah NL. Racial differences in skin resistance. Science. 1963;139:766–9.
11. Corcuff P, Lotte C, Rougier A, Maibach H. Racial differences in corneocytes. Acta Derm Venereol (Stockh). 1991;71:146–8.
12. Sugino K, Imokawa G, Maibach H. Ethnic difference of stratum corneum lipid in relation to stratum corneum function. J Invest Dermatol. 1993;100:597.
13. Meguro S, Arai Y, Masukawa Y, Uie K. Tokimitsu. Relationship between covalently bound ceramides and transepidermal water loss (TEWL). Arch Dermatol Res. 2000;292(9):463–8.
14. Kompaore F, Marty JP, Dupont C. In vivo evaluation of the stra-tum corneum barrier function in Blacks, Caucasians and Asians with two non-invasive methods. Skin Pharmacol. 1993;6:200–7.
15. Wilson D, Berardesca E, Maibach HI. In vitro transepidermal water loss: differences between Black and white human skin. Br J Dermatol. 1988;199:647–52.
16. Berardesca E, Maibach HI. Racial differences in sodium lauryl sulphate induced cutaneous irritation: Black and White. Contact Dermatitis. 1988;18:136–40.
17. Yosipovitch G, Theng CTS. Asian skin: its architecture, function, and differences from Caucasian skin. Cosmet Toiletr. 2002;117(9):57–62.
18. Reed JT, Ghadially R, Elias PM. Effect of race, gender and skin type on epidermal permeability barrier function. J Invest Dermatol. 1994;102:537.
19. Marshall J, Heyl T. Skin diseases in the Western Cape Province. S Afr Med J. 1963;37:1308.
20. Dogliotti M. Skin disorders in the Bantu: a survey of 2000 cases from Baragwanath Hospital. S Afr Med J. 1970;44:670.

21. Scott F. Skin diseases in the South African bantu. In: Marshall J, editor. Essays on tropical dermatology. Amsterdam: Excerpta Medica; 1972.

22. Kligman AM, Epstein W. Updating the maximization test for identifying contact allergens. Contact Dermatitis. 1975;1:231.

23. Fisher AA. Contact dermatitis in black patients. Cutis. 1977;20:303–20.

24. Olumide YM. Contact dermatitis in Nigeria. Contact Dermatitis. 1985;12:241–6.

25. Fregert S, Hjorth N, Magnusson B, et al. Epidemiology of contact dermatitis. Trans St Johns Hosp Dermatol Soc. 1969;55:17.

26. Fisher AA. Vitiligo due to contactants. Cutis. 1976;17:431–7.

27. Kahn G. Depigmentation caused by phenolic detergent germicides. Arch Dermatol. 1970;102:177–87.

28. Verhagen AR. Pomade acne in black patients. Arch Dermatol. 1974;110:465.

29. Plewig G, Fulton JE. Kligman AM:Pomade acne. Arch Dermatol. 1970;101:580.

30. Kaidbey KH, Kligman AM. A human model for coal tar acne. Arch Dermatol. 1974;109:212–5.

31. Berardesca E, Maibach HI. Cutaneous reactive hyperaemia: racial differences induced by corticoid application. Br J Dermatol. 1989;120:787–94.

Biology of Hair

Jessica Dawson and Andrea T. Murina

Introduction

Hair, a defining feature shared by all mammals, serves a variety of critical functions such as social and sexual communication, protection against environmental insults, enhanced sensory perception, temperature homeostasis, and removal of debris from the skin surface [1]. While the basic structure and function of hair is similar among all ethnicities, there are phenotypic variations that are found within ethnic subgroups that can help guide medical and cosmetic management. Human hair has been historically classified into three conventional ethnic subgroups: Asian, African, and Caucasian. This grouping system generalizes hair types and fails to fully illustrate the spectrum of hair phenotypes in humans [2]. Moving away from ethnic categorizations, recent studies found that it is possible to classify hair into non-ethnic types based on curve diameter, curl index, and number of waves [3–5]. While relative curliness of hair may be more important than ethnicity in determining appropriate hair therapies and cosmetic regimens, structural hair differences in this chapter will be compared by ethnicity for the sake of consistency and reader comprehension [6]. This chapter covers the anatomy of hair, hair follicle immune privilege, the hair cycle, hair pigmentation, and the science of hair curl. Alternative methods of classifying hair beyond ethnicity are discussed as well.

Anatomy of Hair

Hair is derived from the epidermis. All hair, regardless of ethnic classification, shares common morphology, chemical makeup, and molecular structure. Hair can be divided into two structures: the follicle and the hair shaft. The hair shaft is more susceptible to environmental damage and cosmetic treatments. The hair shaft is comprised of an outer cuticle, medulla (often absent), and inner cortex. The follicle—the growth structure of hair—is composed of the outer root sheath, inner root sheath, hair bulb, stem cells, and blood supply (Fig. 3.1) [7].

Hair Shaft

Cuticle

The cuticle is the outermost layer of the hair shaft. This layer is made of overlapping flat cells (similar to roof tiles) that are proximally attached

J. Dawson (✉)
University of Washington School of Medicine, Seattle, WA, USA
e-mail: jdawson7@uw.edu

A. T. Murina
Tulane Medical Center, Tulane University, Department of Dermatology, New Orleans, LA, USA

© Springer Nature Switzerland AG 2021
B. S. Li, H. I. Maibach (eds.), *Ethnic Skin and Hair and Other Cultural Considerations*, Updates in Clinical Dermatology, https://doi.org/10.1007/978-3-030-64830-5_3

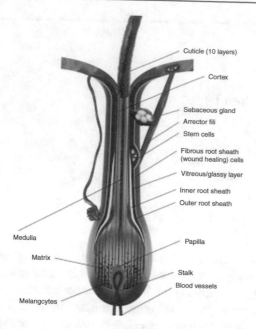

Fig. 3.1 Illustration of anatomy of a hair follicle. (Reprinted from: Park et al. [33], with permission from Elsevier)

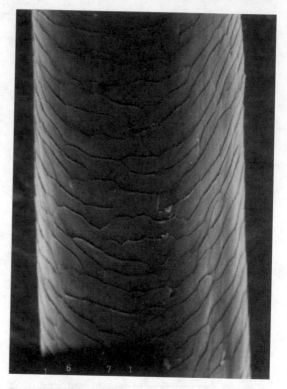

Fig. 3.2 Electron micrograph showing overlapping, roof-like cuticle cells. (Reprinted from: Wolfram [7], with permission from Elsevier)

to the cortex and directed outward and upward in an interlocking fashion with the inner root sheath (Fig. 3.2). The cuticle serves as a follicular anchor to the growing hair and as a self-cleansing mechanism. As the hairs grow and move relative to one another, the outward pointing cuticle cells assist in the removal of trapped debris and desquamated cells [7].

Each cuticle cell is covered by an epicuticle, a thin membrane with a lipid layer that includes the highly studied 18-methyl eicosanoic acid (18-MEA) and free lipids. 18-MEA plays a major role in maintaining the hydrophobicity of hair. Removing the epicuticle 18-MEA by alkaline chemical products can damage hair by increasing hydrophilia [8, 9]. This removal of the cuticle is a form of extreme "weathering" that exposes the inner cortex to environmental damage and increases the likelihood of hair breakage. Weathering refers to excessive chemical treatments, grooming habits, and environmental insults that can damage and break hair. Normal weathering from daily grooming practices results in progressive degeneration from the root to the tip. The use of hair protective agents can increase

hair hydrophobicity, repair cuticle damage, and minimize damage by friction forces [10, 11].

The shape and orientation of cuticle cells determines the effect of friction in hair. The cuticle is formed by 6–8 flat cells thick in Asian hair, slightly less in Caucasian hair, and even less in African hair. This thin cuticle layer contributes to the propensity of African hair to easily break [8]. Cuticle cells become increasingly damaged/weathered toward the tips of the hair in all hair types [12].

Cortex

The cortex is the dominant component of the hair shaft in both weight and volume; it is the primary contributor to the mechanical strength of the hair fibers. Cortical cells contain the melanin granules that give hair its color [6]. Each cortex cell is comprised of spindle-shaped keratin filaments known as microfibrils that are grouped into larger macrofibrils. These macrofibrils make up about 50% of the cortex by mass [7, 8]. Keratin includes large amounts of the sulfur-containing amino acid, cysteine. Cysteine is needed for the formation of disulfide bonds (cystine), which play a pivotal role in mechanical strength, keratin insolubility, and thermal stability of hair. There is no difference in the cystine content of keratin filaments across ethnicities. In all hair types, cystine disulfide bonds can be altered during cosmetic treatments such as perming, bleaching, and straightening. Cystine content decreases as hair gets damaged or weathered.

Keratin proteins are also connected by hydrogen bonds that can be altered with water exposure to create temporary hair styles. An example of hydrogen bond disruption includes the use of rollers on wet hair to make curls known as "wet-setting" [6, 9].

In wool fibers as well as human hair, cortical cells are divided into three regions: the orthocortex, paracortex, and mesocortex. These regions were determined based on the packing of the macrofibrils within the cortical cells within a cysteine matrix [7]. Straight hair tends to have a symmetrical spread of ortho- and paracortices, while curly hair tends to have a non-symmetrical distribution of the cortical cells [13].

Medulla

The medulla is the innermost layer of the hair shaft providing relative resistance to most chemical treatments. It is formed from transparent cells and air spaces. The cells in the medulla contain glycogen-filled vacuoles and citrulline granules. It can be very difficult to identify under light microscopy, and is often entirely absent in certain hair types. It is typically found in courser hair such as gray hair and beard hair. There is a larger medulla in the hair of Asians compared to Caucasians [8]. The medulla is involved in hair splitting as fibers with larger cross-sectional areas have a higher chance of encountering medullary cells that can cause cracks along the fiber axis [14].

Dermal Components

Inner Root Sheath

The inner root sheath (IRS) is comprised of three layers: Henle's layer, Huxley's layer, and the cuticle layer. The IRS cuticle is attached to the cuticle of the hair shaft, gluing the hair shaft to the follicle. The IRS cells produce keratins and trichohyalin that support the developing hair shaft and direct upward and outward movement [15]. Premature desquamation of the inner root sheath in non-inflamed hair follicles is considered a distinctive and specific feature in central centrifugal cicatricial alopecia (CCCA) [16].

Outer Root Sheath

The outer root sheath is a reservoir of multipotent stem cells, including keratinocyte and melanocyte stem cells. It is located in the bulge area between the arrector pili muscle insertion and the duct of the sebaceous gland [15]. Inactive melanocytes in the outer root sheath and in the bulge region of the hair can activate to allow for repigmentation of the hair under certain stimuli [17].

Sebaceous Glands

Sebaceous glands are holocrine glands that can be stimulated by hormones such as androgens, resulting in the secretion of a lipid-rich sebum that conditions hair and provides a protective hydrophobic barrier for the skin [18]. In highly curled hair, it is more challenging for sebum to travel down the hair shaft, resulting in drier hair [6].

Muscle

The arrector pili is a smooth muscle that attaches at the level of the bulge and to the papillary layer of the dermis. It plays an important role in hair follicle integrity. In cold weather, sympathetic innervations cause these muscles to contract resulting in piloerection commonly called "goosebumps" [19, 20]. It was once thought that each hair follicle is attached to a separate arrector pili muscle but this has since been disproven. Now the leading theory is that the arrector pili muscle is associated with all the hair follicles within a follicular unit [21]. Dysfunction of the arrector pili muscle is linked to a variety of hair disorders including androgenetic alopecia. Loss of attachment between the arrector pili muscle and the hair follicle bulge is associated with irreversible or only partially reversible hair loss [22].

Blood Supply

The scalp receives a rich arterial blood supply from the external carotid artery and the ophthalmic artery (a branch of the internal carotid). Throughout the body, arterioles enter the subcutaneous fat and ascend upward into the lower portion of the hair follicle. During the growth phase, anagen, keratinocytes in the outer root sheath, can upregulate expression of vascular endothelial growth factor (VEGF), leading to a notable increase in perifollicular blood flow [15].

Innervation of Hair Follicle

Nerves that innervate the hair follicles originate from the dermis or subcutaneous tissue. At the level of the sebaceous gland, most of the hair follicles are encapsulated by a group of nerves, often called the hair end organ. These nerves are organized in an outer circular layer and an inner longitudinal layer [15]. Differences in nerve supply to hair follicles have been documented with respect to the size of the hair [23].

Hair Cycle

The hair growth cycle can be divided into three phases: anagen (growth), catagen (involution), and telogen (rest) (Fig. 3.3).

The anagen phase is an active growth stage, during which the hair follicle enlarges and produces a hair fiber. Anagen is categorized into six stages (I–VI). In the first five stages (known as proanagen), hair progenitor cells divide, surround the developing dermal papilla, grow downward into the skin, and differentiate into the hair shaft and inner root sheath. The hair shaft begins

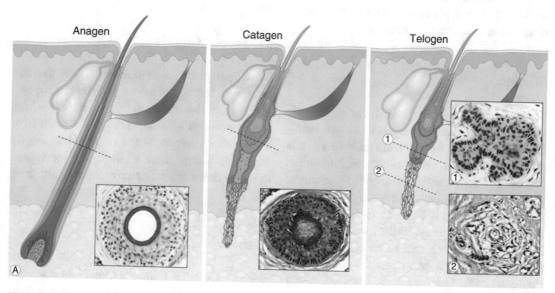

Fig. 3.3 Hair growth cycle with histological cross sections. (Reprinted from: Restrepo and Calonje [42], with permission from Elsevier)

to mature and melanocytes in the hair matrix start to produce the pigment that gives hair its color [15]. Hair follicles in various parts of the body produce different lengths of hair, with the length directly proportional to the duration of anagen. On the scalp, anagen can last for 10 years (median of 3 years), whereas anagen phase of the eyebrow lasts about 70 days [7].

During the catagen phase, metabolic activity slows as follicular keratinocytes undergo apoptosis and melanogenesis ceases. The dermal papilla shrinks and moves upward, eventually to lie immediately underneath the hair-follicle bulge. Catagen lasts approximately 3 months on the scalp.

During the telogen phase, the hair shaft matures into a club hair. As the new growth cycle begins underneath the old hair shaft, the club hair and hair shaft is shed, typically through combing or washing. On the scalp, approximately 50–100 telogen hairs are shed daily. Telogen lasts approximately 3 months. The percentage of follicles in telogen varies dependent on the location of the body. For example, 5–15 percent of scalp follicles are in telogen at a given time, compared to 40–50 percent of hair follicles on the trunk [24]. The majority of sites on the body have a very short anagen and a much longer telogen, resulting in short stable hairs that stay for long periods of time without growing longer [25].

Humans do not shed hair synchronously, like most other animals. Instead, each individual hair follicle undergoes cycles of quiescence and growth. Synchronous disruption of anagen or telogen results in telogen effluvium. Most often, telogen effluvium is due to the synchronized termination of anagen due to physiological stressors such as illness or weight loss [25].

No ethnic differences in the hair growth cycle and number of hairs in anagen or telogen have been found. The average rate of growth is 0.1 mm/day for eyebrow hair and 0.3 mm/day for scalp hair [26]. Differences in the hair growth rate have been observed, particularly that African hair grows slower than Caucasian and Asian hair [27].

Hair Follicle Density

The total lifetime number of hair follicles is determined during embryogenesis, with the exception of injury-mediated hair follicle formation (neogenesis) and experimental induction. Each human has about 2 million hair follicles throughout the body. Disorders of embryogenesis can cause a low density of hair follicle formation (hypotrichosis) that can affect the entire body or specific regions. However, most often, humans undergo appropriate hair follicle embryogenesis and have normal hair follicle density at birth. The hair undergoes various insults later in life, which result in a significant decrease in follicle number with age [26].

Types of Hair Follicles

Human hair can be differentiated into hormone-independent (i.e., eyebrows and eyelashes) and hormone-dependent (i.e., scalp, beard, axilla, pubic). Hormone-dependent hair, known as terminal hair, is long (>2 cm), thick (>60 mm in diameter), and pigmented. Androgen-independent hair, also known as vellus hair, is classically shorter (<2 cm), thinner (<30 mm in diameter), with less or no pigment compared to terminal hair. Vellus hair extends superficially into the subcutaneous fat (<1 mm), while terminal hair typically extends more than 3 mm into subcutaneous fat. Intermediate hair follicles have also been described, which contain characteristics of terminal and vellus forms [26].

Androgenetic alopecia is the most common type of alopecia and is characterized by hair follicle miniaturization on histology (Fig. 3.4). Due to the effects of the testosterone metabolite dihydrotestosterone on hormone-responsive hair, there is a reduction in diameter, length, and pigmentation of the hair. Medications that exert an anti-androgenic affect such as minoxidil and 5-alpha reductase inhibitors can prevent the progression of hair follicle miniaturization [22, 28].

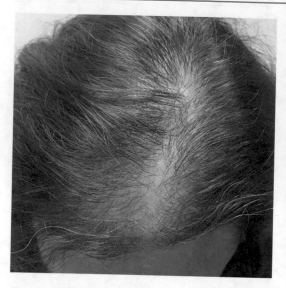

Fig. 3.4 Androgenetic alopecia of hormone-dependent hair

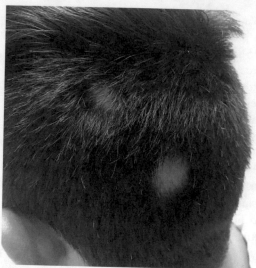

Fig. 3.5 Loss of follicular immune privilege in alopecia areata

The Hair Follicle: An Immune Privileged Site

The hair follicle is considered an immune privileged site—similar to the placenta, brain, testis, and anterior chamber of the eye. Immune privilege is defined as the ability to tolerate antigen introduction without causing an inflammatory immune reaction due to: (i) low or absent major histocompatibility complex (MHC) class 1a/β2 microglobulin expression (making self-peptide presentation virtually impossible); and (ii) creation of an immunosuppressive environment by secreted immune inhibitors [29]. Until recently, immune suppression was thought to occur exclusively in anagen within the hair matrix (where keratinocytes proliferate to form the hair shaft), but studies show that the bulge region (where stem cells reside) has immune shielding throughout the hair cycle. The postulated primary function of anagen hair bulb immune privilege is sequestration of immunogenic antigens, particularly those associated with melanogenesis, from immune recognition. There are two proposed mechanisms for immune-mediated hair dysfunction: (i) immune system's direct attack on the hair follicle; or (ii) disruption of the molecules that create an immunoinhibitory milieu leading to a secondary attack by the immune system [1].

Alopecia areata is a classic disease caused by the loss of follicular immune privilege (Fig. 3.5). Antibodies against melanocyte-associated antigens are associated with alopecia areata. The pathogenesis is linked to upregulation of follicular MHC class I expression allowing self-antigen presentation to the immune system and increased activity of CD8+ T cells and natural killer cells. Moreover, there is also downregulation of mediators that suppress the immune system. IFN-gamma upregulates the expression of MHC class II antigens that trigger an autoimmune response and hair follicle damage. These antigens are typically physiologically absent in the hair follicle matrix and dermal sheath [1]. Genome-wide association studies (GWAS) in patients with alopecia areata suggest mutations in genes that affect cytokine production and regulatory T cell function. These studies have shown areas for promising treatment targets such as the Janus kinase (JAK) pathway. Inhibition of the JAK pathway prevents the upregulation of several cytokines involved in alopecia areata and has been shown to promote substantial hair regrowth [1].

Hair Pigmentation

Hair color is determined by the amount and type of melanin pigment production by cutaneous and follicular melanocytes. In skin and hair, there are two types of melanin pigment: eumelanin and pheomelanin. Eumelanin is a brown-black pigment derived from tyrosine and is found in darker skin and brown or black hair. Pheomelanin is a yellow-red pigment comprised of tyrosine and cystine that predominates in light skin and red or blonde hair [30]. Melanocortin 1 receptor (MC1R) is a key signaling molecule on melanocytes that induces the expression of enzymes responsible for eumelanin synthesis. Mutations in MCR-1 that lead to its inactivation largely account for the red hair phenotype in humans [31]. Melanin is synthesized in melanosomes, derived from the smooth endoplasmic reticulum within neural crest-originating melanocytes, which is then transferred to keratinocytes in skin and hair. Melanocytes in the epidermis rarely proliferate, while the melanocytes in hair follicles repeatedly undergo cell division and differentiate for hair pigmentation in every hair cycle. Melanocytes undergo apoptosis when the hair follicle regresses in telogen and regenerate from melanocyte stem cells located in the hair follicle bulge during anagen [32].

Melanocyte-stimulating hormone (MSH) and corticotropin are formed from proopiomelanocortin, which is synthesized in the pituitary gland and keratinocytes. MSH is thought to cause the dispersion of melanosomes and assists in repairing melanocytic DNA damage from UV radiation by reducing UV-induced hydrogen peroxide formation. Defects in hydrogen peroxide clearance (reduced catalase activity) and increased hydrogen peroxide formation have been linked to premature graying and hair bleaching [33].

Hair color changes can be due to a variety of disease states and exogenous factors. Systemic drugs such as chloroquine, hydroxycholoroquine, sunitinib, pazopanib, dasatinib, phenytoin, phenobarbital, tamoxifen, and low-dose interferon have been reported to cause hair depigmentation. Hair hyperpigmentation has been shown with use of cyclosporine, indinavir, zidovudine, verapamil, and p-aminobenzoic acid. Some, but not all, of these color changes are reversible with drug cessation [33, 34].

Hair can also be dyed using natural (henna, indigo, berries, herbs) or synthetic hair pigments. Temporary dyes cover the cuticle layer only, whereas more permanent dyes add color to the cortex as well. Hydrogen peroxide is the principal ingredient in most hair developers; it penetrates the cortex and oxidizes the melanin, which removes the color to bleach hair [33].

Melanin is the chromophore for laser absorption. Laser hair removal is best suited for people with black, brown, red, or dark blonde hairs. Laser treatments require increased caution in patients with darker skin because the epidermal melanin acts as a competing chromophore to melanin in the hair shaft and can cause epidermal burns. White and gray hairs have no melanin and are not known to respond to lasers. However, externally applied chromophores (dyes) can cause a temporary reduction in white or gray hairs with laser use [35].

Age-Related Hair Changes in Pigmentation

A rule of thumb for hair graying is that by 50 years of age, 50% of people have 50% gray hair [36]. In general, Caucasians start to gray in the mid-30s, Asians in their late-30s, and Africans in mid-40s [33]. The self-renewal of melanocytic stem cells becomes defective during aging resulting in white and gray hairs. Premature hair graying can be found after radiation exposure and several progeria disorders such as Werner syndrome ("adult progeria"), ataxia telangiectasia, and Waardenburg syndrome. These disorders are characterized by DNA damage and instability, which provide insight into the physiologic fate of melanocytic stem cells. By mimicking DNA damage caused by natural aging, ionization radiation exposure in mice models has been shown to cause terminal differentiation of stem cells into mature melanocytes and irreversible hair graying. This suggests that physiologic hair graying is due to melanocytic stem cell dysfunction from accumulating DNA damage [32].

Hair Shaft Shape

Cross-sectional hair shaft shape varies across African, Asian, and Caucasian hair types, see Fig. 3.6 [12]. Asian hair has a round hair shaft with the greatest diameter when compared to African and Caucasian hair types. Caucasian hair is an intermediate in cross-sectional shape and diameter between Asian and African hair. African hair shaft has an elliptical shape with varying diameter throughout the hair shaft and greatest variability among people. The African hair shaft shape has several twists along the longitudinal axis [6]. This makes the hair more susceptible to damage and dry combing more traumatic. While wet combing is more difficult in Caucasian hair types than dry combing, wet combing is preferred

in Afro-textured hair. Wet combing requires less force in African hair because there is decreased torsion and some relaxation of the curl, which reduces the amount of individual hair strand entanglement [7].

The relative hairlessness on most of the human body has evolved to augment eccrine sweating and cooling associated with evaporation. Scalp hair plays an important role in thermoregulation and UV protection. One hypothesis for the evolutionary conservation of Afro-textured hair is that it maintains a boundary layer of cool, dry air near the scalp to prevent overheating [37].

The Science of Hair Curl

Genome-wide association studies (GWAS) show that hair curl is under the complex control of many polymorphic genes [38]. Curliness was previously thought to be a result of the cross-sectional shape of the hair shaft—this has since

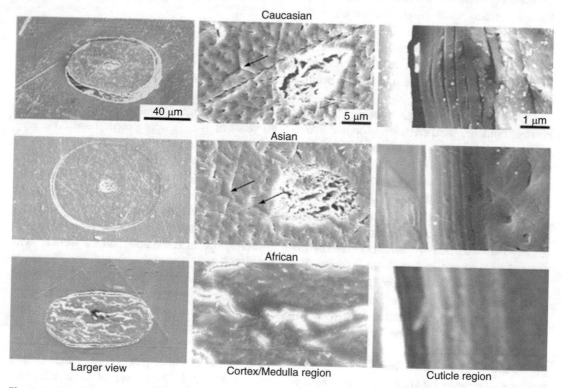

Fig. 3.6 Scanning electron microscope images of virgin hair cross section. (Reprinted from: Wei et al. [12], with permission from Elselvier)

been disproven [39]. Now, the leading hypothesis is that follicular asymmetry leads to coiled hair in all ethnicities/hair types. The exact mechanism of how the curl is formed has yet to be elucidated but there are several hypotheses such as the following: (i) asymmetric distribution of structural keratins in the precortex, (ii) differences in cortical cell shape and keratin fiber orientation, (iii) asymmetry of the outer and inner root sheath cells, (iv) inner root sheath and variations in expression of trichohyalin (a protein associated with curly hair and uncombable hair syndrome), and (iv) dermal papilla asymmetry [38, 40].

Categorizing Hair Curl

Curl patterns have been described subjectively using words such as straight, wavy, curly, frizzy, kinky, woolly, and helical. While these words conjure up global images, these phrases can be confusing due to overlapping characteristics and subjective identification [5]. The popular classification system used widely by consumers and cosmetic companies was developed by a hairdresser, Andre Walker, in the late 1990s. According to Walker, hair can be as follows: straight (Type 1A–1C), wavy (Type 2A–2C), curly (Type 3A–3B), and kinky (Type 4A–4B) [41].

There have been few attempts to objectively categorize hair curl in order to move away from the unscientific references to ethnicity. The first attempt was made by the anthropologist, Hrdy, who assessed hair from seven different populations and measured the average diameter, medullation, scale count, kinking, average curvature, ratio to minimum and maximum curvature, and crimp [4]. Hrdy observed that the average curvature was the most distinctive difference between the population groups and suggested this could be used to create a classification system.

The most recent studies validated a classification system that sorts hair into eight types based on the following: (i) curve diameter, the smallest curve diameter of hair at a given stretched length; (ii) curl index, the ratio between the stretched length to the greatest length occupied by the same piece of hair at rest without applied stress; (iii) the number of twists or kinks of the hair shaft along its main axis; (iv) the number of waves per sample, see Fig. 3.7 [5]. From Type I to Type VIII, the number of waves and twists increases while the diameter of the hair curl decreases. Based on this classification scheme, Asian hair is most

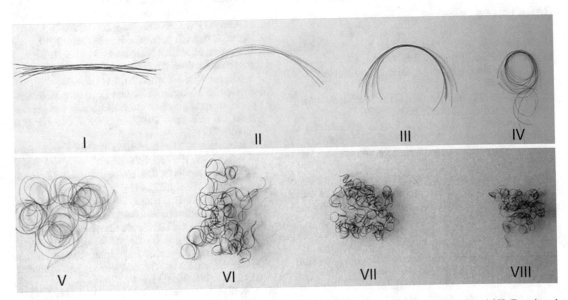

Fig. 3.7 Demographics of sample population across eight hair curl groups proposed by De La Mettri et al.[5] (Reprinted from: Mkentane et al. [4], under Creative Commons Attribution Open Access License)

often type II, Caucasian hair most frequently II and III, and African hair is most often type V to VII [6]. Limitations of this classification system include inter- and intra-rater uniformity and difficulty handling hair to count number of waves for groups V to VIII. The difference between hair group V and VI and hair group VII and VIII when counting waves was minimal. The presence of one extra or less wave could classify hair into a different group resulting in increased inter-rater variability and overall subjectivity [4]. There is still an unmet need for an easy-to-understand, efficient, and consumer-friendly method of classifying hair.

Conclusion

While all hair shares common morphology, basic molecular make up, and molecular structure, there are notable differences in phenotypic presentations. Instead of classifying hair based on unscientific categories of race, scientists continue to test objective measures regarding the qualities of hair and curl. Understanding the physical properties of hair can assist in guiding cosmetic and hair disease management.

References

1. Wang E, de Berker D, Christiano A. Biology of hair and nails. In: Bolognia J, Schaffer J, Cerroni L, editors. Dermatology. 4th ed. Edinburgh: Elsevier; 2018. p. 1144–61.
2. Khumalo N. Beyond "ethnicity" in dermatology. Dermatol Clin. 2014;32(2):9–12.
3. Loussouarn G, Garcel AL, Lozano I, Collaudin C, Porter C, Panhard S, et al. Worldwide diversity of hair curliness: a new method of assessment. Int J Dermatol. 2007;46:2–6.
4. Mkentane K, Van Wyk J, Sishi N, Gumedze F, Ngoepe M, Davids L, et al. Geometric classification of scalp hair for valid drug testing, 6 more reliable than 8 hair curl groups. PLoS One. 2017;12(6):e0172834.
5. De la Mettrie R, Saint-Leger D, Loussouarn G, Garcel A, Porter C, Langaney A. Shape variability and classification of human hair: a worldwide approach. Hum Biol. 2007;79(3):265–81.
6. He A, Chemical OG. Physical properties of hair: comparisons between Asian, Black, and Caucasian Hair.
7. Wolfram L. Human hair: a unique physicochemical composite. J Am Acad Dermatol. 2003;48:S106–14.
8. Dias MF. Hair cosmetics: an overview. Int J Trichol. 2015;7(1):2–15.
9. Robbins C. Chemical and physical behavior of human hair. 4th ed. New York: Springer; 2013.
10. Gavazzoni Dias M. Hair cosmetics: an overview. Int J Trichol. 2015;7(1):2–15.
11. McMichael AJ. Hair breakage in normal and weathered hair: focus on the Black patient. J Investig Dermatol Symp Proc. 2007;12(2):6–9.
12. Wei G, Bhushan B, Torgerson P. Nanomechanical characterization of human hair using nanoindentation and SEM. Ultramicroscopy. 2005;105(1–4):248–66.
13. Yang F, Zhang Y, Rheinstädter M. The structure of people's hair. PeerJ. 2014;2:e619.
14. Kamath YK, Weigmann H. Fractography of human hair. J Appl Polym Sci. 1982;27:2809–3833.
15. Buffoli B, Rinaldi F, Labanca M, Sorbellini E, Trink A, Guanziroli E, et al. The human hair: from anatomy to physiology. Int J Dermatol. 2014;53:331–41.
16. Tan T, et al. Premature desquamation of the inner root sheath in noninflamed hair follicles as a specific marker for central centrifugal cicatricial alopecia. Am J Dermatopathol. 2019;41(5):350–4.
17. Fernandez-Flores A, et al. Histopathology of aging of the hair follicle. J Cutan Pathol. 2019;46:508.
18. Wortsman X, Carreno L, Ferreira-Wortsman C, Poniachik R, Pizarro K, Morales C, et al. Ultrasound characteristics of the hair follicles and tracts, sebaceous glands, Montgomery glands, apocrine glands, and arrector pili muscles. J Ultrasound Med. 2018;38(8):1995–2004.
19. Poblet E, Ortega F, Jimenez F. The arrestor pili muscle and the follicular unit of the scalp: microscopic anatomy study. Dermatol Surg. 2002;28:800–3.
20. Martel J, Badri T. Anatomy, Hair Follicle. 2019.
21. Torkamani N, Rufaut N, Jonas L, Sinclair R. Beyond goosebumps: does the arrector pili muscle have a role in hair loss? Int J Trichol. 2014;6(3):88–94.
22. Sinclair R, Torkamani N, Jones L. Androgenetic alopecia: new insights into the pathogenesis and mechanism of hair loss. F1000Research. 2015;4(F1000 Faculty Rev)
23. Winkelmann R. The innervation of a hair follicle. Ann N Y Acad Sci. 1959;83:400–7.
24. Paus R, Cotsarelis G. The biology of hair follicles. N Engl J Med. 1999;12(7):491–7.
25. James W, Dirk E, Treat J, Rosenbach M, Neuhaus I. Skin: basic structure and function. Andrews' diseases of the skin. 13th ed. Edinburgh: Elsevier; 2020. p. 1–10.
26. Breitkopf T, Leung G, Yu M, Wang E, McElwee K. The basic science of hair biology: what are the causal mechanisms for disordered hair follicle? Dermatol Clin. 2013;31:1–19.
27. Lewallen R, Francis S, Fisher B, Richards J, Li J, Dawson T, et al. Hair care practices and structural

evaluation of scalp and hair shaft parameters in African American and Caucasian women. J Cosmet Dermatol. 2015;14(3):216–23.

28. Piraccini B, Alessandrini A. Androgenetic alopecia. G Ital Dermatol Venereol. 2014;149(1):15–24.

29. Paus R, Bulfone-Paus S, Bertolini M. Hair follicle immune privilege revisited: the key to alopecia areata management. J Investig Dermatol Symp Proc. 2018;19(1):S12–7.

30. McGrath J. The structure and function of skin. In: Calonje J, Brenn T, Lazar A, Billings S, editors. McKee's pathology of the skin. 5th ed. Edinburgh: Elsevier; 2019. p. 1–34.

31. Schaffer J, Bolognia J. The melanocortin-1 receptor: red hair and beyond. Arch Dermatolol. 2001;137(11):1477–85.

32. Nishimura E. Melanocyte stem cells: a melanocyte reservoir in hair follicles for hair and skin pigmentation. Pigment Cell Melanoma Res. 2011;24:401–10.

33. Park AM, Khan S, Rawnsley J. Hair biology: growth and pigmentation. Facial Plast Surg Clin North Am. 2018;26(4):415–24.

34. Ricci F, De Simone C, Del Regno L, Peris K. Drug-induced hair colour changes. Eur J Dermatol. 2016;26(6):531–6.

35. Arsiwala S, Majid I. Methods to overcome poor responses and challenges of laser hair removal in dark skin. Indian J Dermatol Venereol Leprol. 2019;85(1):3–9.

36. Keogh E, Walsh R. Rate of greying of human hair. Nature. 1965;207(999):877–8.

37. Jablonski NG, Chaplin G. The evolution of skin pigmentation and hair texture in people of African ancestry. Dermatol Clin. 2014;32(2):113–21.

38. Westgate G, Ginger R, Green M. The biology and genetics of curly hair. Exp Dermatol. 2017;26(6):483–90.

39. Bernard B. Hair shape of curly hair. J Am Acad Dermatol. 2003;48(6):S120–6.

40. Ü Basmanav F, Cau L, Tafazzoli A, Méchin M, Wolf S, Romano M, et al. Mutations in three genes encoding proteins involved in hair shaft formation cause uncombable hair syndrome. Am J Hum Genet. 2016;99(6):1292–304.

41. Wiltz T, Walker A. Andre talks hair! Simon & Shuster: New York; 1997.

42. Restrepo R, Calonje E. Diseases of the hair. In: Calonje E, Brenn T, Lazar A, Billings S, editors. McKee's pathology of the skin. Edinburgh: Elsevier; 2020. p. 1051–128.

Physiology of Skin Pigmentation

Micah Christine Brown and Chesahna Kindred

Overview of Skin of Color

To dive deep into skin of color, it is first vital to define what skin of color is; in addition to the ethnic races and skin characteristics that are included in this very inclusive and widespread group. People with skin of color come from a wide array of different backgrounds and ethnic groups. These groups include African Americans, Latinos or Hispanics, Native Americans, Pacific Islanders, and Asians [1, 2]. Darker skin is not only a difference in color, it also has differences in presentation of diseases and a certain spectrum of disease that this group of ethnic skin effects. Skin color has been traditionally classified by the Fitzpatrick scale. The Fitzpatrick Skin Photo Types are a skin typing system used to compare skin color and risk of sunburn [3]. However, this long-standing way of categorizing skin color is not an accurate representation because it provides a restricted option for ethnic skin, not taking into consideration the numerous variations of skin color [1, 3]. Since dermatological conditions may pres-

ent differently depending on the ethnicity of the patient, it is important to understand that biologic and pathophysiologic differences are apparent in skin of color [4]. Properly treating a wide array of patients from a culturally competent viewpoint requires a true understanding of the features of ethnic skin. The purpose of this chapter is to highlight the skin and its mechanisms, in addition to shedding light on ethnic skin's unique qualities.

Structure and Function of Skin

The skin is the largest organ in the body and serves many purposes. It serves as a barrier, providing protection from water, microorganisms, mechanical and chemical trauma, and UV light damage [5]. The skin consists of three layers: epidermis, dermis, and hypodermis. The epidermis is the most superficial layer of the skin and consists of well-defined layers of epithelial cells with thickness of each layers depending on body region. Throughout the body, there are areas of thick and thin skin. Thin skin covers most areas of the body, these areas are made up of four layers: from deep to superficial, stratum basale, stratum spinosum, stratum granulosum, and stratum corneum. Hairless skin that inhabits the soles of the feet and palms of the hands is thick and contains an additional layer called the stratum lucidum located between the stratum corneum and stratum granulosum (Table 4.1).

M. C. Brown (✉)
Howard University College of Medicine,
Washington, DC, USA
e-mail: micah.brown@bison.howard.edu

C. Kindred
Kindred Hair and Skin Center, Columbia, MD, USA

Department of Dermatology, Howard University
Hospital, Washington, DC, USA

© Springer Nature Switzerland AG 2021
B. S. Li, H. I. Maibach (eds.), *Ethnic Skin and Hair and Other Cultural Considerations*, Updates in
Clinical Dermatology, https://doi.org/10.1007/978-3-030-64830-5_4

Table 4.1 Layers of the epidermis and characteristics

	Thickness	Cell shape	Cellular components
Stratum basale	1 layer	Cuboidal to columnar	Merkel cells
			Melanocytes
			Hemidesmosomes
Stratum spinosum	8–9 cell layers	Irregular polyhedral	Desmosomes
Stratum granulosum	3–5 cell layers	Polygonal	Dendritic cells
			Keratohyalin granules
			Lamellar granules
Stratum lucidum	2–3 cell layers	Diamond shaped	Eleidin
Stratum Corneum	20–30 cell layers	Dead flattened cells	Corneocytes
			Keratin

Stratum Basale

The stratum basale is the deepest layer of the epidermis separated from the underlying dermis via a basement membrane. The basal layer is connected to the basement membrane by hemidesmosomes. Pathological conditions can arise when these hemidesmosome connections are disrupted (i.e., bullous pemphigoid). This layer contains primarily basal cells. These cuboidal to columnar mitotic stem cells are the precursors of the keratinocytes that inhabit every layer of the epidermis. Merkel cells and melanocytes are among the other cells that make up the basal layer of the epidermis. Merkel cells are oval-shaped epidermal cells predominantly occupying hairless skin areas and functioning as mechanoreceptors for light touch [6]. Merkel cells are adjacently bound by desmosomes with free nerve endings allowing their interaction with various stimuli. Langerhans cells are present in all layers of the epidermis and contribute to the immunologic response by functioning as antigen-presenting cells. Melanocytes are neural crest-derived cells that secrete melanin, the major determinant of skin and hair pigment. Melanosomes, membrane-bound melanin-producing cells in melanocytes, are special structures that contribute to a variety of dermatological conditions and physical differences in ethnic skin.

Stratum Spinosum

The stratum spinosum is the layer superficial to the basal layer and, as the name suggests, is named due to the appearance of the "spines" that the irregular polyhedral cells exhibit histologically [1, 7, 5]. Cells of the stratum spinosum are connected via desmosomes that provide strong adhesion between the 8 and 10 cell layers [6]. Dendritic cells are found in this layer, and they function as antigen-presenting cells, process antigens, and present them to T cells as an essential function of the immune system [8].

Stratum Granulosum

Cells transitioning from the stratum spinosum layer to the stratum granulosum layer undergo physical changes to be efficient. The cell membrane thickens and generates large amounts of fibrous keratin, keratohyalin, and lamellar granules [5]. Keratohyalin secretes keratinous precursor granules that aid in the keratin forming process. Lamellar granules act as a cohesive component that uses glycolipids in the cells to aid in their function [5]. As the keratinocytes travel more superficially, their function changes as well as their morphology. Their cells transition from polygons to flattened cells that are anucleated. Their contents are left behind to aid in the formation of the remaining layers of the epidermis [1].

Stratum Lucidum

The stratum lucidum layer is only present in hairless thick skin of the palms and soles of the feet. This 2–3 cell layer portion of the epidermis contains flattened, diamond-shaped cells containing eleidin, a transformation product of keratohyalin specific to this layer of the epidermis [5].

Stratum Corneum

Most superficially, the stratum corneum is the first layer of defense between the body and the outside world, providing protection from mechanical stresses as well are foreign bodies. Corneocytes, or horny cells, constitute this layer. Corneocytes embedded in a lipid-rich intercellular matrix provide the necessary characteristics that allow the corneum protective nature [6]. The anucelated cells of the stratum corneum signify the death of the keratinocytes. Depending on the area of the body, this layer's thickness is subject to change [5].

Dermis

Underlying the epidermis, the basement layer provides a layer of support and adhesion for the dermis. The two components of the basement layer are the papillary layer that makes direct contact with the epidermis and the reticular layer immediately beneath it [5]. The porous dermal-epidermal junction establishes cell polarity and direction of cell growth, contributing to both structures interacting with it. The dermal layer of the skin is a cohesive system filled with fibrous, filamentous, and amorphous connective tissue, providing a suitable environment for various cells such as hair and hair follicles, sensory neurons, vasculature, sweat glands [9, 5]. While the dermis does not undergo the same progression of cell differentiation as the overlying epidermis, the structure is able to fluctuate in response to external stimuli [9].

Hypodermis

Pigmentation in Skin of Color

The most evident physical differences of skin lie within the pigmentation. As mentioned pre-

viously, the organelle that is responsible for the wide array of skin color, hair color, and eye color is the melanocyte. This neural crest-derived cell has an extensive life cycle as it resides in the deepest layer of the epidermis, the stratum basale. The melanocyte, by way of dendritic cells, communicates with neighboring keratinocytes throughout the epidermis. A specialized lysosomal-related organelle, the melanosome, occupies melanocytes and secretes melanin [10]. Melanin is a tyrosine derivative compound with the sole purpose of providing pigment to hair, skin, and tissues [11]. The melanogenic pathway is initiated by the chemical transformation of tyrosine to dihydroxyphenylalanine (DOPA) by tyrosinase. This cascade yields the two major forms of melanin: eumelanin and pheomelanin [11]. Eumelanin, producing brown/black pigment, is UV absorbent while pheomelanin produces a yellow/red pigment, yielding photo-instability and possible carcinogenesis [11, 12] and many believe that darker skinned individuals have a higher amount of melanocytes, and the opposite for lighter skinned individuals; when in fact, the number of melanocytes does not change from person to person. The difference in pigmentation is a product of the amount of melanin that the particular melanosomes secrete into the epidermis [10]. While the mechanism behind number of melanocytes and their organization is unknown, it is evident that the amount of melanin as well as the type of melanin secreted from melanosomes is the vital determining factor of pigmentation and physical characteristics of dermatological disease (Figs. 4.1 and 4.2).

Hyperpigmentation

Hyperpigmentation is an area of concern predominantly for ethnic skin. Abnormal accumulation of melanin with diseases of the skin exacerbates melanin production, resulting in a darker pigmentation. Another mechanism by which hyperpigmentation can occur is via the sun. Melanin secretion is stimulated when UV radiation from the sun occurs. The long projections of dendritic cells allows for travel of melanin from melanocytes to keratinocytes. Melanin aggregate, around

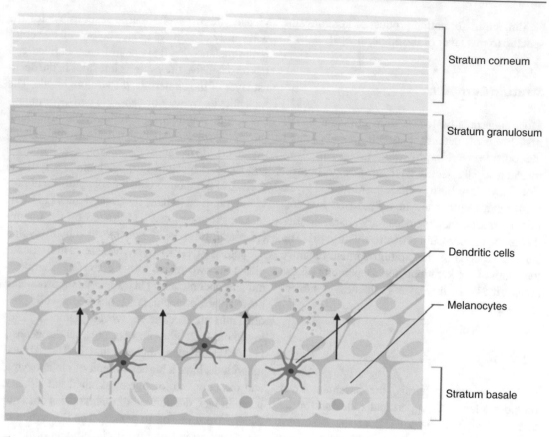

Fig. 4.1 Relationship between melanosomes and keratinocytes in the epidermis

the nucleus of keratinocytes, forms a shield that protects the nuclear contents from damage [1, 12, 13]. Kaidbey et al. suggest that darker skinned individuals possess built-in sun protection of about 13.4 [14], making them less susceptible to actinic damage but more likely to have dyspigmentation. This process coupled with the predisposing factors present in the skin contributes to the skin pigmentation and the differences in presentation of dermatological diseases in skin of color.

Differences in SOC Versus Caucasian Skin

In addition to the obvious differentiation in melanin in ethnic skin versus non-ethnic skin, there are a multitude of variances that contribute to the physiological characteristics of ethnic skin. Understanding these differences can explain cer-

tain ethnic disparities that patients encounter [15]. Skin is a barrier between internal organs and the outside environment, providing protection from foreign objections, pathogens, and maintaining thermoregulation and homeostasis. TEWL measures the amount of water vapor loss via the skin, excluding sweat [1, 15]. Research shows that transepidermal water loss (TEWL) is greater in Black skin when compared to Caucasian skin. While some studies show that Blacks express a higher value of TEWL, other research concludes that Asians have a higher TEWL. While the main components of the epidermis of the skin are overall standard across ethnicities, there are differences that should be addressed. Darker pigmented skin has been found to have more of a resistant barrier function [16] than lighter pigmented skin. This characteristic can attribute to the differences in topical management of certain dermatological diseases. Asian and Black skin

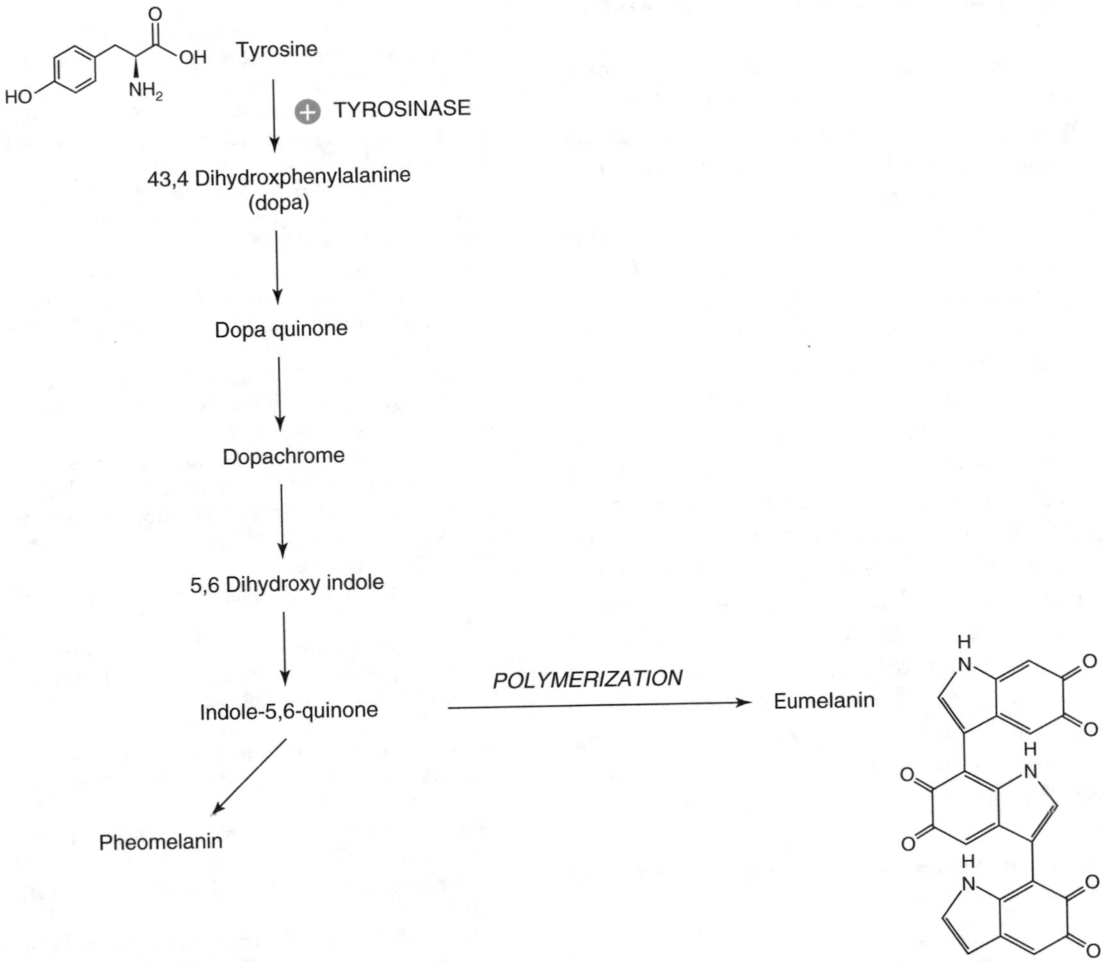

Fig. 4.2 An overview of melanin pigment

has a more compact dermis than White skin [17]. Research findings suggest that maybe degree of pigmentation has an effect on the lipid content of the skin, influencing the ability of the skin to hold water moisture and ceramide [1]. While darker pigmented skin is more resilient, Black skin is more prone to dryness [1]. As mentioned previously, the major structure of the skin remains constant throughout all human races; nevertheless, these minute seeming differences attribute to the physical differences of the skin overtime, pharmacological treatment variation, and a susceptibility to certain dermatological diseases based on type of skin (Table 4.2).

Table 4.2 Differences in ethnic skin and dermatological associations

Dermatological associations	Physiology of skin
Photoprotection, decreased risk of radiation-induced skin damage, increased risk of dyspigmentation	Larger, non-aggregated melanosomes
Thick dermis	Less pronounced photoaging, more resiliency
Higher lipid content	Increased dryness, loss of moisture
Larger, long-lasting fibroblast [18]	Increased prevalence of keloids and atrophic scarring, decreased skin loosening over time

Importance of Ethnic Skin Research

Fortunately, the United States is becoming diverse. According to the United States of America 2018 Census, people of color contribute to about 40% of the population [19]. It is becoming more apparent that cultural competency in medicine is more important than ever. While there is research on skin of color, the research that exists is not nearly enough to confidently and efficiently treat skin of all types. Recently, ethnic skin has become more researched and investigated, providing a conversation for changes in medicine. Moving forward, it is vital that science puts ethnic skin at the forefront of research. For decades, ethnic skin has taken a back seat in research and pharmacology, widening the ethnic disparities gap. Health affects all people, regardless of gender, nationality, and ethnicity; therefore, it is vital that medicine takes a step in the right direction to decrease the disparities associated with ethnic skin. Ultimately, the goal is to properly treat patients not just of Caucasian skin, but patients of all skin types.

Disclosure Statement The authors have nothing to disclose.

References

1. Kindred C, Oreseio C, Halder R. Overview of the structure and function of ethnic skin. In: Nutritional cosmetics: William Andrew, Applied Science Publishers. Elsevier Inc; 2009. p. 47–62.
2. Özdemir BC, Dotto G. Racial differences in cancer susceptibility and survival: More than the color of the skin? Trends Cancer. 2017;3(3):181–97. https://doi.org/10.1016/j.trecan.2017.02.002.
3. Sommers MS, Fargo JD, Regueira Y, Brown KM, Beacham BL, Perfetti AR, et al. Are the fitzpatrick skin phototypes valid for cancer risk assessment in a racially and ethnically diverse sample of women? Ethn Dis. 2019;29(3):505–12. https://doi.org/10.18865/ed.29.3.505.
4. Taylor S. Skin of color: biology, structure, function, and implications for dermatologic disease. J Am Acad Dermatol. 2003;42(6):S41–62.
5. Yousef H, Alhajj M, Sharma S. Anatomy, skin (integument), epidermis. Treasure Island: StatPearls Publishing LLC; 2019.
6. Jackson SM, Williams ML, Feingold KR, Elias PM. Pathobiology of the stratum corneum. West J Med. 1993;158(3):279–85.
7. Betts JG, Johnson E, Wise J, Young K, et al. The integumentary system. Anat Physiol. 2019. https://opentextbc.ca/anatomyandphysiology/chapter/5-1-layers-of-the-skin/
8. Molnar C, Gair J. Somatosensation. Concepts of biology. 2019. https://opentextbc.ca/biology/chapter/17-2-somatosensation/
9. Kolarsick PA, Kolarsick M, Anatomy GC. Physiology of the skin. J Dermatol Nurses Assoc. 2011;3(4):203–13. https://doi.org/10.1097/JDN.0b013e3182274a98.
10. Kaidbey KH, Agin PP, Sayre RM, Kligman AM. Photoprotection by melanin–a comparison of black and Caucasian skin. J Am Acad Dermatol. 1979;1(3):249–60.
11. Ebanks JP, Wickett RR, Boissy RE. Mechanisms regulating skin pigmentation: the rise and fall of complexion coloration. Int J Mol Sci. 2009;10(9):4066–87.
12. Nasti TH, Timares L. MC1R, eumelanin and pheomelanin: their role in determining the susceptibility to skin cancer. Photochem Photobiol. 2015;91(1):188–200.
13. Zaidi KU, Ali SA, Ali A, Naaz I. Natural tyrosinase inhibitors: role of herbals in the treatment of Hyperpigmentary disorders. Mini Rev Med Chem. 2019;19(10):796–808.
14. Vashi NA, de Castro Maymone MB, Kundu RV. Aging differences in ethnic skin. J Clin Aesthet Dermatol. 2016;9(1):31–8.
15. Wesley NO, Maibach HI. Racial (ethnic) differences in skin properties: the objective data. Am J Clin Dermatol. 2003;4(12):843–60.
16. Reed JT, Ghadially R, Elias PM. Skin type, but neither race nor gender, influence epidermal permeability barrier function. Arch Dermatol. 1995;131(10):1134–8.
17. Montagna W, Prota G, Kenney J. Black skin structure and function. Burlington: Elsevier Science; 2012.
18. Nilforoushzadeh MA, Ahmadi Ashtiani HR, Jaffary F, Jahangiri F, Nikkhah N, Mahmoudbeyk M, et al. Dermal fibroblast cells: biology and function in skin regeneration. J Skin Stem Cell. 2017;4(2):e69080.
19. U.S. Census Bureau. Quick facts [online]. 2018. Available at: https://www.census.gov/quickfacts/fact/table/US/PST045218%20census%20

Part II

Skin Diseases and Concerns in Ethnic Skin

Skin Cancer Knowledge, Awareness, and Perception

Karra K. Manier and Howard I. Maibach

Epidemiology

Skin cancer is the most common cancer in the United States [1] with one in five Americans developing the disease in their lifetime [2]. More than 3 million people within the nation are affected yearly and nearly 9,500 diagnoses are made every day [3].

Prevention and Risk Factors

Genetic and environmental factors have been shown to contribute to the pathogenesis of skin cancer. The most common genetic alteration occurring in nearly all skin cancers involves a mutation in the *p53* tumor suppressor gene [4]. *p53* normally functions to repair damaged DNA by arresting the cell cycle and activating the apoptosis pathway. However, this mechanism becomes ineffective when mutated, leading to the inability to protect cells from harmful carcinogens such as ultraviolet radiation (UVR) [4]. Chronic UVR exposure can have detrimental effects on the skin leading to damaged DNA through pyrimidine dimer formation, immunosuppression, reactive oxygen species, and inflammation [5]. Recommendations for skin cancer prevention include wearing protective clothing, broad-spectrum sunscreen, avoiding tanning beds, and performing routine self-examinations [6].

Types of Skin Cancer

Melanoma

Melanoma is the fifth most common cancer in the United States with an increased incidence in Caucasians and males [7]. It affects melanin-producing cells, known as melanocytes, in the epidermal layer of the skin. Patients often identify the lesion themselves due to its abnormal resemblance of a mole that changes in size, shape, or color [8]. The diagnosis of melanoma is made by assessing its characteristic features using the ABCDE criteria: asymmetry, border irregularity, color variegation, diameter greater than 6 mm, and evolution [9]. Other clinical symptoms can include erythema, swelling, pruritus, changes in sensation of the mole, tenderness, pain, or bleeding [10]. Most diagnoses are made between the ages of 65 and 74 years and involve a complete patient history, total-body skin examination, and use of diagnostic tools such as dermoscopy, histological evaluation, or molecular biomarkers to determine if a biopsy

K. K. Manier (✉)
Howard University College of Medicine,
Washington, DC, USA
e-mail: karra.manier@bison.howard.edu

H. I. Maibach
University of California, San Francisco, School of
Medicine, Department of Dermatology,
San Francisco, CA, USA

is needed [10]. The prognosis of melanomas can be assessed using the American Joint Committee on Cancer (AJCC) staging system, which classifies melanomas from Stage 0 to IV based on tumor thickness, involvement of regional lymph nodes, serum lactate dehydrogenase level, and metastasis to other lymph nodes, distant organs, or the central nervous system [10, 11]. The overall 5-year survival rate is estimated at 91.8% [12], making the outcome of melanoma favorable with early detection.

Melanoma is divided into four major subtypes: superficial spreading, nodular, lentigo maligna, and acral lentiginous (Table 5.1). Other uncommon subtypes include desmoplastic, verrucous, and nevoid melanoma. The clinical details of each subtype are described below.

the horizontal phase to its rapid growth in the vertical phase [15]. The lesions present in sun-exposed areas, most commonly on the posterior legs of women and on the trunk of men [16]. Histologically, SSM will present as single cells or nests of epithelioid melanocytes with copious cytoplasm spread throughout the mid and upper level of the epidermis and along the dermal-epidermal junction [10, 17].

Of all subtypes, superficial spreading melanoma is more likely to be associated with a BRAF gene mutation. The disruption of this oncogene causes dysregulation of a signaling pathway resulting in hyperactivation, proliferation, and the transformation of cells [18]. This finding plays an important role in the treatment options for SSM discussed later in this chapter.

Superficial Spreading Melanoma

Superficial spreading melanoma (SSM) is the most common subtype, being responsible for nearly 70% of all cases [13, 14]. It is generally diagnosed in patients between the ages of 40 and 60 years old and occurs more often in males and Caucasians [10, 13, 15]. The majority of SSM arise from a pre-existing nevus [15]. It initially appears as a light brown to black, irregular bordered macule that progresses into a plaque or nodule with variegated pigmentation [10, 15]. The changes in appearance reflect the transition from its localization to the epidermis during

Nodular Melanoma

Nodular melanoma (NM) is the second most common subtype of melanoma. It makes up 10–15% of all melanomas [14], typically occurring in patients within their sixth decade of life [15], and frequently presenting on the head, neck, and trunk [16]. NM is the most rapidly growing subtype, often resulting in a diagnosis at later stages and association with a poor prognosis [19]. It appears as a firm papule or nodule with minor color variegation and possible ulceration [10, 19]. Because of its irregular color characteristics, the typical ABCD criteria cannot be used for the

Table 5.1 Major subtypes of melanoma

Melanoma	Common Location	Characteristics	Histology
Superficial spreading	Posterior legs (women) and trunk (men)	Light brown to black, irregular bordered macule that progresses into a plaque or nodule with variegated pigmentation	Single cells or nests of epithelioid melanocytes with copious cytoplasm spread throughout the mid and upper level of the epidermis and along the dermal-epidermal junction
Nodular	Head, neck, and trunk	A firm papule or nodule with minor color variegation and possible ulceration	An in situ component that lacks extension beyond three rete ridges of the mass
Lentigo maligna	Head and neck	An asymmetric macule of mottled or variegated pigmentation with irregular borders	Spindled, epithelioid, or desmoplastic melanocytes in single cells or nests along the epidermal-dermal junction
Acral lentiginous	Nail beds, palms, and soles	An asymmetric, brown to black macule or papule with irregular borders	An acanthotic epidermis with atypical, hyperchromatic melanocytes along the epidermal-dermal junction

diagnosis. Rather, the melanoma is assessed with an EFG mnemonic for its elevation, firm consistency, and rapid growth [10].

In contrast to other melanomas, nodular melanoma does not have a radial growth phase. It directly enters a vertical growth phase upon invasion of the dermis, thus explaining its rapid growth rate and nodular appearance [17]. NM is histologically characterized by an in situ component that lacks extension beyond three rete ridges of the mass [20].

Lentigo Maligna Melanoma

Lentigo maligna (LM) is the initial presentation of lentigo maligna melanoma and is often referred to as the "in situ" form. LM becomes malignant when the atypical melanocytes are no longer confined to the epidermal layer and invade the dermis with potential for metastasis [21]. Around 5% of the in situ lesions will progress into invasive melanoma [22]. This subtype is one of the least common, representing 4–10% of melanomas. The diagnosis of the slow-growing tumor is regularly made in males and individuals over the age of 40 with a peak between 60 and 80 years old [21]. An asymmetric macule of mottled or variegated pigmentation with irregular borders in sun-exposed areas including the face and neck will be seen on presentation [10, 23]. LM can be evaluated using the ABCD criteria; however, a full-thickness biopsy and analysis of the dermatopathological features is critical to differentiate from the in situ form [21]. The in situ phase appears on histology as an atrophic epidermis with solar elastosis and proliferation of atypical melanocytes in the arrangement of single cells or nests along the epidermal-dermal junction and within adnexal structures [10, 20, 23]. The malignant melanoma will have spindled, epithelioid, or desmoplastic melanocytes [20, 24].

Acral Lentiginous Melanoma

Acral lentiginous melanoma (ALM) is the least common subtype, accounting for 4–10% of melanoma cases [10]. Acral refers to peripheral body parts, where the tumor most commonly occurs – the palms of the hands, soles of the feet, and nail beds. The uncommon locations are often the reason for its late diagnosis and poor survival rate [10]. Even in the setting of early detection, ALM is often initially misdiagnosed leading to a significant delay and an advanced stage at the time of the correct diagnosis [25]. The mean age at diagnosis is 62.8 years old [26] and the tumor often presents as an asymmetric, brown to black macule or papule with irregular borders on the palms and soles [10]. Subungual ALM features differ with longitudinal hyperpigmented streaks that extend beyond the proximal or lateral nail fold, known as the Hutchinson sign (Fig. 5.1) [15]. An acanthotic epidermis with atypical, hyperchromatic melanocytes along the epidermal-dermal junction will be seen on histology [20].

Other rare melanoma subtypes include amelanotic, desmoplastic, nevoid, and verrucous.

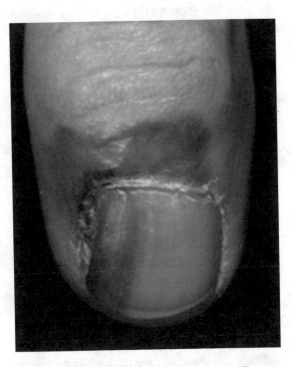

Fig. 5.1 Hutchinson's sign (Reprinted from Teramo, Martinez-Said, Guo, and Garbe with permission from Springer Nature

Non-melanoma Skin Cancer

Basal Cell Carcinoma

Basal cell carcinoma (BCC) is the most common skin cancer. It affects the stratum basale layer of the epidermis, which contains proliferative cells that produce keratinocytes for the other differentiated layers [27]. The incidence is steadily increasing with more than 4 million people diagnosed in the United States each year [28]. BCC most commonly presents on the face, but can also arise on the trunk, extremities, and genital mucosa [29]. The tumor can arise de novo or as an autosomal dominant disorder known as nevoid basal cell carcinoma syndrome. The inherited condition is caused by a *PTCH* gene mutation, affecting the sonic hedgehog pathway and manifesting as numerous basal cell carcinomas, pits of the palms and soles, and jaw keratocysts [29]. BCC is a locally aggressive tumor and rarely metastasizes.

The three main subtypes include nodular, superficial, and morpheaform. Nodular BCC is the most common subtype, making up 50–79% of all cases [29]. Its classic appearance involves a papule or nodule with pearly telangiectasias that may contain crust surrounding a central depression [30]. These lesions typically occur on the head with a preference for the forehead, eyelids, nasolabial folds, and cheek [29]. Superficial BCC is the second most common subtype, representing up to 15% of diagnoses. The tumor appears as a well-demarcated, scaly, and erythematous patch or plaque [29]. Unlike the other subtypes, superficial BCC predominates on the trunk and extremities rather than the head and neck [29]. Morpheaform BCC is the least common subtype, approximated at 5–10% of cases. It is also referred to as sclerosing or infiltrating BCC due to its clinical resemblance to scleroderma and its aggressive characteristics [29]. A lesion typically presents as pink, pearly, scar-like, indurated plaques or depressions with irregular borders [29]. Nodular and superficial BCCs have indolent-growth characteristics, while morpheaform BCCs show aggressive-growth with focal extensive destruction and a higher recurrence

rate [29]. All BCC tumors have a common histological feature including clusters of basaloid with surrounding stromal tissue and peripheral palisading nuclei [29]. However, biopsies are still required to confirm the diagnosis, identify distinguishing characteristics, and determine suitable treatment.

Squamous Cell Carcinoma

Squamous cell carcinoma (SCC) is estimated to cause 20% of skin cancer cases. The tumor arises from cells in the stratum spinosum layer, where keratin is produced and antigen-presenting immune cells known as Langerhans cells are found [31]. SCCs often emerge from an actinic keratosis, a carcinoma in situ lesion that is common in chronically sun-exposed individuals. The precursor presents as a scaly palpable, skin colored, pink or brown lesion on the head and neck, chest, and upper extremities [32]. Those with numerous actinic keratoses have a 6–10% overall risk of developing SCC [32]. Other precursors include bowenoid papulosis, epidermodysplasia verruciformis, Bowen's disease, and erythroplasia of Queyrat [33]. As SCC develops, it presents as a scaly, erythematous patch with a central depression and possible crusting and ulceration [32]. The aggressive tumor has an increased propensity to recur and metastasize, particularly if the lesion developed from injured or chronically scarred skin [32, 33].

Dermatofibrosarcoma Protuberans

Dermatofibrosarcoma protuberans (DFSP) is a rare, slow growing soft tissue tumor that most commonly presents in adults during the third to fifth decade of life [34]. The tumor arises within the dermis and infiltrates into the subcutaneous tissue or less commonly, can arise within the subcutaneous tissue without dermal involvement [35]. DFSP has a predominance for the trunk, extremities, and head and neck. Other uncommon sites include the breast, vulva, and penis [34, 35]. The lesion initially appears as an indurated plaque or nodule that develops overtime into reddish-blue, brown, or violaceous prominent nodules [33, 35]. Though DFSP is relatively a low-grade sarcoma, it has a high recurrence rate and low potential for metastasis with the lungs as the most common site [33, 35]. Recurrent or chronic tumors can cause extensive local destruction with invasion into multiple structures including the bone [35]. Uniformed spindle cells with thin nuclei and unclear cell borders will be visualized on histology [35].

Merkel Cell Carcinoma

Merkel cell carcinoma (MCC) is a cutaneous neuroendocrine tumor commonly associated with polyomavirus. It typically affects males and peaks in individuals within their seventh decade of life [36]. The head, neck, and extremities are the usual sites of presentation [36]. The clinical features can vary depending on the presence of the Merkel cell polyomavirus with positive tumors having unspecified characteristics or pink-red to violaceous dome-shaped nodules [36]. The classic round blue cell tumor will be visualized histologically with circular nuclei, diffuse chromatin, and multiple mitoses with nuclear fragmentation [36]. Cytokeratin (CK20), neuroendocrine (neuron-specific endolase, synaptophysin, chromogranin, CD56), and neurofilament markers are often underutilized but should be used to confirm the diagnosis [36, 37].

Treatment

Treatment of skin cancer involves a wide variety of therapeutic options that is dependent on tumor features and patient preference. Clinical and histopathological characteristics, involvement of lymph nodes or distant metastasis, and the presence of genetic mutations are all factors that are considered in the selection of the most appropriate treatment [38]. Local melanomas are primarily treated with surgical excision [39]. Regional melanomas receive surgical intervention with lymph node dissection in addition

to adjuvant immunotherapy or radiation [40]. Tumors containing *BRAF* mutations can be targeted with combination therapy involving *BRAF* (vemurafenib/dabrafenib) and *MEK* (trametinib/cobimetinib) inhibitors. Those without BRAF mutations can be treated solely with PD-1 inhibitors (nivolumab) or in combination with a CTLA-4 inhibitor, ipilimumab [40].

Most non-melanoma tumors are treated with surgical procedures including Mohs micrographic surgery, local excision, radiation, and electrodessication and curettage [41]. Of these options, MMS is highly preferred because of its high cure rate and sparing the removal of unaffected tissue; however, it is only indicated for tumors in areas with a high risk of recurrence or for cosmesis and functionality [41, 42]. Other therapeutic options include photodynamic therapy, cryotherapy, radiation or topical therapy, and laser treatment [43, 44]. Advanced disease can be managed with chemotherapy and targeted therapies such as hedgehog pathway inhibitors and epidermal growth factor receptor inhibitors for BCC and SCC, respectively [43, 44].

Skin Cancer in Skin of Color

Skin cancer occurs less frequently in individuals with skin of color, arising in fewer than 20% of Hispanics, Asians, and African Americans combined [45]. These populations contain an increased amount of melanin in comparison to Caucasians, allowing for protection against ultraviolet radiation, and a lower incidence in skin cancer [33]. Although skin cancer is not as common in skin of color, there is an increased association of morbidity and mortality due to its atypical clinical presentation and delayed diagnosis [45]. Considering that more than half of the US population will be represented by those of color by the year 2060, it is crucial to understand the characteristic features of skin cancer in skin of color in effort to promptly identify and effectively treat this population [45]. Clinical features of skin cancer are listed in Table 5.2 and described in detail below.

Table 5.2 Skin cancer in skin of color

Non-melanoma	Frequency	Location	Characteristics
Basal cell carcinoma	Most common in Hispanics and Asians	Face, trunk, and extremities	Pigmented, pearly appearance
Squamous cell carcinoma	Most common in African Americans	Lower extremities and anogenital region	Pigmented papule or nodule
Malignant melanoma	Most common in African Americans, Asians, and Hispanics	Nail beds, palms and soles, and mucosal membranes	Varies based on subtype

Basal Cell Carcinoma in Skin of Color

Basal cell carcinoma is the most frequently diagnosed skin cancer in Hispanics and Asians, but the second most in African Americans [45]. In all races, UVR exposure is the most common contributing factor for BCC [46], underscoring the need for sun protection for every population. Additional risk factors include chronic scars and infection, immunosuppression, radiation, and thermal burns. Albinism, xeroderma pigmentosum, and nevoid basal cell carcinoma can also play a role in the pathogenesis of these tumors, particularly in African Americans [33, 45]. Most BCC tumors present with pigmentation and difficulty identifying the classic telangiectasias and pearly appearance (Fig. 5.2) [45]. Consequently, pigmented tumors are frequently misdiagnosed as seborrheic keratosis, melanoma, or nevus sebaceous [33, 45]. Although there is limited literature regarding BCC in Hispanics, reports have shown that this population is likely to be diagnosed with multiple BCC tumors rather than a solitary lesion [45]. Asians with BCC have shown to present with a "black pearly appearance" particularly surrounding the border of the tumor [45]. Chinese patients have specifically been shown to develop BCC at a later age and more likely to have tumors associated with pruritus [45]. Differences between the anatomical sites or metastatic rate in those of skin of color and in Caucasians have not been reported [33, 45].

Squamous Cell Carcinoma in Skin of Color

Squamous cell carcinoma is the most common skin cancer in African Americans and second

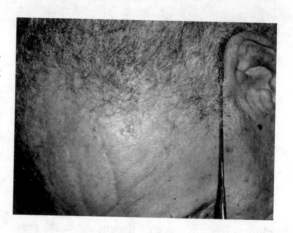

Fig. 5.2 Basal cell carcinoma on frontal scalp of African American man (Reprinted from Jackson with permission from Springer Nature)

most common in Asians and Hispanics. The tumor is responsible for at least 30% of skin cancers in African Americans, Black Indians, and the Japanese. The risk factors for SCC differ for each race with chronic inflammation being the greatest predisposition in African Americans [33]. Osteomyelitis, hidradenitis suppurativa, and lupus vulgaris are common causes of chronic scarring [33] and can cause a higher rate of metastasis than in Caucasians if SCC develops from these lesions [45]. Actinic keratosis and seborrheic keratosis have been reported as risk factors for Chinese Asians and the Japanese [46]. In both African Americans and Asians, SCC can develop in areas of chronic discoid lupus erythematous with a higher potential to metastasize than SCC progressing from other previous lesions [33, 45]. Similar to BCC, other predisposing factors for individuals with skin of color involve leg ulcers, exposure to radiation, and immunosuppression [33]. The tumors primarily occur on anatomical

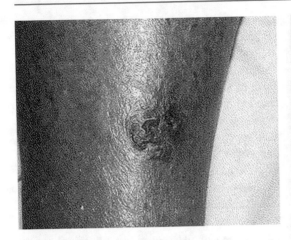

Fig. 5.3 Squamous cell carcinoma on the lower leg of a Black male (Reprinted from Gloster and Neal with permission from Elsevier)

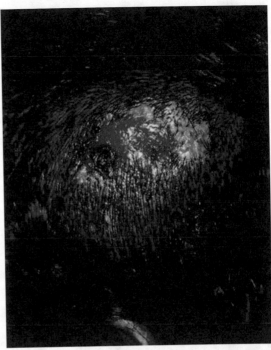

Fig. 5.4 An Indian female with SCC in nevus sebaceous of scalp. (Photograph courtesy of June K. Robinson, M.D. Reprinted with permission from Springer Nature)

sites that receive less sun exposure such as the lower extremities and can present as a pigmented papule or nodule (Fig. 5.3) [45]. Patients with these lesions may report clinical symptoms of leg warmth, hypopigmented, depigmented, or hyperpigmented macules [46].

SCC can develop in the anogenital region, specifically on the anus, penis, or vulva [46]. Penile SCC is considerably rare in the United States in comparison to other geographic areas [47]. Although there is a low incidence, Hispanics in the United States have a 72% higher rate than in other ethnic populations [47] and tend to have larger and hyperpigmented tumors [45]. Caucasians and African Americans are reported to be equally affected; however, African Americans generally present at younger ages with more advanced disease, and thus have a decreased survival period [45, 46] (Fig. 5.4).

Malignant Melanoma in Skin of Color

Melanoma is the third most common skin malignancy in all populations and has the highest rate of mortality [33]. Following along with BCC and SCC, risk factors for melanomas in skin of color include albinism, burns, trauma, radiation therapy, immunosuppression, and previous pig-

mented lesions [46]. The clinical appearance of melanomas varies in minorities with a predominance on nonexposed skin such as the nail beds (Fig. 5.5), palms and soles, and mucosal membranes in Asians and Blacks, and in sun-exposed areas in Hispanics (Fig. 5.6) [33]. As previously mentioned, melanoma has a relatively high 5-year survival rate, yet this prognosis does not apply for individuals with skin of color. African Americans and Hispanics present with a lower survival rate and thicker, Stage IV tumors [33, 48, 49]. Socioeconomic and cultural factors both contribute to the poor prognosis among these minorities [48]. For instance, patients with limited insurance coverage were more likely to be diagnosed with a melanoma at an advanced stage due to lack of access to preventive services [48]. Language barriers have also been shown to hinder access to skin cancer screenings and follow-up care for those who have a preferred language other than English [48].

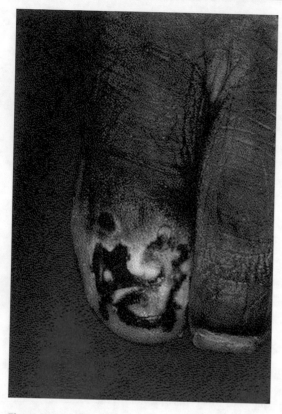

Fig. 5.5 Melanoma of the nail bed in a black male. (Reprinted from Gloster and Neal with permission from Elsevier)

Dermatofibrosarcoma Protuberans in Skin of Color

Dermatofibrosarcoma protuberans occurs in up to 10% of skin cancer cases in African Americans, making their incidence nearly double the rate than in Caucasians [33]. DFSP has a similar clinical appearance in all racial groups. The lesion can resemble a keloid, a lesion typically found in African Americans that rapidly forms after exposure to skin trauma [50]. Therefore, any uncommon appearing keloid occurring in abnormal areas or those without recent trauma should be biopsied in patients with skin of color [33] (Fig. 5.7).

Awareness and Perception of Skin Cancer

Skin cancer risk perception plays an integral part in the prognosis and outcome of skin cancer in minorities. Educational, cultural, and psychological factors all contribute to an individual's

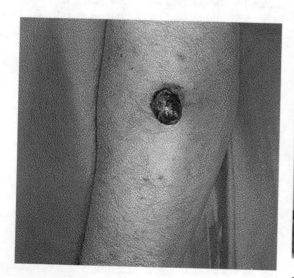

Fig. 5.6 Nodular melanoma in a Hispanic male. (Reprinted from Gloster and Neal with permission from Elsevier)

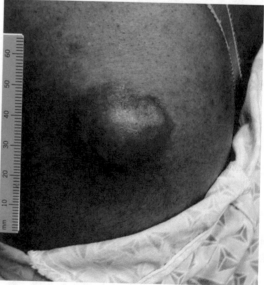

Fig. 5.7 Dermatofibrosarcoma protuberans. A large firm pink-brown nodule on the shoulder (Reprinted from Al-Haseni and Sahni with permission from Springer Nature)

knowledge and perceived risk. Many minorities, particularly older adults and the educationally disadvantaged, lack basic knowledge of skin cancer and are at greater risk of having inaccurate perceptions about the disease [51]. Their misconceptions involve being less susceptible to developing skin cancer, disbelieving the importance of conducting regular skin examinations to identify lesions, and thinking that not much can be done to decrease the risk of skin cancer [51]. These misunderstandings illustrate the critical need for skin cancer education in all races.

Currently, skin cancer screenings are not routinely recommended for adults without any signs, symptoms, or history of skin cancer. On account of this guideline, many individuals go without receiving or learning about a total body skin examination unless there is a specific concern. Reports have shown that in comparison to Caucasians, minorities are less likely to receive [52], or learn how to perform a skin self-examination by a physician or health care professional [53]. Furthermore, minorities that are aware of skin cancer screenings are more likely to conduct skin self-examinations if they perceive themselves as high risk and have a personal history of skin cancer [53]. In effort to change the narrative of skin cancer and encourage preventative behavior among low- or high-risk patients, physicians should consider teaching skin self-examinations during the standard physical examination and assist patients with identifying alarming signs that may go unnoticed.

Individuals primarily obtain skin cancer knowledge from multimedia sources, whose messages often target individuals who are most at risk with fair skin complexions or excessive sun exposure [53]. As a result, those from ethnic backgrounds and without these risk factors may not consider this information useful and can be less likely to utilize the preventive measures that are being highlighted. Moving forward, media sources should consider inclusivity and accounting for all racial groups to help raise awareness of skin cancer.

Next Steps

Addressing the disparity in perception and prevention is necessary to improve the diagnosis and prognosis of skin cancer in skin of color. For both patients and physicians, understanding and identifying the clinical variations of skin cancer in minorities will allow for early detection and appropriate treatment. In addition, improving social resources for these individuals by increasing access to preventive services will provide underinsured patients with cancer screenings and education on regular skin self-examinations, and ultimately aiding in a timely diagnosis. Finally, increasing patient education through media resources and physician visits should be emphasized and focused on the risk factors for skin cancer, the aberrant anatomical sites where tumors can arise, and preventive techniques.

References

1. Guy GP, et al. Vital signs: melanoma incidence and mortality trends and projections – United States, 1982–2030. MMWR. 2015;64(21):591–6.
2. Stern RS. Prevalence of a history of skin cancer in 2007: results of an incidence-based model. Arch Dermatol. 2010;146(3):279–82.
3. Skin cancer. 2018 [cited 2018 December 21]; Available from: https://www.aad.org/media/stats/conditions/skin-cancer.
4. Benjamin CL, Ananthaswamy HN. p53 and the pathogenesis of skin cancer. Toxicol Appl Pharmacol. 2007;224(3):241–8.
5. Narayanan DL, Saladi RN, Fox JL. Ultraviolet radiation and skin cancer. Int J Dermatol. 2010;49(9):978–86.
6. Prevent skin cancer. 2018 [cited 2018 December 21]; Available from: https://www.aad.org/public/spot-skin-cancer/learn-about-skin-cancer/prevent.
7. Surveillance, Epidemiology, and End Results (SEER) Program. 2018.
8. Avilés-Izquierdo JA, et al. Who detects melanoma? Impact of detection patterns on characteristics and prognosis of patients with melanoma. J Am Acad Dermatol. 2016;75(5):967–74.
9. What to look for: ABCDEs of melanoma. 2018 [cited 2018 December 22].
10. Rotte A, Bhandaru M. Melanoma—diagnosis, subtypes and AJCC stages. In: Immunotherapy of

melanoma, vol. 21-47. Cham: Springer International Publishing; 2016.

11. Gershenwald, J.E. and R.A.J.A.o.S.O. Scolyer, Melanoma Staging: American Joint Committee on Cancer (AJCC) 8th Edition and Beyond. 2018. 25(8): p. 2105–2110.

12. Surveillance, Epidemiology, and End Results (SEER) Program 2018, National Cancer Institute: Bethesda

13. Singh P, Kim HJ, Schwartz RA. Superficial spreading melanoma: an analysis of 97 702 cases using the SEER database. Melanoma Res. 2016;26(4): 395–400.

14. Types of Melanoma. 2018 [cited 2018 December 22, 2018].

15. Garbe C, Bauer J. In: Bolognia JL, Schaffer JV, Cerroni L, editors. Melanoma. 4th ed: Elsevier; 2018.

16. Kibbi N, Kluger H, Choi JN. Melanoma: clinical presentations. In: Kaufman HL, Mehnert JM, editors. Melanoma. Cham: Springer International Publishing; 2016. p. 107–29.

17. Smoller BR. Histologic criteria for diagnosing primary cutaneous malignant melanoma. Mod Pathol. 2006;19:S34–40.

18. Dhomen N, Marais R. New insight into BRAF mutations in cancer. Curr Opin Genet Dev. 2007;17(1):31–9.

19. Menzies SW, et al. Dermoscopic evaluation of nodular melanoma. JAMA Dermatol. 2013;149(6): 699–709.

20. Brinster NK, et al. Melanoma. In: Brinster NK, et al., editors. Dermatopathology: high-yield pathology. Philadelphia: Elsevier; 2011. p. 355–63.

21. Charifa A, Chen CSJ. Cancer, melanoma, lentigo maligna: StatPearls; 2018. [cited 2018 December 23, 2018].

22. Weinstock MA, Sober AJ. The risk of progression of lentigo maligna to lentigo maligna melanoma. Br J Dermatol. 1987;116(3):303–10.

23. Cohen LM. Lentigo maligna and lentigo maligna melanoma. J Am Acad Dermatol. 1995;33(6): 923–36.

24. Elston DM. Melanocytic neoplasms. In: Elston DM, Ferringer T, editors. Dermatopathology: Elsevier. p. 101–31.

25. Metzger S, et al. Extent and consequences of physician delay in the diagnosis of acral melanoma. Melanoma Res. 1998;8(2):181–6.

26. Bradford PT, et al. Acral lentiginous melanoma: incidence and survival patterns in the United States, 1986-2005. Arch Dermatol. 2009;145(4):427–34.

27. Chu DH. Structure and function of the skin. In: Goldman L, Schafer AL, editors. Goldman-cecil medicine. Philadelphia: Elsevier; 2016. p. 2632–7.

28. Basal cell carcinoma. 2018 [cited 2018 December 21]; Available from: https://www.skincancer.org/skin-cancer-information/basal-cell-carcinoma.

29. Marzuka AG, Book SE. Basal cell carcinoma: pathogenesis, epidemiology, clinical features, diagnosis, histopathology, and management. Yale J Biol Med. 2015;88(2):167–79.

30. Ortel B, Bolotin D. Cancer of the skin. In: Kellerman RD, Bope ET, editors. Conn's current therapy 2018. Philadelphia, PA: Elsevier; 2018.

31. SEER training modules, layers of the skin. 2018 [cited 2018 December 22]; Available from: https://training.seer.cancer.gov/melanoma/anatomy/layers.html.

32. Alam M, Ratner D. Cutaneous squamous-cell carcinoma. N Engl J Med. 2001;344(13):975–83.

33. Bradford PT. Skin cancer in skin of color. Dermatol Nurs. 2009;21(4):170–206.

34. Reha J, Katz SC. Dermatofibrosarcoma protuberans. Surg Clin N Am. 2016;96(5):1031–46.

35. Thway K, et al. Dermatofibrosarcoma protuberans: pathology, genetics, and potential therapeutic strategies. Ann Diagn Pathol. 2016;25:64–71.

36. Pulitzer M. Merkel cell carcinoma. Surg Pathol Clin. 2017;10(2):399–408.

37. Cassler NM, et al. Merkel cell carcinoma therapeutic update. Curr Treat Options Oncol. 2016;17(7):36.

38. Gandhi SA, Kampp J. Skin cancer epidemiology, detection, and management. Med Clin. 2015;99(6):1323–35.

39. Swetter SM, et al. Guidelines of care for the management of primary cutaneous melanoma. J Am Acad Dermatol. 2019;80(1):208–50.

40. Network, N.C.C. Melanoma. 2018 April 30, 2019]; Available from: https://www.nccn.org/patients/guidelines/melanoma/files/assets/common/downloads/files/melanoma.pdf.

41. Shriner DL, et al. Mohs micrographic surgery. J Am Acad Dermatol. 1998;39(1):79–97.

42. Divine J, et al. A comprehensive guide to the surgical management of nonmelanoma skin cancer. Curr Probl Cancer. 2015;39(4):216–25.

43. Bichakjian C, et al. Guidelines of care for the management of basal cell carcinoma. J Am Acad Dermatol. 2018;78(3):540–59.

44. Alam M, et al. Guidelines of care for the management of cutaneous squamous cell carcinoma. J Am Acad Dermatol. 2018;78(3):560–78.

45. Higgins S, et al. Review of nonmelanoma skin Cancer in African Americans, hispanics, and asians. Dermatol Surg. 2018;44(7):903–10.

46. Gloster HM, Neal K. Skin cancer in skin of color. J Am Acad Dermatol. 2006;55(5):741–60.

47. Morrison BF. Risk factors and prevalence of penile cancer. West Indian Med J. 2014;63(6):559–60.

48. Wich LG, et al. Impact of socioeconomic status and sociodemographic factors on melanoma presentation among ethnic minorities. J Community Health. 2011;36(3):461–8.

49. Jacobsen AA, et al. Defining the need for skin cancer prevention education in uninsured, minority, and immigrant communities. JAMA Dermatol. 2016;152(12):1342–7.

50. Marneros AG, et al. Clinical genetics of familial keloids. Arch Dermatol. 2001;137(11):1429–34.

51. Buster KJ, et al. Skin cancer risk perceptions: a comparison across ethnicity, age, education, gender, and income. J Am Acad Dermatol. 2012;66(5):771–9.

52. Korta DZ, Saggar V, Wu TP, Sanchez M. Racial differences in skin cancer awareness and surveillance practices at a public hospital dermatology clinic. J Am Acad Dermatol. 2013;70(2):312–7.

53. Pipitone M, et al. Skin cancer awareness in suburban employees: a Hispanic perspective. J Am Acad Dermatol. 2002;47(1):118–23.

54. Teramoto Y, Martinez-Said H, Guo J, Garbe C. (2019) Acral Lentiginous Melanoma. In: Balch C. et al. (eds) Cutaneous Melanoma. Springer, Cham. https://doi-org.libproxy2.usc.edu/10.1007/978-3-319-46029-1_67-1.

55. Jackson BA, Jackson BA. (2013) Skin Cancers in Skin of Color. In: Alexis A, Barbosa V. (eds) Skin of Color. Springer, New York, NY. https://doi-org.libproxy2.usc.edu/10.1007/978-0-387-84929-4_11.

56. Al-Haseni A, Sahni D. (2017) Skin Cancer. In: Vashi N, Maibach H. (eds) Dermatoanthropology of Ethnic Skin and Hair. Springer, Cham. https://doi-org.libproxy2.usc.edu/10.1007/978-3-319-53961-4_16.

Other Effects of Ultraviolet Light: Photosensitivity, Photoreactivity, and Photoaging

Umer Ansari and Valerie M. Harvey

The Electromagnetic Spectrum: UVA, UVB, and VL

Solar radiation encompasses a continuum of wavelengths including ultraviolet radiation (UVR; 280–400 nm), visible light (VL; 400–760 nm), and infrared radiation (IR; 760 nm – 1 mm) [1]. The classification scheme most widely utilized in dermatology further separates UVR into UVB (290–320 nm) and UVA (340–400 nm). UVA is further subdivided into UVA1 (340–400 nm) and UVA2 (320–340 nm) [2]. Because the majority of wavelengths are absorbed by the ozone layer, only a fraction of UVR reaches the earth's surface, accounting for only 3% of terrestrial radiation [3]. At ground level, UVA is 20 times more abundant than UVB, as its longer wavelengths can more efficiently penetrate the ozone layer [4]. VL accounts for 44% of solar radiation at ground level, with IR accounting for the remaining portion [3, 5].

The Biological Effects of Ultraviolet Radiation

UVA

The cellular and molecular impact of UVR on cutaneous structures is well documented. The long wavelengths of UVA facilitate its penetration to the deeper portions of the dermis [6]; 20–50% of UVA reaches the depth of melanocytes, and approximately 30% of UVA is capable of infiltrating the dermis [4, 7].

One major way by which UVA provokes epidermal and dermal injury is through the formation of free radicals and reactive oxygen species (ROS) [4, 8]. UVA is absorbed by chromophores (light absorbing molecules) including melanin, DNA, RNA, and aromatic amino acids, triggering photochemical reactions that produce the ROS [1, 9]. Following UVA exposure, keratinocytes and fibroblasts increase their expression of biomarkers related to oxidative damage such as ferritin, lysozyme, matrix metalloproteinase-1 (MMP-1), heme oxygenase-1, and superoxide dismutase-2 [4, 10]. A recent study using human skin constructs showed that UVA exposure modulated the expression of genes implicated in oxidative stress and extracellular matrix modeling. Sixty of 74 genes were expressed after minimal amounts of UVA exposure, suggesting that the threshold for UVA-induced change is quite low [10].

U. Ansari
University of Maryland Medical Systems, Baltimore, MD, USA

V. M. Harvey (✉)
Hampton Roads Center for Dermatology, The Hampton University Skin of Color Research Institute, Hampton University, Hampton, VA, USA

© Springer Nature Switzerland AG 2021
B. S. Li, H. I. Maibach (eds.), *Ethnic Skin and Hair and Other Cultural Considerations*, Updates in Clinical Dermatology, https://doi.org/10.1007/978-3-030-64830-5_6

Reactive oxygen species elicit a number of detrimental effects, including mitochondrial and cellular membrane injury, and apoptosis [7, 11, 12]. Structural sequelae of UVA-induced ROS are evident by the destruction of dermal elastin and collagen, and the effacement of the dermal-epidermal junction [4, 9, 10, 13]. ROS also mediate the release of cytokines and inflammatory mediators such as histamine, prostaglandins, and kinins [14], which cause dilatation of the vasculature in the subpapillary plexus [14, 15].

UVA causes direct damage to DNA through the formation of pyrimidine dimers [12]. Recent data suggest that UVA-induced dimers may be more mutagenic than those caused by UVB [12]. Runger et al. showed that UVA-irradiated primary human fibroblasts possess less effective DNA repair and cell cycle arrest mechanisms compared to human fibroblasts exposed to equimutagenic doses of UVB [12].

There is evidence to suggest that melanin and its intermediaries exacerbate UVA-mediated damage. Eniko et al. demonstrated that cultured human type VI melanocytes exposed to UVA experience higher levels of DNA single-strand breaks compared to type I melanocytes, presumably secondary to the higher melanin content of the former [16]. Marrot et al. also found a correlation between DNA damage and cellular melanin content; breakage was more intense within melanocytes than in fibroblasts, and in cells with high vs. low melanin content following melanogenic stimulation [17]. Together, these findings suggest that individuals with darker skin are also susceptible to UVA-induced phototoxicity, and strengthen the rationale for sun protection in those with darker skin types.

UVB

In contrast to UVA, UVB less effectively penetrates the epidermis; 9–15% of UVB reaches the melanocytes, and 10% of UVB contacts the dermis [4, 7]. Because most of UVB is absorbed

in the epidermis, much of its biological sequelae occur there. The relatively short wavelength of this light spectrum renders it more potent, imparting its deleterious effects at much lower doses [1]. UVB directly injures DNA, causing the formation of cyclobutane-pyrimidine and pyrimidine-pyrimidine dimers within keratinocytes and melanocytes [1]. As mutagenesis progresses, cells gain the ability to evade the regulatory mechanisms of apoptosis [18]. Subsequent clonal expansion of genomically modified cells leads to carcinogenesis with the development of squamous cell carcinomas, basal cell carcinomas, or melanomas [18].

DNA dimer formation is associated with upregulation of melanogenic genes [6]. After UVB exposure, keratinocytes express the p53 protein, which in turn activates transcription of proopiomelanocortin (POMC). POMC is processed into several different biologically active hormones, including alpha melanocyte stimulating hormone (alpha-MSH). Alpha-MSH then binds to melanocortin-1 receptors on melanocytes and activates melanin redistribution, melanocyte proliferation, and de novo melanin synthesis [19]. This cascade of events is accompanied by elevated levels of tyrosinase mRNA [20]. The newly produced melanin is transferred to the superficial layers of the epidermis [7, 19, 20]. UVB-generated melanogenesis, in combination with epidermal acanthosis, provides broad-spectrum coverage against subsequent UVA, UVB, and VL exposure [1, 12].

UVB is also integral to vitamin D3 production (cholecalciferol). UVB converts dehydrocholesterol (provitamin D) to previtamin D3 in the basal and spinous layers of the epidermis [9]. Previtamin D3 is then heat converted to vitamin D3. Due to the increased absorbance of UVB by epidermal melanocytes, darker skinned individuals are less efficient producers of vitamin D and therefore more susceptible to vitamin D deficiency [21]. A detailed discussion on the formation and function of vitamin D is provided in a review by Goring and Koshuchowa [22].

Biological Effects of UVB in Darker Skin

A number of factors provide darker skin with relative protection against the harmful effects of UVB. Melanin, an avid absorber and deflector of UVB [23, 24], serves as a physical shield for UVB exposed cells [12, 23], effectively diminishing the proportion of keratinocytes, melanocytes, and dermal fibroblasts exposed to UVB radiation [23, 24]. Furthermore, wavelengths less than 310 nm are preferentially absorbed by the stratum corneum (SC). Studies have shown that the SC of black skin has a greater number of layers [25, 26]. Although the SC of black and white skin are of equal thickness, an increase in layers makes black skin more compact and cohesive, conferring increased relative protection to UVB. Together, these factors may account for the lower levels of UVB-propagated DNA damage observed in darker skin compared to lighter skin [27, 28].

Visible Light

VL has recently been identified as a potential contributor to photodamage. Similar to UVR, VL is absorbed by a number of chromophores including melanin, B-carotene, and protoporphyrin [15]. VL triggers free radical damage, inflammatory reactions, and the activation of matrix metalloproteinases, leading to subsequent dermal damage [15, 29]. A recent study by Chiarelli-Neto et al. [28] showed that VL generated singlet oxygen free radicals via interaction with melanin [28]. Cells expressing higher melanin levels developed more necro-apoptosis, suggesting that VL-induced phototoxicity may be more severe among darker skin types. The effects of VL are significant, since the majority of currently available proprietary sunscreens are ineffective against this spectrum of light [29].

Skin Classification Systems

The Fitzpatrick skin phototype system (SPS), based on a self-reported tendency to sunburn and ability to tan, was initially developed as a method to assess one's tolerance to UVR exposure [1]. It was originally created to classify skin phototype in Caucasians, (types I to IV), with higher gradation correlating to darker skin. Skin types V and VI were later added in order to include individuals with brown and black skin, respectively. Although widely employed by dermatologists, the SPS has notable shortcomings [27]. First, studies have shown a poor correlation between skin photo-type, constitutive pigmentation, and minimum erythema dose (MED) [30, 31]. Second, burning and tanning are subjective assessments with inter-individual differences in connotation [32]. Third, the classification is particularly unreliable in classifying black skin, and clinical trials have shown inconsistent correlation between skin phototype classification and sun sensitivity [33–35]. Finally, although people of color are commonly categorized into types IV–VI based on ethnicity, ethnic skin spans the entire spectrum of skin color [36].

Bino et al. proposed an alternate classification to the Fitzpatrick-SPS system, based on the Individual Typology Angle (ITA), as determined by colorimetric properties of skin L* (luminance) and b* (yellow/blue component) [27]. Bino et al. created six groups of skin color in which the ITA corresponded to relative melanin concentration, with lower ITA values signifying darker skin [27]. They were able to validate the ITA measurements in ex vivo skin samples and showed consistent correlations between ITA measurements and constitutive pigmentation [27]. Furthermore, ITA correlated with the dose needed for skin to burn, with lower ITAs requiring higher doses to burn. While the ITA values were fairly consistent in white and African subjects across geographic regions, values ranged widely among Hispanics and Asians [27]. The ITA may provide a more accurate and objective measurement of constitutive pigmentation than the Fitzpatrick system and may prove to be more predictive of the physiological sequelae of UV exposure [27].

The Clinical Effects of UVA, UVB, and VL

UVA and Erythema

UVA radiation is one-thousand-fold less effective than UVB in causing erythema [4, 37]. UVA-induced erythema follows a biphasic pattern [1, 14]. Immediate erythema, typically present in skin types I/II, occurs within seconds to minutes of exposure [1, 14]. Delayed erythema, which occurs within minutes to hours, is experienced irrespective of skin type [1, 14, 38]. However, the dose required to produce UVA-delayed erythema increases with constitutive pigmentation, suggesting a protective role for melanin [7, 14].

UVA and Pigmentation

Numerous studies have shown UVA to be more melanogenic than erythemogenic [15, 38]. The pigmentary effects of UVR are classified based on the timing of onset and duration of exposure [39]. UVA causes immediate pigment darkening (IPD), which occurs immediately after light exposure, is gray in color and fades within minutes to hours [14, 40]. With increased or repetitive exposure, UVA can also produce persistent pigment darkening (PPD), which is brown in color and can persist for as long as 1 day. IPD and PPD both result from the oxidation and redistribution of pre-existing melanin [1, 15]. Both IPD and PPD are more pronounced in dark vs. fairly complexed individuals [7].

UVA and Photoaging

Lifelong sun exposure contributes to as much as 95% of the visible signs of aging [36].

Photoaging is characterized by patchy/mottled pigmentation, rhytid formation, laxity, sagging, and xerosis. Histologically, there is altered dermal collagen and elastin, epidermal atrophy, and pigmentary changes [4, 41, 42]. These changes occur less frequently and with less severity among darker skin types [43–45]. Photoaging manifests uniquely in different skin types. Due to its melanogenic properties [15, 38, 46], UVA has been suspected to exacerbate the prominent pigmentary component of aging in ethnic skin. Multiple studies have shown that photoaging in Asians and African Americans is first evidenced as pigmentary changes, including lentigines, dyschromias, and keratoses [47–49]. Compared to their white counterparts, Chinese subjects show a 10-year delay in the development of rhytides [50, 51].

UVA-mediated pigmentary lesions are markedly diminished when sunscreen contents are altered, such that the ratio UVA protection factor (UVAPF) to SPF (which provides UVB coverage) is increased [46]. Products with a UVAPF to SPF ratio greater than three are most effective in preventing pigmented lesions caused by exposure to sunlight [46]. In vitro studies show that sunscreens meeting this ratio provide better protection against dermal damage, produce fewer photoaging-related biomarkers, and result in fewer clinically apparent pigmentary lesions [4, 52, 53].

UVB and Erythema

Sunburn, the most well-known consequence of excessive sun exposure, is largely attributed to UVB injury, which triggers the release of cytokines and inflammatory mediators causing local inflammatory responses [6] leading to capillary dilation within the superficial dermis [15]. UVB is more erythemogenic than melanogenic, with a MED much lower than its minimal melanogenic dose (MMD) [38]. UVB produces erythema as its first cutaneous effect at relatively low quantities [1]. The MED increases linearly with the level of pigmentation [32]. Both constitutive pigmentation and delayed tanning (DT) pigmentation from prior UVB exposure protect against erythema and DNA damage from all forms of UV radiation [14, 54]. Immediate erythema, which preferentially occurs in lighter skin types, typically manifests 6–24 hours postexposure [14]. Darkly pigmented individuals are relatively protected in regard to the intensity and duration of UVB erythema. The time frame for subsequent fading and desquamation depends on baseline pigmentation. It may last for 1–2 weeks in lighter skin types (Fitzpatrick I/II), while in darker skinned individuals, erythema often resolves within 72 hours [14, 54].

UVB-Induced Pigmentation

Delayed tanning (DT) occurs 3–5 days after UVB exposure, may persist for weeks to months, and results from newly synthesized melanin [69, 79]. UVB-induced pigmentation is always preceded by erythema in lighter skin types, but this process is less common in darker skin [14]. The UVB dose needed to cause DT is dependent on constitutive skin pigmentation, with darker skin types possessing higher MMDs [55]. The absolute pigmentary increase is independent of constitutive skin pigmentation but increases linearly with UVB dosage [56]. Thus, once the MMD dose of UVB is achieved, additional increases in tanning depend only on UVB dosage, irrespective of baseline skin color.

The Impact of VL on Erythema and Pigmentation

At very high doses, VL is capable of causing erythema [7]. In vivo studies have shown that exposure to increasing amounts of VL results in increasing degrees of erythema associated with IPD in darker skin types [15]. Because VL penetrates to the deep dermis, VL-mediated erythema is thought to occur by a similar mechanism to that of UVA [15]. It has been hypothesized that, in darker skin types, VL causes heat, generation of which leads to vasodilation and subsequent erythema [57].

In the absence of UVR, VL can induce IPD, PPD, and DT [58, 59]. IPD and PPD caused by VL reveal similar photometric action spectra to UVA, and arise from the oxidization and redistribution of pre-existing melanin [57, 60]. Skin specimens obtained 24 hours after VL irradiation demonstrated a redistribution of melanin to the spinous layer of the epidermis [5]. The ability to develop IPD and PPD is skin-type dependent. Mahmood et al. were unable to illicit IPD or PPD in their subjects with skin type II, whereas VL induced sustained pigmentation in subjects with skin types IV–VI [15, 59]. After repeated exposure, VL can produce DT in all skin types [5] via neomelanogenic pathways [13].Within the VL spectrum, the pro-pigmenting affect of blue/violet line (415 nm) appears strongest [61]. A recent study has shown that VL-induced hyperpigmentation is mediated by Opsin 3. Opsin 3 is a G-protein-coupled receptor which when activated triggers a cascade of events initiated by calcium influx that ultimately results in melanogeneis [62]. In order for melanogenesis to occur, the skin may require priming via multiple VL exposures [57]. Therefore, depending on the circumstances of exposure, VL may generate pigmentation via mechanisms analogous to either UVA or UVB.

Photodermatoses

Photodermatoses are a group of disorders that are either caused or exacerbated by sun exposure. A clue to their presence lies in their distribution, with localization of symptoms to photoexposed body sites. Photodermatoses are broadly classified into four major categories: (1) idiopathic or immunologically mediated (see Table 6.1); (2) drug-induced photodermatoses (Table 6.2); (3) photo aggravation of pre-existing cutaneous conditions (Table 6.3); and (4) disorders of defective DNA repair disorders. Phytophotodermatitis is an additional subset of photodermatoses that deserves brief mention. This self-limited phototoxic inflammatory eruption is caused by UVA activation of furcoumarins, present in foods such as lemons, limes, parsley, and celery [63, 64].

Table 6.1 Characteristics of immunologically mediated or idiopathic photodermatoses

Photodermatoses	Pathogenesis	Epidemiology	Clinical features	Histopathology	UV action spectrum	Treatment[a]
Actinic lichen planus (synonyms: lichen planus subtropicus, lichen planus tropicus, and summertime actinic lichenoid eruption) [64]	Altered expression of self-antigens leading to recruitment of cytotoxic T cells	Commonly presents in third decade of life [65, 72] but can also occur during childhood. No sexual predilection. Increased prevalence in tropical countries, including Middle East, Egypt, Tunisia, India [66, 73]	Non-pruritic. Well-demarcated light brown to slate blue annular or discoid patches with peripheral hypopigmentation [66, 73]. Involves exposed areas of the face, dorsal hands, and extensor forearms. Typically occurs during spring and summer, improves during fall and winter [65, 72]	Interface dermatitis. Vacuolar degeneration. Perivascular lymphocytic infiltrate. Pigment incontinence [65, 72]	UVB (evidence for photo-induction is lacking)	Topical and intralesional corticosteroids. Hydroxychloroquine [65, 72]. Acitretin with topical corticosteroids [67]
Actinic prurigo (synonyms: hereditary polymorphous light eruption, solar prurigo)	Delayed hypersensitivity reaction to UV-induced auto-antigen. Lesional skin shows activated CD4 positive T cells and memory T lymphocytes	Childhood to young adulthood. Often resolves in adolescence or early adult life [68, 75]. Adult-onset variant (age >21) is more common in Asian populations [66, 73, 68, 75]	Intense pruritus. Erythematous papules that may become crusted, excoriated, and lichenified plaques secondary to scratching [68, 75, 69, 76]. Sun-exposed areas of the face, forearms, hands, and legs	Hyperkeratosis. Acanthosis. Spongiosis. Dense lymphocytic infiltrate in the superficial and mid dermis, papillary dermal edema [68, 75, 70, 77]	UVA, UVB [68, 75]	Topical corticosteroids. Topical calcineurin inhibitors. Tetracycline with vitamin E [70, 77]. Oral corticosteroids. Desensitization with narrow-band UVB. Thalidomide for more recalcitrant disease [71, 78]. Cyclosporine. Azathioprine. Pentoxifylline

(continued)

Increased risk associated with HLA DRB1ª 0407 allele among Mexican and Columbian AP patients [66, 73] Cases of progression between PLE and AP suggest that the two may share mutual pathogenesis	In children, no gender predilection Female predilection in adults [69, 76] In Asian patients, there is a reported male predominance [68, 75] Commonly seen in North, Central and South America, Native Indian, Latin American mestizos [66, 70, 73, 77] and ethnic Chinese [66, 73]	Unexposed areas may be affected in up to 20% of cases [70, 77]. 30–50% of cases have labial and conjunctival involvement Chronic course with spontaneous improvement Adult-onset variant follows a milder course [70, 77] Ethnic manifestations: chelitis and conjunctivitis with increased prevalence among Native Americans [69, 76]. Adult variant is more common in Asian populations and is associated with longer disease duration [68, 75]. In Thailand, this variant was described in Fitzpatrick skin type IV and V [66, 73]. Mucosal involvement is less common in Asians [68, 75]

Table 6.1 (continued)

Photodermatoses	Pathogenesis	Epidemiology	Clinical features	Histopathology	UV action spectrum	Treatment[a]
Chronic actinic dermatitis	Contact dermatitis-like delayed type hypersensitivity reaction against endogenous photo-induced cutaneous antigen [66, 73] (DNA suspected candidate) Photo-induced immunosuppression is altered [72, 79]	Older than 50 years of age [69, 73, 76, 80] Male predominance [69, 76] In the United States, commonly observed in Fitzpatrick skin types V–VI [73, 80] Additional notes: uncommon association with HIV infection [74, 81]	Pruritus [73, 80] Lichenified papules and plaques in photo-exposed regions of chest, neck, face, scalp, and arms [66, 69, 73, 76]. Sparing of the upper eyelids, retro auricular, and submental areas [69, 75, 76, 82] Secondary alopecia Leonine facies in severe and chronic cases [69, 75, 76, 82] Reported associations with contact allergy to compositae (UK patients), sesquiterpene lactone mix, metals, rubber, topical medications, and sunscreens [69, 75, 76, 82] Ethnic variations: lichenified plaques most common morphology observed in the Indian population [66, 73]. Mean age of onset in this population is 44 years [66, 73]	Spongiosis, and acanthosis with mixed infiltrate of lymphohistiocytes, eosinophils, and plasma cells [66, 69, 73, 76]	UVA, UVB, and visible light [69, 73, 76, 80]	Avoidance of contact allergens [69, 76] Oral and topical corticosteroids, topical tacrolimus [69, 76] Resistant cases may consider: low-dose PUVA, azathioprine, danazol, cyclosporine, mycophenolate mofetil [69, 75, 76, 82]

Juvenile spring eruption (Synonyms: dermatitis pustularis vernalis aurium, perniosis juvenilis vernalis aurium)	Considered a variant of polymorphic light eruption [76, 77, 83, 84]	Onset in childhood to young adulthood Male predilection Additional notes: commonly associated with lack of hair covering the ears and large ears	Localized to the helices Onset after 12–24 hours after exposure to cold weather in the spring Papulovesicular lesions +/–crusting Bullae in severe cases Resolution with minimal scarring after 1–3 weeks [76, 77, 83, 84]	Spongiosis with scattered apoptotic keratinocytes Mononuclear cell infiltrate in the papillary and reticular dermis [77, 84]	UVA	Many cases are self-limited Moderate to severe episodes: topical emollients, topical corticosteroids, and oral antihistamines [77, 84]
Lichen planus pigmentosus	Etiology unknown, potential triggers include contact with amla oil and mustard oil [78, 85]	Onset in third or fourth decade of life [79, 86] Slight female predilection [79, 86] Initially described in Indian patients, but has been described in other groups [79, 86]	Usually asymptomatic; 1/3–1/2 of cases report mild pruritus and burning Poorly defined diffuse or reticular slate grey-brown-black macules and patches. Symmetrical distributed in exposed areas, most commonly affecting the face and neck. Extremities and back may also be affected Rare inverse variant affects intertriginous areas Subset of patients have concurrent lichen planus Follows chronic course [79, 86]	Vacuolar degeneration of basal epidermis Perivascular lymphohistiocytic infiltrate Melanophages in the upper dermis	UVR	Topical tacrolimus 0.1% [80, 87] Topical corticosteroids Neodymium: yttrium–aluminum–garnet laser [81, 88]

(continued)

Table 6.1 (continued)

Photodermatoses	Pathogenesis	Epidemiology	Clinical features	Histopathology	UV action spectrum	Treatment[a]
Polymorphous light eruption	Reduced UVR-induced immunosuppression and/or a delayed-type hypersensitivity response to a photoantigen [76, 83]. Possible mechanisms include decreased expression of apoptotic cell clearance genes in keratinocytes or deficits in free radical clearance [69, 76] Autosomal dominant with reduced penetrance in 3–56% of patients [73, 80]	Mean onset during the second and third decades of life [69, 76, 83, 88, 89] Female predominance [69, 76, 83, 88, 89], 4 times more often than men [76, 83] Frequently seen in higher latitudes and temperate climates [66, 69, 73, 76, 83, 88, 89]. Most commonly occurs in Fitzpatrick skin types I-IV [66, 73, 76, 83] Seasonal exacerbation has been reported in Indian patients during March–September [66, 73] Additional notes: PMLE patients may have reduced tendency toward skin cancer development [89, 90]	Pruritic Develop within hours to days after sun exposure. Localized to sun-exposed skin, including extensor arms, forearms, and chest, sparing the face. Presents with variable morphology, most commonly papular [73, 80], but may in include macular, papulovesicular, plaque-like, vesiculobullous, and erythema multiforme-like Monomorphic lesions within individual patients [76, 83] Infrequent association with systemic symptoms of malaise, headache, fever, and nausea [69, 76] Spontaneous resolution in days if further exposure is avoided [66, 69, 73, 75, 76, 82, 88, 89] Worse in spring and summer months [69, 76, 88, 89] Ethnic variation: A pinpoint papular variant has been described in men of African, African American, and Asian descent [66, 73, 76, 83, 88, 89, 90, 91]	Nonspecific dependent on individual clinical morphology. Common presentation includes parakeratosis and spongiosis in the epidermis. Lymphocytic perivascular infiltrate, containing eosinophils and neutrophils, in the dermis with subepidermal edema [73, 80] Erythema multiforme variant: liquefaction degeneration at the dermo-epidermal junction with vacuolar changes [76, 80] Pinpoint variant: spongiosis, red blood cell extravasation, and focal vesicular formation. Perivascular and interstitial lymphocytic infiltrate	Most commonly UVA, but UVB-induced lesions have been reported [69, 75, 76, 82, 83]	Affected individuals may experience natural hardening and develop an increased tolerance Iatrogenic photo hardening to controlled exposures of UV doses to promote photoadaption Topical corticosteroids Oral antihistamines Oral corticosteroids prophylactically and/or for flares [69, 76, 83] Antimalarials, azathioprine, thalidomide, and/or cyclosporine for severe/refractory cases [69, 75, 76, 82, 83]

Solar urticaria	IgE-mediated hypersensitivity reaction to photo-induced allergen [73, 80, 91, 92] Mast-cell degranulation mediates symptoms	Second and third decades of life [69, 76] Female predilection [69, 73, 75, 76, 80, 82] Additional notes: 21–48% of patients have atopic diathesis [69, 76, 92, 93]	Pruritus, erythema, and wheals form within 30 minutes of sun exposure on the upper chest, and arms [69, 76] Burning sensation may precede onset of symptoms [75, 82] Resolves within 24 hours [69, 76] Severe cases may develop anaphylactoid reaction accompanied by light-headedness, nausea, bronchospasm, syncope [69, 76] Ethnic variation: a Singapore study showed a male predilection, later age of onset, and reaction to visible light [66, 73]	Vasodilation, dermal edema Perivascular infiltrate of lymphocytes and eosinophils [73, 80]	UVR, less commonly visible light [73, 75, 80, 82]	Oral antihistamines taken regularly or prophylactically prior to sun exposure [69, 73, 75, 76, 80, 82] Graduated exposure therapy of UVA or PUVA [69, 76] Resistant cases may consider omalizumab, plasmapheresis, IVIG [69, 76]

aFirst-line treatment should include prophylactic photoprotective measures, including minimizing sun exposure, use of broad-spectrum sunscreens, and wearing protective clothing

Table 6.2 Causes of drug-induced photosensitivity reactions

Phototoxic agents	Photoallergic agents
Amiodarone	Amantadine
Antineoplastic agents: 5-FU, dacarbazine, vinblastine	Antimalarials: chloroquine, hydroxychloroquine, quinidine, quinine
Antimalarials: chloroquine, hydroxychloroquine, quinidine, quinine	Antimicrobials: chloramphenicol, pyrimethamine, quinolones
Antimicrobials: ceftazidime, griseofulvin, ketoconazole, quinolones, tetracyclines, trimethoprim	Benzodiazepines: chlordiazepoxide
Atorvastatin	Dapsone
Calcium channel blockers: diltiazem	Diphenhydramine
Nonsteroidal anti-inflammatory drugs (NSAIDS)	Flu amide
Oral: proprionic acid derivatives	Griseofulvin
Chlorpromazine	Nonsteroidal anti-inflammatory drugs (NSAIDs)
Porphyrins	Oral:
Psoralens	Piroxicam
Retinoids: isotretinoin, etretinate	Celecoxib
Sulfur-containing medications: hydrochlorothiazide, furosemide, sulfonamides, sulfonylureas	Topical:
	Oxicams
	Proprionic acid derivatives
	Phenothiazine
	Pilocarpine
	Pyridoxine
	Ranitidine
	Sulfur-containing medications: hydrochlorothiazide, furosemide, sulfonamides, sulfonylureas
	Tricyclic antidepressants

Table 6.3 Common photoaggravated dermatoses

Atopic dermatitis
Chronic cutaneous lupus erythematosus
Darier disease (synonyms: Darier-White disease, dyskeratosis follicularis, keratosis follicularis)
Dermatomyositis
Pellagra
Pemphigus erythematosus

The characteristic "streaky" linear rash can present with erythema, vesicle, and blister formation, involving affected sites within 24–48 hours of exposure. Patients can subsequently develop hyperpigmentation that may take months to resolve. Notably, the inflammatory stage may go unnoticed and patients may present only after pigmentary changes develop.

The approach to the patient suspected of suffering from photodermatoses includes a thorough history and physical exam, as well as phototesting. Additional laboratory testing may be necessary based on the clinical findings, and may include skin biopsies, screening for antinuclear antibodies, porphyrins, a comprehensive metabolic panel, and a urine analysis. While the medical treatment of these conditions may vary, meticulous photoprotective measures—including minimizing sun exposure, the use of broad-spectrum sunscreens, and wearing protective clothing—are mandatory.

Sun Protection

The sun protection factor (SPF) measures how well a product protects against UVB radiation. The Food and Drug Administration defines SPF as the ratio of MED with an applied product to the MED unprotected [65]. For example, skin applied with a sunscreen of SPF 30 will sustain 30 times more sunlight before burning compared to unprotected skin. Sunscreens with an SPF 30 prevent 97% of the sun's rays from penetrating the skin. There is no data to indicate significant additional benefit from applying sunscreen with an SPF greater than 50 [65]. SPF does not provide information on a products' efficacy in protection from UVA or VL [66].

Chemical sunscreens are composed of organic compounds that work by absorbing UV radiation. Commonly used organic ingredients are avobenzone, oxybenzone, ensulizole, octinoxate, and octisalata [66]. However, depending on the compound, the degree and spectrum of UVA and UVB protection varies [66]. These compounds are also vulnerable to photodegradation and may be prone to generating free radicals [66]. They can subsequently cause photosensitizing or photoirritating reactions in susceptible individuals [66]. Newer ingredients such as ecamsule, bemotrizinol, and bisoctrizole have been added to formulations as they protect against both UVB and UVA and function as photostabilizers when paired with avobenzone [66].

Physical sunscreens are composed of inorganic compounds and protect skin by absorbing, deflecting, and scattering solar radiation [66]. They are composed of inorganic compounds such as iron oxide (FeO), titanium dioxide (TiO2), and zinc oxide (ZnO) [66]. Their spectrum of action covers UVB, UVA, and VL. Iron oxide specifically has been shown to be more effective than the other inorganic compounds in preventing the erythema and irritation caused by VL [67]. These inorganic compounds are generally safe for use and are favored by consumers due to their transparency upon application [68].

The American Academy of Dermatology (AAD) recommends that all individuals apply sunscreen prior to outdoor exposure regardless of age, gender, or race [69]. The AAD recommends water-resistant sunscreens with an SPF of 30 or higher [69]. However, a recent split face study demonstrated the sunscreens with an SPF 100 were significantly more effective than sunscreens with SPF 50 at protection against sunburns [70]. Sunscreens should be applied 15 minutes prior to sun exposure, and reapplied approximately every 2 hours, or after swimming or sweating [69]. Guidelines also recommend usage of protective clothing such as a long-sleeved shirt, pants, and a wide brimmed hat.

Conclusion

Human skin experiences both immediate and delayed effects as a consequence of exposure to UVR and VL. These effects vary in magnitude and degree across skin types. Although higher levels of melanin confer darker skin with some protection against UVB-induced erythema, studies show that darker skin may be more susceptible to the cellular toxicity and subsequent photoaging caused by UVA. Emerging data also show that the toxic effects of VL may be more pronounced in darker skin types. Additional studies characterizing the effects of UV and VL on photodermatoses and photoaging are warranted in order to optimize the treatment and management of all patients.

References

1. Sklar LR, Almutawa F, Lim HW, Hamzavi I. Effects of ultraviolet radiation, visible light, and infrared radiation on erythema and pigmentation: a review. Photochem Photobiol Sci. 2013;12(1):54–64. https://doi.org/10.1039/c2pp25152c.
2. Diffey B. What is light? Photodermatol Photoimmunol Photomed. 2002;18(2):68–74.
3. Qiang F. Radiation (Solar). In: Holton JR editor. Encyclopedia of atmospheric sciences. 5th ed.; 2003:1859–1863.
4. Battie C, Jitsukawa S, Bernerd F, Del Bino S, Marionnet C, Verschoore M. New insights in photoaging, UVA induced damage and skin types. Exp Dermatol. 2014;23(Suppl 1):7–12. https://doi.org/10.1111/exd.12388.
5. Randhawa M, Seo I, Liebel F, Southall MD, Kollias N, Ruvolo E. Visible light induces melanogenesis in human skin through a photoadaptive response. PLoS One. 2015;10(6):e0130949. https://doi.org/10.1371/journal.pone.0130949.
6. Marrot L, Meunier JR. Skin DNA photodamage and its biological consequences. J Am Acad Dermatol. 2008;58(5 Suppl. 2):139–48. https://doi.org/10.1016/j.jaad.2007.12.007.
7. Maddodi N, Jayanthy A, Setaluri V. Shining light on skin pigmentation: the darker and the brighter side of effects of UV radiation. Photochem Photobiol. 2012;88(5):1075–82. https://doi.org/10.1111/j.1751-1097.2012.01138.x.
8. Ou-Yang H, Stmatas G, Saliou C, Kollias N. A chemiluminescence study of UVA-induced oxida-

tive stress in human skin in vivo. J Invest Dermatol. 2004;122(4):1020–9.

9. Romanhole RC, Ataide JA, Moriel P, Mazzola PG. Update on ultraviolet A and B radiation generated by the sun and artificial lamps and their effects on skin. Int J Cosmet Sci. 2015;37(4):366–70. https://doi.org/10.1111/ics.12219.

10. Marionnet C, Pierrard C, Lekuene F, Bernerd F. Modulations of gene expression induced by daily ultraviolet light can be prevented by a broad spectrum sunscreen. Photochem Photobiol Sci. 2012;116:37–47.

11. Agar N, Young AR. Melanogenesis: a photoprotective response to DNA damage? Mutat Res. 2005;571(1–2 SPEC.ISS):121–32. https://doi.org/10.1016/j.mrfmmm.2004.11.016.

12. Rünger TM, Farahvash B, Hatvani Z, Rees A. Comparison of DNA damage responses following equimutagenic doses of UVA and UVB: a less effective cell cycle arrest with UVA may render UVA-induced pyrimidine dimers more mutagenic than UVB-induced ones. Photochem Photobiol Sci. 2012;11(1):207. https://doi.org/10.1039/c1pp05232b.

13. Bernerd F, Asselineau D. UVA exposure of human skin reconstructed in vitro induces apoptosis of dermal fibroblasts: subsequent connective tissue repair and implications in photoaging. Differ Cell Death. 1998;5(9):792–802.

14. Hönigsmann H. Erythema and pigmentation. Photodermatol Photoimmunol Photomed. 2002;18:75–81. https://doi.org/10.1034/j.1600-0781.2002.180204.x.

15. Mahmoud BH, Hexsel CL, Hamzavi IH, Lim HW. Effects of visible light on the skin. Photochem Photobiol. 2008;84(2):450–62. https://doi.org/10.1111/j.1751-1097.2007.00286.x.

16. Wenczl E, Van Der Schans GP, Roza L, et al. (Pheo)melanin photosensitizes UVA-induced DNA damage in cultured human melanocytes. J Invest Dermatol. 1998;111(4):678–82. https://doi.org/10.1046/j.1523-1747.1998.00357.x.

17. Marrot L, Belaidi JP, Meunier JR, Perez P, Agapakis-Causse C. The human melanocyte as a particular target for UVA radiation and an endpoint for photoprotection assessment. Photochem Photobiol. 1999;69(6):686–93.

18. Brash DE. Roles of the transcription factor p53 in keratinocyte carcinomas. Br J Dermatol. 2006;154(Suppl):8–10. https://doi.org/10.1111/j.1365-2133.2006.07230.x.

19. Cui R, Widlund HR, Feige E, et al. Central role of p53 in the suntan response and pathologic hyperpigmentation. Cell. 2007;128(5):853–64. https://doi.org/10.1016/j.cell.2006.12.045.

20. D'Orazio J, Jarrett S, Amaro-Ortiz A, Scott T. UV radiation and the skin. Int J Mol Sci. 2013;14(6):12222–48. https://doi.org/10.3390/ijms140612222.

21. Jablonski NG. The evolution of human skin colouration and its relevance to health in the modern world. J R Coll Physicians Edinb. 2012;42(1):58–63.

22. Göring H, Koshuchowa S. Vitamin D – the sun hormone. Life in environmental mismatch. Biochem Biokhimiâ. 2015;80(1):8–20. https://doi.org/10.1134/S0006297915010022.

23. Antoniou C, Lademann J, Schanzer S, et al. Do different ethnic groups need different sun protection? Skin Res Technol. 2009;15(3):323–9. https://doi.org/10.1111/j.1600-0846.2009.00366.x.

24. Kaidbey K, Agin P, Sayre R. A K. Photoprotection by melanin--a comparison of black and Caucasian skin. J Am Acad Dermatol. 1979;1:249–60.

25. Thomson M. Relative efficiency of pigment and horny layer thickness in protecting the skin of Europeans and Africans against solar ultraviolet radiation. J Physiol. 1955;127:236–46.

26. Weigand D, Haygood C, Gaylor J. Cell layers and density of negro and Caucasian stratum corneum. J Invest Dermatol. 1974;62(6):563–8.

27. Del Bino S, Bernerd F. Variations in skin colour and the biological consequences of ultraviolet radiation exposure. Br J Dermatol. 2013;169(Suppl 3):33–40. https://doi.org/10.1111/bjd.12529.

28. Chiarelli-Neto O, Ferreira AS, Martins WK, et al. Melanin photosensitization and the effect of visible light on epithelial cells. PLoS One. 2014;9(11):1–9. https://doi.org/10.1371/journal.pone.0113266.

29. Liebel F, Kaur S, Ruvolo E, Kollias N, Southall MD. Irradiation of skin with visible light induces reactive oxygen species and matrix-degrading enzymes. J Invest Dermatol. 2012;132(7):1901–7. https://doi.org/10.1038/jid.2011.476.

30. Youn J, Oh J, Kim B, et al. Relationship between skin phototype and MED in Korean, brown skin. Photodermatol Photoimmunol Photomed. 1997;13(5–6):208–11.

31. Leenutaphong V. Relationship between skin and cutaneous response to UV radiation in Thai. Photodermatol Photoimmuno. 1995;11:198–203.

32. Eilers S, Bach DQ, Gaber R, et al. Accuracy of self-report in assessing fitzpatrick skin phototypes I through VI. JAMA Dermatol. 2016;60611(11):1289–94. https://doi.org/10.1001/jamadermatol.2013.6101.

33. Pichon L, Landrine H, Corral I, Hao Y, Mayer J, Hoerster K. Measuring skin cancer risk in African Americans: is the Fitzpatrick Skin Type Classification Scale culturally sensitive? Ethn Dis. 2010;20(2):174–9.

34. Kelser E, Linos E, Kanzler M, Lee W, Sainani K, Tang J. Reliability and prevalence of digital image skin types in the United States: results from National Health and Nutrition Examination Survey 2003–2004. J Am Acad Dermatol. 2012;66(1):163–5.

35. Sanclemente G, Zapata JF, García JJ, Gaviria Á, Gómez LF, Barrera M. Lack of correlation between minimal erythema dose and skin phototype in a colombian scholar population. Skin Res Technol. 2008;14(4):403–9. https://doi.org/10.1111/j.1600-0846.2008.00306.x.

36. Agbai ON, Buster K, Sanchez M, et al. Skin cancer and photoprotection in people of color: a review and

recommendations for physicians and the public. J Am Acad Dermatol. 2014;70(4):748–62. https://doi.org/10.1016/j.jaad.2013.11.038.

37. Ravnbak MH, Philipsen PA, Wiegell SR, Wulf HC. Skin pigmentation kinetics after exposure to ultraviolet A. Acta Derm Venereol. 2009;89(4):357–63. https://doi.org/10.2340/00015555-0635.

38. Kollias N, et al. Erythema and melanogenesis action spectra in heavily pigmented individuals as compared to fair-skinned Caucasians. Photodermatol Photoimmunol Photomed. 1996;12:183–8. https://doi.org/10.1111/j.1600-0781.1996.tb00197.x.

39. Wolber R, Schlenz K, Wakamatsu K, et al. Pigmentation effects of solar simulated radiation as compared with UVA and UVB radiation. Pigment Cell Melanoma Res. 2008;21(4):487–91. https://doi.org/10.1111/j.1755-148X.2008.00470.x.Pigmentation.

40. Roh K, Kim D, Ha S, Ro Y, Kim J, Lee H. Pigmentation in Koreans : study of the differences from caucasians in age, gender and seasonal variations. Br J Dermatol. 2001;144(1):94–9.

41. Kotrakaras R, Kligman A. The effect of topical tretinoin on photodamaged facial skin: the Thai experience. Br J Dermatol. 1993;129:302–9.

42. Beradesca E, Leveqe J-L, Maibach H. Ethnic skin and hair; 2006.

43. Halder R, Ara C. Skin cancer and photoaging in ethnic skin. Dermatol Clin. 2003;21(4):725–32.

44. Taylor S. Enhancing the care and treatment of skin of color, part 2: understanding skin physiology. Cutis. 2005;76(5):302–6.

45. Zastrow L, Ferrero L, Herrling T, Groth N. Sun protection under Asian light. Asian soc Cosm Sci. 2007;4:62–8.

46. Fourtanier A, Moyal D, Seite S. UVA filters in sunprotection products: regulatory and biological aspect. Photochem Photobiol Sci. 2012;11:81–9.

47. Griffiths C, Wang T, Hamilton T, Voorhees J, Ellis C. A photonumeric scale for the assesment of cutaneous photodamage. Dermatol Arch. 1992;128(3):347–51.

48. Larnier C, Ortonne J, Venot A, et al. Evaluation of cutaneous photodamage using photographic scale. Br J Dermatol. 1994;130(2):167–73.

49. Vierkotter A, Krutmann J. Environmental influences on skin aging and ethnic-specific manifestations. Dermatoendocrinology. 2012;4(3):227–31.

50. Nouveau-Richard S, Yang Z, Mac-Mary S, et al. Skin ageing: a comparison between Chinese and European populations: a pilot study. J Dermatol Sci. 2005;40(3):187–93. https://doi.org/10.1016/j.jdermsci.2005.06.006.

51. Chan H, Jackson B. Laser treatment on ehtnic skin. In: Lim HW, Hoenigsmann H, Hawk JL, editors. Photodermatol New York Inf Healthc; 2007.

52. Lejeune F, Christiaens F, Bernerd F. Evaluation of sunscreen products using a reconstructed skin model exposed to simulated daily ultraviolet radiation: relevance of filtration profile and SPF value for daily photoprotection. Photodermatol Photoimmunol Photomed. 2008;24(5):249–55.

53. Marionnet C, Grether-Beck S, Seite S, et al. A broad-spectrum sunscreen prevents UVA radiation-induced gene expression in reconstructed skin in vitro and in human skin in vivo. Exp Dermatol. 2011;20(6):466–82.

54. Miyamura Y, Coelho SG, Schlenz K, et al. The deceptive nature of UVA tanning versus the modest protective effects of UVB tanning on human skin. Pigment Cell Melanoma Res. 2011;24(1):136–47. https://doi.org/10.1111/j.1755-148X.2010.00764.x.

55. Ravnbak MH, Wulf HC. Pigmentation after single and multiple UV-exposures depending on UV-spectrum. Arch Dermatol Res. 2007;299(1):25–32. https://doi.org/10.1007/s00403-006-0728-3.

56. Ravnbak MH, Philipsen PA, Wiegell SR, Wulf HC. Skin pigmentation kinetics after UVB exposure. Acta Derm Venereol. 2008;88(3):223–8. https://doi.org/10.2340/00015555-0431.

57. Mahmoud BH, Ruvolo E, Hexsel CL, et al. Impact of long-wavelength UVA and visible light on melanocompetent skin. J Invest Dermatol. 2010;130(8):2092–7. https://doi.org/10.1038/jid.2010.95.

58. Kollias N, Baqer A. An experimental study of th changes in pigmentation in human skin in vivo with visible and near infrared light. Photochem Photobiol. 1984;39(5):651–9.

59. Rosen CF, Jacques SL, Stuart ME, Gange RW. Immediate pigment darkening: visual and reflectance spectrophotometric analysis of action spectrum. Photochem Photobiol. 1990;51(5):583–8. https://doi.org/10.1111/j.1751-1097.1990.tb01969.x.

60. Ramasubramaniam R, Roy A, Sharma B, Nagalakshmi S. Are there mechanistic differences between ultraviolet and visible radiation induced skin pigmentation? Photochem Photobiol Sci. 2011;10(12):1887–93. https://doi.org/10.1039/c1pp05202k.

61. Duteil L, Cardot-Leccia NQ-R, C Maubert Y, Harmelin Y, et al. Differences in visible light-induced pigmentation according to wavelengths: a clinical and histological study in comparison with UVB exposure. Pigment Cell Melanoma Res. 2014;27(5):822–6.

62. Regazzetti C, Sormani L, Debayle D, et al. Melanocytes sense blue light and regulate pigmentation through Opsin-3. J Invest Dermatol. 2018;138(1):171–8. https://doi.org/10.1016/j.jid.2017.07.833.

63. Marcos LA, Kahler R, Quaak MS, et al. Phytophotodermatitis. Int J Infect Dis. 2015;38:7–8. https://doi.org/10.1016/j.ijid.2015.07.004.

64. Raam R, DeClerck B, Jhun P, et al. Phytophotodermatitis: the other "lime" disease. Ann Emerg Med. 2016;67(4):554–6. https://doi.org/10.1016/j.annemergmed.2016.02.023.

65. Al-Jamal MS, Griffith JL, Lim HW. Photoprotection in ethnic skin. Dermatol Sin. 2014;32(4):217–24. https://doi.org/10.1016/j.dsi.2014.09.001.

66. Morabito K, Shapley NC, Steeley KG, Tripathi A. Review of sunscreen and the emergence of non-

conventional absorbers and their applications in ultraviolet protection. Int J Cosmet Sci. 2011;33(5):385–90. https://doi.org/10.1111/j.1468-2494.2011.00654.x.

67. Bissonnette R, Nigen S, Bolduc C, Méry S, Nocera T. Protection afforded by sunscreens containing inorganic sunscreening agents against blue light sensitivity induced by aminolevulinic acid. Dermatol Surg. 2008;34(11):1469–74. https://doi.org/10.1111/j.1524-4725.2008.34311.x.

68. Nohynek G. Nanotechnology, cosmetics and the skin: is there a health risk? Skin Pharmacol Physiol. 2008;21(3):136–49.

69. American Academy of Dermatology – Sunscreen FAQs.

70. Williams J, Prithwiraj M, Atillasoy E, Wu M, Farberg A, Rigel D. SPF 100+ sunscreen is more protective against sunburn than SPF 50+ in actual use: results of a randomized, double-blind, split-face, natural sunlight exposure clinical trial. J Am Acad Dermatol. 2018;78(5):902–10.

71. Kim GH, Mikkilineni R. Lichen planus actinicus. Dermatol Online J. 2007;13(1):404–11. http://eprints.cdlib.org/uc/item/98k4v2zx. Accessed 26 May 2016.

72. Salman SM, Kibbi A-G, Zaynoun S. Actinic lichen planus. J Am Acad Dermatol. 1989;20(2):226–31. https://doi.org/10.1016/S0190-9622(89)70026-8.

73. Sharma VK, Sahni K, Wadhwani AR. Photodermatoses in pigmented skin. Photochem Photobiol Sci. 2013;12(1):65–77. https://doi.org/10.1039/c2pp25182e.

74. Jansen T, Gambichler T, von Kobyletzki L, Altmeyer P. Lichen planus actinicus treated with acitretin and topical corticosteroids. J Eur Acad Dermatol Venereol. 2002;16(2):174–5. https://doi.org/10.1046/j.1468-3083.2002.00392_3.x.

75. Ker KJ, Chong WS, Theng CTS. Clinical characteristics of adult-onset actinic prurigo in Asians: a case series. Indian J Dermatol Venereol Leprol. 2013;79(6):783–8. https://doi.org/10.4103/0378-6323.120726.

76. Lim H, Hawk J. Photodermatologic disorders. In: Dermatology. 3rd ed: Saunders; 2012. p. 1467–86.

77. Sanchez MR. Cutaneous diseases in Latinos. Dermatol Clin. 2003;21(4):689–97. https://doi.org/10.1016/S0733-8635(03)00087-1.

78. Lovell CR, Hawk JLM, Calnan CD, Magnus IA. Thalidomide in actinic prurigo. Br J Dermatol. 1983;108(4):467–71. https://doi.org/10.1111/j.1365-2133.1983.tb04601.x.

79. Paek SY, Lim HW. Chronic actinic dermatitis. Dermatol Clin. 2014;32(3):355–61., viii-ix. https://doi.org/10.1016/j.det.2014.03.007.

80. González E, González S. Drug photosensitivity, idiopathic photodermatoses, and sunscreens. J Am Acad Dermatol. 1996;35(6):871–85. https://doi.org/10.1016/S0190-9622(96)90108-5.

81. Tan AW-M, Lim K-S, Theng C, Chong W-S. Chronic actinic dermatitis in Asian skin: a Singaporean experience. Photodermatol Photoimmunol Photomed. 2011;27(4):172–5. https://doi.org/10.1111/j.1600-0781.2011.00589.x.

82. Srinivas CR, Sekar CS, Jayashree R. Photodermatoses in India. Indian J Dermatol Venereol Leprol. 2012;78 (Suppl 17):S1–8. https://doi.org/10.4103/0378-6323.97349.

83. Gruber-Wackernagel A, Byrne SN, Wolf P. Polymorphous light eruption: clinic aspects and pathogenesis. Dermatol Clin. 2014;32(3):315–34, viii. https://doi.org/10.1016/j.det.2014.03.012.

84. Lava SAG, Simonetti GD, Ragazzi M, Guarino Gubler S, Bianchetti MG. Juvenile spring eruption: an outbreak report and systematic review of the literature. Br J Dermatol. 2013;168(5):1066–72. https://doi.org/10.1111/bjd.12197.

85. Kanwar AJ, Dogra S, Handa S, Parsad D, Radotra BD. A study of 124 Indian patients with lichen planus pigmentosus. Clin Exp Dermatol. 2003;28(5):481–5. https://doi.org/10.1046/j.1365-2230.2003.01367.x.

86. Kanwar A, Dogra S. A study of 124 Indian patients with lichen planus pigmentosus. Clin Exp Dermatol. 2003;28(5):481–5. https://doi.org/10.1046/j.1365-2230.2003.01367.x/full. Accessed 27 Mar 2016.

87. Al-Mutairi N, El-Khalawany M. Clinicopathological characteristics of lichen planus pigmentosus and its response to tacrolimus ointment: an open label, non-randomized, prospective study. J Eur Acad Dermatol Venereol. 2010;24(5):535–40. https://doi.org/10.1111/j.1468-3083.2009.03460.x.

88. Kim J-E, Won C-H, Chang S, Lee M-W, Choi J-H, Moon K-C. Linear lichen planus pigmentosus of the forehead treated by neodymium:yttrium-aluminum-garnet laser and topical tacrolimus. J Dermatol. 2012;39(2):189–91. https://doi.org/10.1111/j.1346-8138.2011.01233.x.

89. Bansal I, Kerr H, Janiga JJ, et al. Pinpoint papular variant of polymorphous light eruption: clinical and pathological correlation. J Eur Acad Dermatol Venereol. 2006;20(4):406–10. https://doi.org/10.1111/j.1468-3083.2006.01482.x.

90. Lembo S, Fallon J, O'Kelly P, Murphy GM. Polymorphic light eruption and skin cancer prevalence: is one protective against the other? Br J Dermatol. 2008;159(6):1342–7. https://doi.org/10.1111/j.1365-2133.2008.08734.x.

91. Chiam LYT, Chong W-S. Pinpoint papular polymorphous light eruption in Asian skin: a variant in darker-skinned individuals. Photodermatol Photoimmunol Photomed. 2009;25(2):71–4. https://doi.org/10.1111/j.1600-0781.2009.00405.x.

92. Leenutaphong V, Hölzle E, Plewig G. Pathogenesis and classification of solar urticaria: a new concept. J Am Acad Dermatol. 1989;21(2):237–40. https://doi.org/10.1016/S0190-9622(89)70167-5.

93. Uetsu N, Miyauchi-Hashimoto H, Okamoto H, Horio T. The clinical and photobiological characteristics of solar urticaria in 40 patients. Br J Dermatol. 2000;142(1):32–8. https://doi.org/10.1046/j.1365-2133.2000.03238.x.

Inflammatory Disorders: Acne Vulgaris, Atopic Dermatitis, Seborrheic Dermatitis, Lupus Erythematosus, Dermatomyositis, and Scleroderma

Andrew F. Alexis and Whitney A. Talbott

Acne Vulgaris

Acne vulgaris is a common inflammatory disorder of the pilosebaceous unit affecting 85% of the population between 12 and 24 years old. Although acne is thought to be a disease of adolescence, it frequently continues into adulthood, especially among adult women [1]. Acne is a top presenting concern in the dermatologist office among white, black, Hispanic, and Asian individuals [2, 3]. Several factors identified in the development of acne include increased sebum production, follicular hyperkeritinization, presence of *Propionibacterium acnes* (*C. acnes*) and inflammation.

Clinical Presentation

Acne has a wide clinical presentation, and is typically found in areas with high density of sebaceous glands such as the face, chest, and back. Non-inflammatory acne consists of open and closed comedones. Inflammatory acne begins with the microcomedone and subsequently develops into papules, pustules, nodules, and cysts. Acne conglobata is a severe variant of nodulocystic acne and is referred to as acne fulminans when patients develop associated fever, arthritis, and systemic symptoms.

Acne variants frequently seen in skin of color include pomade acne and acne cosmetica. Follicle occluding hair products and cosmetics, respectively, can cause a primary comedonal facial acne. Pomade acne usually affects the forehead and temples, where hair products may have contact with the skin. Patients should be counseled on use of non-comedogenic skin care products or silicone-based hair styling products [4]. Hair products should be applied only to the scalp, 1 inch behind the hairline [4].

Erythema or hyperpigmentation can persist despite treatment of acne lesions, and nodulocystic acne can leave pitted scars, hypertrophic scars, and keloids even after resolution. For skin of color, post-inflammatory hyperpigmentation (PIH) is a major concern, and frequently more distressing than actual acne lesions [5–7] (Fig. 7.1). Hyperpigmentation can have a long duration, even greater than 1 year for some patients [7]. Acne sequelae have also been found to disproportionately affect patients of darker skin types [8]. This may be explained by the marked level of subclinical inflammation seen in biopsy specimens of African American women with acne [4]. In a comparison to other ethnicities,

A. F. Alexis (✉)
Mount Sinai Morningside and Mount Sinai West, Department of Dermatology, Mount Sinai Doctors, New York, NY, USA

W. A. Talbott
Icahn School of Medicine at Mount Sinai, Department of Dermatology, New York, NY, USA

© Springer Nature Switzerland AG 2021
B. S. Li, H. I. Maibach (eds.), *Ethnic Skin and Hair and Other Cultural Considerations*, Updates in Clinical Dermatology, https://doi.org/10.1007/978-3-030-64830-5_7

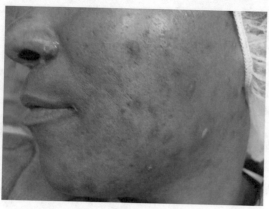

Fig. 7.1 Post-inflammatory hyperpigmentation secondary to acne. Note central hypopigmentation with surrounding hyperpigmentation secondary to excoriation

Asian patients showed the highest negative impact on self-perception and social functioning [9]. However across all ethnicities, over one third of patients reported anxiety and depression symptoms [9]. Acne therefore should be treated quickly to avoid long-term sequalae and impact on social development.

Treatment

The overall treatment for skin of color is similar to that in lighter skin phototypes; however, the increased prevalence of PIH in darker skin types – both iatrogenic and secondary to acne – should help direct treatment. This requires providers to initiate aggressive acne therapy to reduce the number of acne lesions and subsequent PIH, while limiting potential of skin irritation [4]. Patients should be encouraged to refrain from picking at lesions, as mechanical insults from excoriation can further exacerbate hyperpigmentation. Sunscreen and photoprotection are also recommended to further PIH.

The Global Alliance to Improve Outcomes in Acne recently released a practical management guideline with current standards in acne therapy [10]. Options include topical and oral retinoids, topical and oral antibiotics, oral contraceptive agents, hormonal therapies, and procedural therapy.

First-line therapy for patients with comedonal acne or inflammatory acne is a topical retinoid in combination with benzoyl peroxide (BPO). Together these normalize keratinization and kill *C. acnes*, thereby reducing formation of the microcomedone and further inflammatory lesions. Topical retinoids (tretinoin, adapalene, tazarotene) are safe and efficacious in skin of color, and are all more effective at higher concentrations [11, 12]. Topical retinoids also have the added benefit of treating scaring, hyperpigmentation, and overall skin texture [13]. In one study comparing tazarotene 0.1% cream and adapalene 0.3% gel, both showed reduction in post-inflammatory hyperpigmentation; however, tazarotene was significantly more effective [14]. Other studies have found adapalene to be better tolerated than tazarotene; however, in clinical practice, vehicle, concentration, and dosing regimen affect tolerability and should therefore be titrated for a given patient [15]. In a study comparing tretinoin 0.025% gel and adapalene 0.1% gel, both were equally effective and adapalene was again less irritating [16]. Combination products that include a retinoid and BPO such as adapalene 0.1%/BPO2.5% gel can simplify treatment regimens and have been proven effective in all skin types [17]. Patients should titrate retinoid dose at initiation and be counseled on retinoid-induced irritation during the first 2–4 weeks of treatment. Of note, ethanolic gel vehicles tend to be more irritating than cream, foam, or lotion formulations. However, newer sophisticated formulations utilizing aqueous gels and microsphere or micodispersed technologies are well tolerated across the spectrum of skin types. Irritation is further reduced without sacrificing efficacy, by applying a moisturizer before application of the retinoid [18]. As the retinoid becomes more tolerable, the concentration can be titrated up as needed.

In combination with a topical retinoid, BPO is the top antimicrobial choice for reducing the concentration of *C. acnes* and limiting the potential for microbial resistance. Patients should start with lower concentrations as investigators have found no significant difference between BPO 2.5% gel compared to BPO 5% gel with respect to inflammatory lesion reduction [19, 20]. In addition, BPO 10% was associated with higher rates on irritation [20]. Topical antibiotics including clindamycin and erythromycin are not recommended as monotherapy; however, they can be used in combination with BPO for inflammatory acne [10].

Additional topical anti-inflammatory medications that have been effective in skin of color include azelaic acid and dapsone. In addition to anti-inflammatory affects, azelaic acid reversibly inhibits tyrosinase, which makes it safe and effective for patients with acne and associated PIH [21, 22]. Topical dapsone 5% and 7.5% gel has been proven safe and effective in comedonal and inflammatory acne in skin of color patients [23, 24].

Inflammatory acne non-responsive to topical therapies or more widespread disease affecting the trunk can be treated with an oral antibiotic. The oral tetracyclines are most commonly used. To limit bacterial resistance, systemic therapy should be limited to 3–4 months, and topical therapy should be continued for maintenance [10]. In skin of color, the threshold for starting systemic antibiotics should be low, given increased risk of PIH and cosmetic disfigurement in these populations [25].

In patients with severe acne, isotretinoin is highly effective. Isotretinoin is an oral retinoid that is FDA approved for nodulocystic acne and recalcitrant acne with risk of scarring. It is safe and effective in skin of color patients and may also hasten the resolution of PIH (AFA, clinical observation) [26, 27]. The standard counseling and laboratory evaluation should be done with all patients due to risks of systemic toxicities.

For individual inflamed or nodulocystic lesions, low-dose intralesional corticosteroid injections (triamcinolone acetonide 2.5–3.3 mg/ml) can be used to reduce local inflammation [25]. Higher concentrations should be avoided in darker skinned patients due to increased risk of hypopigmentation. However, if keloids have developed, higher concentrations may be necessary.

Acne affecting the lower third of the face in adult women is usually driven by hormonal abnormalities. OCPs, other estrogen containing contraceptives (patch, ring), and hormonal therapies such as spironolactone can be considered. These patients should also be continued on maintenance therapy with a topical retinoid and BPO [10].

Laser and light therapy have shown some benefit in Asian populations; however, more studies are needed to evaluate their utility among all ethnicities – especially among those with Fitzpatrick skin types IV–VI [10, 26].

Chemical peels can also aid in the treatment of acne and improve PIH. In skin of color, superficial chemical peels with salicylic acid or glycolic acid have shown the most efficacy while minimizing risk of PIH. In a study comparing glycolic acid and salicylic-mandelic acid (SMP) peels, both were effective therapies; however, SMPs were better tolerated and had higher efficacy in reducing acne lesions and hyperpigmentation [28].

Atopic Dermatitis

Atopic dermatitis (AD) is a common chronic inflammatory skin disease characterized by pruritus. It is frequently accompanied by other atopic disorders such as allergic rhinitis, asthma, and food allergies. Patients typically present in childhood and exhibit a chronic and relapsing course.

Epidemiology

The prevalence of AD differs based on the population studied. In the United States, the prevalence is estimated at 15.6% and rates vary among different ethnic groups [29]. AD is more frequently seen in African American populations (19.3%), followed by Caucasians (16.1%), and Hispanics (7.8%) [29]. The increased prevalence of AD in black patients is observed in Europe as well [30]. Few population studies have compared prevalence rates in Asian populations. However higher incidence rates have been demonstrated in Chinese infants compared to Caucasians [31]. Worldwide AD appears to have higher rates in Africa and Oceania when compared to the Indian subcontinent and Northern and Eastern Europe [32].

Genetics and Pathophysiology

AD involves a complex interplay of genetic and environmental factors. Key determinants of disease include genetic predisposition, skin barrier dysfunction, immune-related genes, and environmental triggers. Thirty-one distinct genetic loci have been identified in a diverse population of patients and likely represent a multifactorial basis for development of AD [33]. The filaggrin gene encodes for an essential structural component of the stratum corneum, and loss of function mutation is widely associated with AD. It is suggested that decreased integrity of the epithelium allows environmental allergens to more easily penetrate the skin leading to inflammation and sensitization. Filaggrin mutations are significantly more prevalent of European ancestry compared to populations of African or Asian ancestry [34, 35]. However, when a population of predominately African Americans was studied, authors identified a loss-of-function mutation in filaggrin-2, which was associated with more persistent disease [36]. Of note, patients without filaggrin mutations, may still develop an acquired filaggrin deficiency because of the upregulation of TH2 cytokines, IL4 and IL-13, which downregulate filaggrin expression [37]. Other structural components of the epidermis such as variations of claudin 1, upregulation of loricrin, and downregulation of involucrin have also been associated with disease [37]. Additional immune-related genes identified in AD development include IL-31, STAT6, thymic stromal lymphopoietin (TSLP), interferon regulatory factor 2 (IRF2), toll-like receptor 2 (TLR2), FcepsilonRI alpha (FCER1A), and B-defensin 1 (DEFB1) [37]. IL-31 is an essential component of pruritis seen in AD.

There have been several environmental factors shown to contribute to disease. AD is frequently found in higher rates among urban and higher income populations. This may be related to varying rates of pollution, cigarette smoke, exposure to infectious agents, diet, breastfeeding, and hygiene practices [37]. Supporters of the "hygiene hypothesis" suggest decreased exposure to infectious agents in early life may predispose individuals to allergic diseases [38]. In a Chinese study, AD was seen at significantly higher rates in children with prenatal exposure to household mold or home renovation [39]. Protective factors for AD may include subtropical climates with higher temperatures and humidity and use of topical emollients during the neonatal period [40, 41].

Clinical Presentation

The clinical presentation of AD varies based on age and chronicity of disease; however, pruritus dominates at all stages. In the acute form, lesions present as erythematous papules or plaques, typically with eroded vesicles, serous drainage, and crust. Subacute lesions include erythematous scaly excoriated plaques. Chronic lesions show thickened lichenified papules and plaques with scale and excoriation. In severe cases, an erythroderma can occur characterized by generalized erythema, severe pruritus, and systemic signs or symptoms (hypothermia, peripheral edema, fluid and electrolyte imbalance).

AD in skin of color may appear more hyperchromic with red-brown, dark brown, purple, or gray hues in lesional skin. Associated edema, warmth, or scale may help identify lesions [37]. Darkly pigmented patients may show follicular prominence. Also known as papular eczema, this presents with small papules or "goose bump-like" skin, commonly on the trunk and extensor surfaces. In Asian populations, eczematous lesions may present with a psoriasiform morphology with lesions that are well demarcated with increased lichenification and scale compared to white populations [42]. This may be linked to studies that suggest gene expression in Asian populations with AD show parallels to European AD and psoriasis profiles [42].

In infantile AD (0–2 years), symptoms usually present at 2 months of age and frequently affects the cheeks, scalp, neck, trunk, and extensor surfaces. Childhood AD affects children 2–12 years old and is typically seen in the antecubital and popliteal fossa. Other common locations include the periorificial face, neck, wrists, hands, ankles, and feet. In children, eczema lesions are typically lichenified. Adolescent and adult AD is usually a persistence of childhood AD; however, sites of predilection may change. Adults may show primarily face or hand disease.

Additional skin findings that may accompany AD include ichthyosis vulgaris, keratosis pilaris, palmar and plantar hyperlinearity, Dennie-Morgan lines (marked horizontal folds inferior to lower eyelid), periorbital darkening, anterior neck folds, and Hertoghe sign (thinning of lateral eyebrows).

Patients with AD are at increased risk of infections due to impaired skin barrier function. Providers should have a high level of suspicion for bacterial impetiginization with *S. aureus* and *S. pyogenes*, and eczema herpeticum in AD patients [43]. Patients are also at risk for molluscum contagiosum and warts [43].

Treatment

Treatment of AD is driven by disease severity and is largely similar across ethnicities. For limited disease, topical steroids and topical calcineurin inhibitors (tacrolimus, pimecrolimus) are frequently used. Crisaborole, a topical phosphodiesterase 4 inhibitor, can also be used for mild-moderate disease. Patients should be counseled on potential side effects of topical steroids including risk of hypopigmentation in darker skin types.

For more widespread, moderate-severe disease, phototherapy and systemic medications should be considered. The most common phototherapy regimen uses narrowband UVB and typically requires higher doses for more deeply pigmented skin types [44]. Skin of color patients should be counseled on increased risk of tanning (which may be culturally undesirable for some subsets of patients of color) and post-inflammatory hyperpigmentation with phototherapy [45]. Beyond phototherapy, systemic options include cyclosporine, mycophenolate mofetil, azathioprine, methotrexate – all of which have potential end-organ toxicities and require serological monitoring, and biologic therapy with

dupilumab [37], which has a more favorable safety profile compared to the aforementioned oral agents. Dupilumab is a human monoclonal antibody, which targets the alpha subunit of the IL-4 and IL-13 receptors and thereby blocks signaling of the IL-4 and IL-13 pathway. The most common side effects reported include conjunctivitis and injection site reactions.

Avoidance of aggravating factors is an essential component of treatment. Potential triggers include environmental allergens (pollen, dust mites, animal dander), sweating, harsh soaps, fragrances, wools, tobacco smoke, and stress [38]. Mattress and pillow covers, frequent vacuum cleaning, and miticide sprays may help decrease exposure to allergens in the home [29]. Gentle skin care should be employed even during inactive disease. Patients should take quick shower/baths with lukewarm water and mild cleansers. Topical anti-inflammatory agents or bland emollients should be applied immediately after bathing. All scented products should be avoided. There has been conflicting evidence on the utility of bleach baths in AD [46]. Since many AD patients are colonized with *S. aureus* or susceptible to bacterial superinfection, some authors suggest using bleach baths (0.5 cup of household bleach in full bathtub) twice weekly and periodic intranasal mupirocin for reduction of bacterial load [47].

Seborrheic Dermatitis

Seborrheic dermatitis is a chronic and relapsing eczematous disorder that occurs in areas of the skin with a large density of active sebaceous glands. It is most commonly seen on the scalp but frequently affects the central regions of the face, and less commonly, the chest and intertriginous areas. The infantile form is usually self-limited to the first 3 months of life. The adult form is often a chronic course that peaks in the fourth and sixth decades; however, it can first present in adolescence. Men are affected more than females. The pathogenesis of seborrheic dermatitis is linked to immune dysregulation of high levels of the commensal yeast, *Malassezia*, and abnormalities of sebum composition [48]. Patients with seborrheic dermatitis were found to have high levels of triglycerides and cholesterol and low levels of squalene and free fatty acids in sebum when compared to controls [49].

Clinical Presentation

Seborrheic dermatitis presents as red to red-brown patches with greasy scale in highly sebaceous areas such as scalp, eyebrows, nasolabial folds, beard area, forehead, ears, retroauricular space, mid-chest, and intertriginous areas. Pityriasis simplex capillitii refers to dandruff or fine white greasy scaling without the erythema and is thought to be a mild form of seborrheic dermatitis. Depending on the level of irritation, underlying skin ranges from mild scaly patches to think plaques with adherent crust, and more rarely exfoliative erythroderma. It is often itchy, particularly in the scalp, which can lead to hair breakage and loss. In skin of color, *Malassezia* infections often produce pigmentary changes. *Malassezia furfur* has been reported to produce azelaic acid, which inhibits tyrosinase and impedes melanin production [38]. Clinically, this may appear as hypopigmented patches in active areas of active seborrheic dermatitis (Fig. 7.2). Petaloid seborrheic dermatitis refers to a presentation characterized by pink or hypopigmented

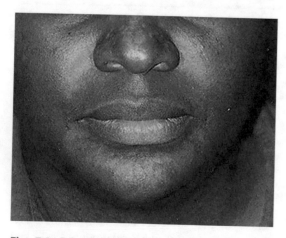

Fig. 7.2 Seborrheic dermatitis. Note hypopigmented macules and patches on nasal bridge, nasolabial folds, and chin

polycyclic coalescing rings in seborrhea areas of the face [50]; this less common presentation is more frequently seen in populations with skin of color compared to populations of European ancestry. An additional unusual variant was reported in an African American woman with progressive hyperpigmented facial papules in typical seborrhea areas of the face [51]. Lesions of seborrheic dermatitis can be aggravated by stress, sun/heat, febrile illness, seasonal changes, and aggressive topical therapy.

Infantile seborrheic dermatitis appears similarly to the adult form in the scalp and face. Infants frequently present with "cradle cap," in which inflammation results in an adherent scaly and crusted plaques on the scalp vertex. In body creases, such as axillae and inguinal folds, plaques may appear sharply demarcated with maceration, oozing, and satellite lesions.

While seborrheic dermatitis frequently occurs in healthy individuals, severe presentations or flares can be associated with HIV infection and neurologic disease such as Parkinson disease or stroke. Extensive or severe seborrheic dermatitis should raise the suspicion for these underlying disorders.

Treatment

Treatment for infantile seborrheic dermatitis is aimed at loosening the adherent scale with use of emollients such as mineral oil or petroleum jelly. One study demonstrated equal therapeutic response with the use of ketoconazole 2% cream compared to hydrocortisone 1% cream, with clearance of all lesions at 2 weeks [52]. Authors recommended the use of ketoconazole cream given better long-term safety profile when compared to topical steroids.

Topical antifungals, particularly azoles and corticosteroids, are mainstay of therapy in adolescent and adult seborrheic dermatitis. For scalp disease, over-the-counter dandruff shampoos with coal tar, selenium sulfide, and zinc pyrithione have been shown to control symptoms. Ketoconazole 2% shampoo and ciclopirox 1% shampoo can also be used [48]. Difference in hair care practices and hair morphology in the African American community may pose difficulty with treatment [53]. Patients should be encouraged to wash hair at least once weekly. Shampoos should be applied directly to scalp to minimize dryness to hair shaft and remain on scalp for 10–15 minutes before rinsing clean. Moisturizing conditioners to be used post-shampooing are frequently recommended to prevent drying the hair shafts and associated breakage (which is a higher risk in populations with Afro-textured hair). Topical steroids can be a beneficial addition in treatment. Fluocinolone 0.01% solution and betamethasone valerate 0.12% foam were shown to reduce pruritus and inflammation of the scalp [54]. A pilot trial using 1% pimecrolimus cream demonstrated improvement in seborrheic dermatitis and associated hypopigmentation in African American adults [55]. Calcineurin inhibitors, mainly pimecrolimus 1% cream and tacrolimus 0.1% ointment, may improve symptoms as well as topical steroids with lower adverse side-effect profiles [48]. Seborrheic dermatitis affecting the face and body benefit from topical antifungals, corticosteroids, and calcineurin inhibitors as well. Ketoconazole 2% cream and hydrocortisone 1% have been shown to be equally effective in reducing symptoms [56].

Lupus Erythematosus

Lupus erythematosus is a multi-organ system autoimmune disease characterized by a variety of serologic markers and clinical manifestations. Cutaneous lupus erythematosus (CLE) presents with a broad spectrum of skin findings and may be the first sign of systemic lupus erythematosus (SLE).

Epidemiology

Women are significantly more affected that men with a ratio of 6:1 in SLE and 3:1 in CLE [38]. Lupus most often presents during childbearing years, with a distinct racial predilection. The prevalence of CLE is three to four times higher in African American women as compared to Caucasian women, and the same holds true for SLE [57]. Hispanics and Asian/Pacific Islander populations show a higher prevalence of SLE when compared to Caucasians, but still less than that of blacks [58]. Worldwide, specific ethnic populations tend to have higher rates of lupus as well. In a New Zealand population study, Pacific and Maori (indigenous Polynesian) people have a greater risk of all types of cutaneous lupus compared to the European population [59]. Similarly, in the United Kingdom, the highest prevalence of SLE is seen in people of black Caribbean ethnicity [60].

Pathogenesis

The pathogenesis of lupus involves a complex interplay of genetic factors and environmental triggers, which initiate a multifaceted inflammatory cascade. Potential environmental triggers are ultraviolet radiation, medication, and virus infection. The most strongly associated genes include major histocompatibility complex HLA-DR, PTPN22, STAT4, IRF5, TREX1, and C1Q [61]. Using these genes, genomic studies in ethnic populations have identified polymorphisms associated with disease incidence, severity, and systemic manifestations [62]. Few studies exist for CLE specifically. One such genome-wide association study in Asia attributed the low prevalence of subacute cutaneous lupus in Asian populations when compared to Caucasians, due to the lack of the HLA-DR3 allele in the Asian population [63].

Clinical Presentation

Cutaneous lupus lesions are classified into three major subtypes: acute cutaneous lupus (ACLE), subacute cutaneous lupus (SCLE), and chronic cutaneous lupus, which includes discoid lupus (DLE), lupus erythematosus tumidus, lupus panniculitis, and chilblain lupus. These classifications however are not fixed as DLE can be short lived and features of ACLE or SCLE may persist. One patient can also present with more than one subtype.

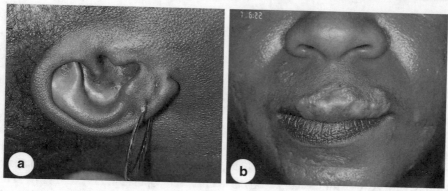

Fig. 7.3 Discoid lesions most frequently occur on the face, scalp, and ears (**a**, **b**). Lesions may occasionally appear hypertrophic (**b**)

DLE is the most common form of chronic cutaneous lupus and presents with intensely inflamed plaques resulting in dyspigmentation and disfiguring scarring (Fig. 7.3). Due to the level of inflammation, the adnexa are often involved resulting in follicular plugging and scarring alopecia. Lesions tend to have a central area of hypopigmentation with hyperpigmentation at the borders. It most often occurs on the head and neck including mucosal surfaces. It is rare for discoid lesions to occur below the neck. When lesions are very hyperkeratotic, it is referred to as hypertrophic DLE, commonly on the extensor arms. Sun exposure is believed to promote discoid lesions, and squamous cell carcinoma can develop in chronic DLE scars. The lower lip is the most frequently affected site [64, 65]. In DLE, disease is usually limited to the skin; however, 5–15% of patients will later develop SLE [38]. In one study, early onset DLE was associated with a decreased likelihood of renal disease in Latin American populations who later developed SLE [66].

SCLE is a photosensitive eruption typically presenting with annular plaques with raised borders and central clearing. Lesions may also be papulosquamous in nature. Most common areas affected include the sides if the face, neck, upper trunk, and extensor arms. The mid-face is often spared. These lesions do not scar but can resolve with dyspigmentation. Numerous medications have been associated with the development of SCLE. These include hydro-

chlorothiazide, calcium channel blockers, terbinafine, angiotensin-converting-enzyme inhibitors, NSAIDs, griseofulvin, and anti-tumor necrosis factor agents [67]. Lesions sometimes persist despite discontinuing the offending medication. Only 10–15% of these patients develop internal disease [38]. Anti-Ro autoantibodies are associated with SCLE, which may result in an overlap with Sjogren's syndrome [68].

ACLE is characterized by bilateral malar erythema and/or edema also known as the "butterfly rash." The nasolabial fold is classically spared. It often occurs after sun exposure, is transient, and resolves without scarring. The presentation is strongly associated with internal disease [38]. A severe variant of ACLE known as Rowell's syndrome may present with widespread erythema multiforme-like lesions [69].

When assessing skin of color for lupus lesions, erythema is sometimes masked by deeply pigmented normal skin. Physicians must keep in mind, for darker skin tones, erythema and inflammation may present as hyperpigmentation or hyperchromia rather than redness [70].

Systemic lupus erythematosus (SLE) affects multiple organ systems beyond the skin, including joints, hematologic, pulmonary, renal, and central nervous system. The American College of Rheumatology uses 11 criteria to classify SLE [71]. Four out of 11 are cutaneous manifestations: malar rash, discoid, rash, photosensitivity, and oral ulcers. The remaining seven include non-erosive arthritis, pleuritis/pericarditis, renal

Table 7.1 Non-specific cutaneous manifestations of SLE [38, 62]

Non-specific cutaneous manifestations of SLE
Vascular lesions
Raynaud's phenomenon
Livedo reticularis
Palmar erythema
Periungal telangiectasia
Vasculitis
Livedoid vasculopathy and atrophie blanche
Diffuse non-scarring alopecia
Papular and nodular mucinosis

disorder, neurologic disorder, hematologic disorder, positive ANA, and an immunologic disorder (presence of Anti-DNA, Anti-smith, or antiphospholipid antibodies). Although not present in the official criteria, non-specific cutaneous lesions that may warrant an evaluation for SLE are listed in Table 7.1.

Several population studies have shown an association between ethnicity and disease severity. Evidence supports that compared to their Caucasian counterparts, African American and Hispanic populations present at an earlier age, have a higher incidence of organ dysfunction, and demonstrate a higher mortality rate [72]. A combination of genetic and environmental factors is thought to drive this, as Hispanic Americans show more severe disease than Hispanics from Puerto Rico [73]. This is further supported by similar SLE prevalence rates in native Asians, Latin Americans, and Caucasian Americans, despite differences within US emigrant populations [38, 74]. Lupus nephritis, a strong factor of morbidity and mortality, is more prevalent in skin of color populations, and Chinese populations have shown the highest rates [75].

Treatment

Given photosensitivity in lupus, sun protection is imperative with protective clothing and broad-spectrum, high SPF sunscreens. This is especially important to review in darker skinned patients who often do not traditionally use sun protection [76]. In addition to sun avoidance, topical and intralesional corticosteroids are first-line therapies and traditionally very effective. For discoid lesions, including those on the face, high-potency topical steroids are the most effective [38]. Patients should be counseled on appropriate application and the cutaneous effects of over use. Intralesional triamcinolone can be performed monthly. Topical calcineurin inhibitors can be used for their steroid-sparing effects [77].

There are no drugs currently approved for the specific treatment of cutaneous lupus. However, several of the medications used for SLE show benefit in skin lesions. Antimalarials (hydroxychloroquine [HCQ], chloroquine [CQ], and quinacrine) are first-line systemic therapies. Quinacrine (100 mg/day) can be added to HCQ (200 mg twice daily) or CQ for synergistic effect. Response is typically slow, and patients may need to continue therapy 2–3 months before noticing effect. Combination therapy with topicals is therefore also used. Patients should be counseled on smoking cessation, as studies have found decreased therapeutic benefit in smokers [38]. An important side effect to monitor while on antimalarials is ocular toxicity. Baseline ophthalmologic exam should be performed within 1 year of starting HCQ/CQ. Annual screening should be done in high-risk patients (renal disease, tamoxifen use, dose greater than 5/mg/kg total body weight); however, some authors recommend that annual exams can be postponed until year 5 of treatment in low-risk patients [78]. In a cohort of Latin American patients, long-term antimalarials (>2 years) were associated with a decrease in mortality and a 38% delay in death [79]. Antimalarial-resistant patients tend to be unresponsive to other immunosuppressive agents; however, alternative options include oral retinoids, thalidomide, high-dose prednisone, methotrexate, mycophenolate mofetil, dapsone, and azathioprine [63]. Since many lupus patients are women of childbearing potential, safety profile and teratogenicity should be considered. Skin of color patients are more likely to receive treatment with immunosuppressive drugs when compared to Caucasians, likely due to higher rates of severe disease [79].

Currently, there are little data on biologic therapies for cutaneous lupus. Belimumab has shown some efficacy; however, Black/African American patients show mixed results [80, 81]. Rituximab has shown favorable responses in ACLE and bullous lupus specifically [80]. Drugs recently studied in SLE that show improvement in cutaneous symptoms include sifalimumab and anifrolumab [82].

Cosmetic camouflage can also be used for chronic dyspigmented lesions.

Dermatomyositis

Dermatomyositis (DM) is an idiopathic inflammatory myopathy that presents with symmetric inflammation of the proximal extensor muscles, characteristic skin manifestations, and a variety of systemic findings. When the typical cutaneous features of DM are present without evidence of muscle inflammation, it is referred to as amyopathic dermatomyositis. The etiology of dermatomyositis remains unclear. It is speculated to be the result of an immune-mediated process in genetically predisposed individuals after exposure to environmental triggers such as infection, medications, and malignancy [83]. Autoimmune antibodies are identified in most cases, and recently myositis-specific antibodies have been suggested to correlate with distinct clinical presentations within the DM spectrum [84]. In addition, certain HLA alleles are thought to confer a risk for the development of DM [85]. DM can occur concurrently with other autoimmune connective tissue diseases including lupus erythematosus, Sjogren's syndrome, scleroderma, rheumatoid arthritis, and mixed connective tissue disease.

DM has a bimodal age distribution. Juvenile dermatomyositis (JDM) most commonly occurs in children between 10 and 15 years old; however, it can occur as early as 2 years. It is typically a milder disease as compared to adult DM. Adult DM is most commonly seen in individuals between 45 and 60 years old with a female to male 2:1 predominance. Prevalence of DM in African Americans patients is 2–4 times higher than in Caucasians [62]. Up to 40% of patients with adult DM have an associated malignancy, and some authors consider DM to be a paraneoplastic event [86]. Common accompanying malignancies include colon, ovarian, breast, pancreatic, lung, and gastric cancers and lymphoma [86]. Nasopharyngeal carcinoma should be considered in Asian populations with DM [87]. In some populations, there is a weaker association with malignancy. Afro-Caribbean patients with DM for instance, show lower rates on malignancy, likely related to younger age at onset and associated connective tissue diseases in the Caribbean [88].

Clinical Presentation

Pathognomonic features of DM include heliotrope rash and Gottron papules. Heliotrope rash is periorbital edema and erythema usually affecting the upper eyelid. Gottron papules are erythematous-violaceous papules or plaques overlying the dorsal joint extensors of the hand. These lesions characteristically involve the dorsal aspect of metacarpophalangeal joints, proximal interphalangeal joints, and/or distal interphalangeal joints When just erythema is present, it is called Gottron's sign and can affect the hand as well as the elbows. In skin of color, these symptoms typically appear hyperpigmented. Other characteristic skin findings in DM include malar erythema, mechanic's hands (hyperkeratosis, scaling, and fissuring of fingers), and periungal changes such as dilated capillary loops and ragged cuticles. Poikiloderma is also characteristic and can be seen in distinctive locations including the upper back (shawl sign), upper chest (V sign), and lateral thighs (Holster sign). Lesions are often associated with pruritus, which may help distinguish itself from lupus erythematosus. Features commonly found in JDM include calcinosis cutis and small vessel vasculitis. In most patients, skin manifestations will precede the development of muscle inflammation. DM typically effects the proximal muscle groups, and patients will report difficulty performing certain maneuvers such as rising from a chair, climbing stairs, brushing their hair, or reaching for something above their head. Systemic disease frequently associated with DM includes calcinosis, pulmonary disease, notably diffuse interstitial fibrosis, cardiac disease, and previously mentioned malignancies [89]. Systemic symptoms may include malaise, loss of energy, arthralgias, dysphagia, dyspnea, and palpitations.

Laboratory tests to evaluate for objective muscle inflammation include aldolase and creatine kinase (CK). These muscle enzymes are elevated in approximately 95% of patients with classic DM during their disease [90]. CK and aldolase levels can also be used to asses for disease flares. Other muscle enzymes less frequently tested include lactate dehydrogenase, alanine, and aspartate transaminases. In addition to elevated muscle enzymes, imaging studies used to confirm muscle disease include MRI and ultrasound. MRI is highly sensitive for detecting inflammation. While, ultrasound provides a more accessible and cheaper option, it is not as sensitive. More traditional procedures used to confirm DM include muscle biopsy, typically of the triceps and electromyography (EMG) on a proximal muscle. If the abovementioned tests are negative on two occasions, and muscle enzymes are not elevated, a diagnosis of amyopathic DM is given. However, given cutaneous lesions sometimes occur before muscle disease, repeat muscle examinations and laboratory testing should be done at 2–3 month intervals for the next 2 years.

Several autoantibodies have been associated with DM and can confer clinical phenotype. Autoantibodies to M-i2 nuclear antigen have been associated with classic proximal muscle involvement and hallmark skin rash. Anti-SRP usually denotes severe muscle involvement with no skin lesions. Anti-Jo-1 is one of many autoantibodies directed against aminoacyl transfer RNA synthetases (antisynthetase syndrome), and correlates with polymyositis and DM with higher rates of Raynaud's phenomenon, mechanic's hands, and ILD. Some autoantibodies have been shown to correlate with the most severe ILD such as Anti-MDA-5, Anti-PL-7, and Anti-PL-12 [83]. There have been few studies comparing the rates of specific autoantibodies in ethnic populations. In an Indian population, the studied DM autoantibodies replicated the common associated phe-

notypes [91]. In a Korean study, Anti-p140 and anti-p155/140 antibodies were associated with rapidly progressive ILD and cancer-associated myositis, respectively [92]. In a cohort study data from patients with antisynthetase syndrome demonstrated African American populations had a higher prevalence of Anti-PL2 and, independent of antisynthetase antibody status, had more severe lung involvement than white patients [93].

Treatment

Treatment for DM must address cutaneous and muscle disease. Immunosuppressive agents are mainstay with corticosteroids being first-line. Authors recommend high-dose prednisone with slow taper based on clinical judgment [83]. With few clinical trials, there is no formal consensus on corticosteroid dosage and duration. Traditionally, prednisone is dosed 1 mg/kg per day with taper to 50% at 6 months and slow taper over 2–3 years [94]. Other immunosuppressive drugs used include methotrexate (MTX, 5–20 mg/weekly), azathioprine (2–3 mg/kg per day), mycophenolate mofetil (2–3 g per day), cyclosporine (3–5 mg/kg per day), tacrolimus (0.06 mg/kg per day), and IVIG (2 g/kg per month) [83]. Biologic agents (rituximab, abatacept, tocilizumab) can be considered for refractory disease. Comorbidities may drive the selection of corticosteroid-sparing agents. Patients with myositis-associated interstitial lung disease, for instance, should avoid MTX, due to risk of lung toxicity [95]. Mycophenolate mofetil can improve myositis-associated ILD in addition to cutaneous symptoms [96]. Cyclophosphamide is also used in setting of severe ILD [97]. In addition to pharmacologic treatment, adjunctive physical therapy programs have shown to improve strength and reduce disability [83].

Cutaneous symptoms are more difficult to treat and for many patients persist despite resolution of muscle disease. As ultraviolet light exposure is thought to exacerbate disease, all patients should be counseled on photoprotection and sunscreen. For limited skin involvement, topical steroids can be used especially for associated pruritus. However, studies documenting the efficacy of this therapy are lacking. Few case reports and observational studies have demonstrated favorable response with topical calcineurin inhibitors [98]. Antimalarials have demonstrated the most convincing treatment response, with 40–75% of patients with cutaneous symptoms showing improvement [89]. One study found that patients who do not respond to HQ or HQ + quinacrine show therapeutic effect when switched to CQ [99]. Panniculitis-associated DM may also respond to antimalarials. In cutaneous DM recalcitrant to antimalarials, MTX is often substituted. This has the added benefit of treating myositis. MTX (5–15 mg/week) should be given with folic acid to reduce potential for adverse effects such as gastrointestinal upset, malaise, and mucositis. Mycophenolate mofetil may help control symptoms; however, routine laboratory monitoring should be done with attentiveness to opportunistic infections and risk of malignancy. High-dose IVIG (2 g/kg over 2 days) has shown favorable response as monotherapy or in combination with treatments listed above. Additional agents proposed include azathioprine, dapsone, etanercept, infliximab, rituximab, calcineurin inhibitors (cyclosporin A, tacrolimus), rapamycin, thalidomide, and cyclophosphamide [89]. Recently, tofacitinib has shown favorable response in cutaneous DM [100].

Patients with JDM should be monitored closely while on immunosuppressive agents with regular monitoring by a pediatrician. Calcinosis cutis is often unresponsive or recurrent after treatment [101]. Therapies used include surgical excision, laser therapy, extracorporeal shock wave lithotripsy, and pharmacological management with diltiazem [101, 102].

Scleroderma

Scleroderma is an autoimmune connective tissue disorder characterized by fibrosis of the skin and internal structures. Two major clinical subsets are localized scleroderma also known as morphea and systemic sclerosis. Molecular studies in morphea and systemic sclerosis have shown that while these processes show similarities in inflammatory pathways, they are likely biologically distinct entities.

Morphea

Morphea is more prevalent in women than in men and affects children and adults. The racial distribution has not been well studied; however, in a retrospective review, morphea was most common in Caucasians [103]. It has three major clinical variants that include plaque-type morphea, linear morphea, and generalized morphea. Less common variants include deep, guttate, and nodular or keloid morphea. Autoantibodies, notably ANA and ssDNA, are most frequently seen in linear and generalized morphea.

Clinical Presentation

Plaque-type morphea is the most common (56%) and presents with a slightly raised, erythematous plaque typically on the trunk [38]. It is frequently asymptomatic and over time peripherally expands as the center of the lesions becomes sclerotic. Active disease will typically have an inflammatory margin characterized by a lilac or violaceous ring. However, this is not always appreciated. In the later stages, post-inflammatory pigmentation usually dominates. Adnexal structures including sweat glands and hair follicles are often destroyed.

Linear morphea presents as a linear erythematous streak or multiple small plaque-type morphea that coalesce to form a line. Lesions tend to involve underlying structures including fascia, muscle, and tendons, which can lead to muscle weakness, joint immobility, and limb asymmetry. Linear morphea frequently presents in childhood and when it occurs on the forehead or scalp, it is referred to as en coup de sabre. En coup de sabre morphea can involve underlying bone, meninges, and brain, which may put the child at risk for neurologic and ocular involvement.

Generalized morphea presents first as plaque-type morphea; however, lesions rapidly progress and continue to expand until the entire trunk or limb is affected. It often does not respond well to therapy.

Morphea can undergo spontaneous resolution after 3–5 years; however, some patients have a more relapsing disease course. It does not increase mortality, but patients experience significant morbidity.

Treatment

Treatment of morphea is guided by the subtype, activity of disease, area of involvement, and symptoms. Topical and systemic immunosuppression can be used to treat active morphea lesions; however, burned-out morphea is unresponsive to such therapies. Early treatment is ideal, as treatment of active disease is usually most successful. While topical corticosteroids are the most common treatment, phototherapy is the best studied treatment modality for morphea. Of the phototherapy studies performed, strongest support is demonstrated for the use narrow-band ultraviolet B, broadband ultraviolet A, and ultraviolet A-1 [104]. It is proposed that NBUVB should be used for superficial lesions and BB UVA and UVA-1 is more suitable for deeper lesions [104]. Less convincing evidence supports the use of PUVA and extracorporeal phototherapy. Notably, a retrospective review demonstrated that the efficacy of UVA1 phototherapy is not significantly influenced in Fitzpatrick skin types I–V [105]. Topical therapies are useful for individual lesions; however, they do not suppress overall disease progression. Topical immunosuppressive medications that have been proven efficacious in plaque-type morphea include twice-daily tacrolimus, calcipotriene when applied twice daily under occlusion, and a case series in imiquimod when applied three to five times a week [104, 106, 107]. Topical steroids are frequently used anecdotally; however, there are no studies to date evaluating its efficacy. Of the immunomodulators, monotherapy with oral methotrexate and combination therapy with methotrexate and pulse corticosteroids have been the most efficacious. Clinical improvement has also been seen with mycophenolate mofetil, infliximab, and imatinib [104].

Systemic Sclerosis

Systemic sclerosis (SSc) presents with limited or diffuse disease. There is a female predominance and age of onset is usually between 30 and 50 years. In the United States, blacks have a higher prevalence of systemic sclerosis than whites and greater associated morbidity and mortality [108]. Black patients tend to present at an earlier age and have a higher likelihood of diffuse disease [109].

The pathogenesis of systemic sclerosis is only somewhat understood. Factors known to contribute to the disease include immune dysregulation and autoimmunity, vascular dysfunction, and systemic tissue fibrosis [38]. Limited and diffuse forms will have positive antinuclear antibodies (ANA); anti-centromere antibodies are associated with limited SSc, whereas anti-topoisomerase I (anti-Scl70) or anti-RNA polymerase III antibodies are more closely associated with diffuse SSc. Black patients are more likely to have anti-SCL70 serologies, which supports the higher probability of diffuse disease and anti-U1-RNP antibodies, which are associated with autoimmune overlap syndromes [110]. Multiple studies have demonstrated increased disease severity in Black patients [109–112]. Black patients show a higher incidence of skin, lung, and renal involvement and overall mortality [109]. When compared to Caucasians, Black and Hispanic populations are more likely to show diffuse skin disease, pigmentary changes of the skin, digital ulcerations, and more severe pulmonary hypertension [113]. In a Han Chinese cohort, authors also found higher rates of diffuse disease and pulmonary fibrosis in Han Chinese compared to US Caucasians [114].

Clinical Presentation

Early manifestations of systemic sclerosis include Raynaud's phenomenon, nail fold capillary changes, and autoantibodies. Patients with limited systemic sclerosis usually develop sclerosis on the face and distal extremities, while diffuse sclerosis involves the distal limbs, proximal limbs, and/or trunk. Skin fibrosis usually occurs in three stages. In the early edematous phase, skin appears puffy, followed by the indurated phase when the skin hardens and appears taut and shiny, and lastly the late atrophic phase with thinning of the skin. Associated findings include flexion contractures and ulceration of the digits. Sclerosis of the face results in microstomia due to fibrosis of perioral skin and a beaked nose. Additional cutaneous findings include photo-distributed hyperpigmentation or hypopigmentation, leukoderma of scleroderma (also known as salt-and-pepper sign; area of depigmentation with sparing of the perifollicular skin), telangiectasias, and dystrophic calcinosis usually of the extremities (Fig. 7.4).

Limited systemic sclerosis and diffuse systemic sclerosis show variations in internal organ involvement. Limited systemic sclerosis can present as CREST syndrome. CREST is an acronym for its clinical features that includes calcinosis, Raynaud's phenomenon, esophageal dysmotility, sclerodactyly, and telangiectasias. While limited and diffuse systemic sclerosis can develop interstitial lung disease, the limited subtype has a higher likelihood of pulmonary artery hypertension. Diffuse scleroderma tends to involve internal organs earlier in the disease with a worse prognosis. Common organs affected comprise the pulmonary, gastrointestinal, renal, and cardiac systems.

The American College of Rheumatology (ACR) published criteria for the classification of systemic sclerosis that can help guide diagnosis [115]. The clinical criteria and scoring system can be found in Table 7.2. A score of 9 or more indicates a patient with systemic sclerosis.

Treatment

Treatment for systemic sclerosis is directed against the patient's comorbid conditions. Comprehensive screening should be performed with referrals to the appropriate specialists for pulmonary, renal, gastrointestinal, and cardiac manifestations [116]. Patients with Raynaud's phenomenon should be counseled to avoid triggers such as cold temperatures and smoking. It can pharmacologically be managed with calcium channel blockers such as nifedipine and alpha-adrenergic antagonists (Prazosin) [117]. A topical gel preparation of nitroglycerin was also

Table 7.2 ACR classification criteria for systemic sclerosis

Clinical and laboratory features	Subcategory	Score
Skin	Skin thickening of fingers of both hands proximal to MCPs	9
	Puffy fingers	2
	Whole finger, distal to MCP	4
Fingertip lesions	Ulcers on digital tip	2
	Pitting scars	3
Telangiectasia		2
Abnormal nail fold capillaries		2
Pulmonary artery hypertension ± interstitial lung disease		2
Raynaud's phenomenon		3
Scleroderma-related antibodies[a]		3

[a]anticentromere, anti-Scl70, anti-RNA polymerase 3 [115]

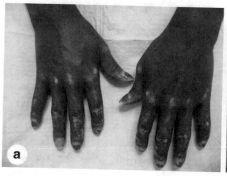
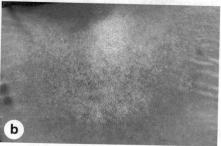

Fig. 7.4 Leukoderma of scleroderma (**a**, **b**). Note depigmentation with sparing of perifollicular skin (**b**)

found to be effective if used immediately before or after an attack [118]. In cases with associated digital ulcerations, intravenous iloprost and phosphodiesterase inhibitors, including sildenafil, vardenafil, and tadalafil can be used [117]. Bosentan has been shown to limit the development of new ulcers but does not affect the rate of ulcer healing. Novel approaches that have shown efficacy include atorvastatin and the Rho kinase inhibitor fasudil [117]. Surgical management with thoracic sympathectomy or digital artery sympathectomy can be considered in refractory cases; however, this comes with risk and have fallen out of favor [117].

Skin involvement in systemic sclerosis is frequently guided by comorbidities as most therapies have proven ineffective. Anecdotally, topical corticosteroids and topical calcineurin inhibitors can be helpful in diminishing cutaneous signs/symptoms, but efficacy tends to be limited. Patients with overlap autoimmune syndromes and myositis have shown favorable response to methotrexate [116]. Mycophenolate mofetil and cyclophosphamide particularly in ILD have also shown some benefit [116, 119]. In severe cases, few studies have suggested hematopoietic stem cell transplantation as a treatment option [50].

References

1. Collier CN, Harper JC, Cafardi JA, Cantrell WC, Wang W, Foster KW, et al. The prevalence of acne in adults 20 years and older. J Am Acad Dermatol. 2008;58(1):56–9.
2. Alexis AF, Sergay AB, Taylor SC. Common dermatologic disorders in skin of color: a comparative practice survey. Cutis. 2007;80(5):387–94.
3. Davis SA, Narahari S, Feldman SR, Huang W, Pichardo-Geisinger RO, McMichael AJ. Top dermatologic conditions in patients of color: an analysis of nationally representative data. J Drugs Dermatol: JDD. 2012;11(4):466–73.
4. Lawson CN, Callender VD. Acne and rosacea. In: Vashi NA, Maibach HI, editors. Dermatoanthropology of ethnic skin and hair. Cham: Springer International Publishing; 2017. p. 103–28.
5. Callender VD, Alexis AF, Daniels SR, Kawata AK, Burk CT, Wilcox TK, et al. Racial differences in clinical characteristics, perceptions and behaviors, and psychosocial impact of adult female acne. J Clin Aesthet Dermatol. 2014;7(7):19–31.
6. Rendon MI, Rodriguez DA, Kawata AK, Degboe AN, Wilcox TK, Burk CT, et al. Acne treatment patterns, expectations, and satisfaction among adult females of different races/ethnicities. Clin Cosmet Investig Dermatol. 2015;8:231–8.
7. Abad-Casintahan F, Chow SK, Goh CL, Kubba R, Hayashi N, Noppakun N, et al. Frequency and characteristics of acne-related post-inflammatory hyperpigmentation. J Dermatol. 2016;43(7):826–8.
8. Perkins AC, Cheng CE, Hillebrand GG, Miyamoto K, Kimball AB. Comparison of the epidemiology of acne vulgaris among Caucasian, Asian, Continental Indian and African American women. J Eur Acad Dermatol Venereol: JEADV. 2011;25(9):1054–60.
9. Gorelick J, Daniels SR, Kawata AK, Degboe A, Wilcox TK, Burk CT, et al. Acne-related quality of life among female adults of different races/ethnicities. J Dermatol Nurses Assoc. 2015;7(3):154–62.
10. Thiboutot DM, Dréno B, Abanmi A, Alexis AF, Araviiskaia E, Barona Cabal MI, et al. Practical management of acne for clinicians: an international consensus from the Global Alliance to Improve Outcomes in Acne. J Am Acad Dermatol. 2018;78(2):S1–S23.e1.
11. Pariser DM, Thiboutot DM, Clark SD, Jones TM, Liu Y, Graeber M. The efficacy and safety of adapalene gel 0.3% in the treatment of acne vulgaris: a randomized, multicenter, investigator-blinded, controlled comparison study versus adapalene gel 0.1% and vehicle. Cutis. 2005;76(2):145–51.
12. Thielitz A, Helmdach M, Ropke EM, Gollnick H. Lipid analysis of follicular casts from cyanoacrylate strips as a new method for studying therapeutic effects of antiacne agents. Br J Dermatol. 2001;145(1):19–27.
13. Leyden J, Stein-Gold L, Weiss J. Why topical retinoids are mainstay of therapy for acne. Dermatol Ther. 2017;7(3):293–304.
14. Tanghetti E, Dhawan S, Green L, Del Rosso J, Draelos Z, Leyden J, et al. Randomized comparison of the safety and efficacy of tazarotene 0.1% cream and adapalene 0.3% gel in the treatment of patients with at least moderate facial acne vulgaris. J Drugs Dermatol: JDD. 2010;9(5):549–58.
15. Thiboutot D, Arsonnaud S, Soto P. Efficacy and tolerability of adapalene 0.3% gel compared to tazarotene 0.1% gel in the treatment of acne vulgaris. J Drugs Dermatol: JDD. 2008;7(6 Suppl):s3–10.
16. Tu P, Li GQ, Zhu XJ, Zheng J, Wong WZ. A comparison of adapalene gel 0.1% vs. tretinoin gel 0.025% in the treatment of acne vulgaris in China. J Eur Acad Dermatol Venereol: JEADV. 2001;15(Suppl 3):31–6.
17. Alexis AF, Johnson LA, Kerrouche N, Callender VD. A subgroup analysis to evaluate the efficacy and safety of adapalene-benzoyl peroxide topical gel in black subjects with moderate acne. J Drugs Dermatol: JDD. 2014;13(2):170–4.
18. Zeichner J. Strategies to minimize irritation and potential iatrogenic post-inflammatory pigmenta-

tion when treating acne patients with skin of color. J Drugs Dermatol: JDD. 2011;10(12 Suppl):s25–6.

19. Kawashima M, Sato S, Furukawa F, Matsunaga K, Akamatsu H, Igarashi A, et al. Twelve-week, multicenter, placebo-controlled, randomized, double-blind, parallel-group, comparative phase II/III study of benzoyl peroxide gel in patients with acne vulgaris: a secondary publication. J Dermatol. 2017;44(7):774–82.

20. Mills OH Jr, Kligman AM, Pochi P, Comite H. Comparing 2.5%, 5%, and 10% benzoyl peroxide on inflammatory acne vulgaris. Int J Dermatol. 1986;25(10):664–7.

21. Kircik LH. Efficacy and safety of azelaic acid (AzA) gel 15% in the treatment of post-inflammatory hyperpigmentation and acne: a 16-week, baseline-controlled study. J Drugs Dermatol: JDD. 2011;10(6):586–90.

22. Woolery-Lloyd HC, Keri J, Doig S. Retinoids and azelaic acid to treat acne and hyperpigmentation in skin of color. J Drugs Dermatol: JDD. 2013;12(4):434–7.

23. Alexis AF, Burgess C, Callender VD, Herzog JL, Roberts WE, Schweiger ES, et al. The efficacy and safety of topical dapsone gel, 5% for the treatment of acne vulgaris in adult females with skin of color. J Drugs Dermatol: JDD. 2016;15(2):197–204.

24. Taylor SC, Cook-Bolden FE, McMichael A, Downie JB, Rodriguez DA, Alexis AF, et al. Efficacy, safety, and tolerability of topical dapsone gel, 7.5% for treatment of acne vulgaris by Fitzpatrick skin phototype. J Drugs Dermatol: JDD. 2018;17(2):160–7.

25. Alexis AF. Acne vulgaris in skin of color: understanding nuances and optimizing treatment outcomes. J Drugs Dermatol: JDD. 2014;13(6):s61–5.

26. Davis EC, Callender VD. A review of acne in ethnic skin: pathogenesis, clinical manifestations, and management strategies. J Clin Aesthet Dermatol. 2010;3(4):24–38.

27. Kelly AP, Sampson DD. Recalcitrant nodulocystic acne in black Americans: treatment with isotretinoin. J Natl Med Assoc. 1987;79(12):1266–70.

28. Garg VK, Sinha S, Sarkar R. Glycolic acid peels versus salicylic-mandelic acid peels in active acne vulgaris and post-acne scarring and hyperpigmentation: a comparative study. Dermatol Surg. 2009;35(1):59–65.

29. Fu T, Keiser E, Linos E, Rotatori RM, Sainani K, Lingala B, et al. Eczema and sensitization to common allergens in the United States: a multiethnic, population-based study. Pediatr Dermatol. 2014;31(1):21–6.

30. Williams HC, Pembroke AC, Forsdyke H, Boodoo G, Hay R, Burney P. London-born black Caribbean children are at increased risk of atopic dermatitis. J Am Acad Dermatol. 1995;32(2):212–7.

31. Mar A, Tam M, Jolley D, Marks R. The cumulative incidence of atopic dermatitis in the first 12 months among Chinese, Vietnamese, and Caucasian infants born in Melbourne, Australia. J Am Acad Dermatol. 1999;40(4):597–602.

32. Odhiambo JA, Williams HC, Clayton TO, Robertson CF, Asher MI. Global variations in prevalence of eczema symptoms in children from ISAAC Phase Three. J Allergy Clin Immunol. 2009;124(6):1251–8.e23.

33. Paternoster L, Standl M, Waage J, Baurecht H, Hotze M, Strachan DP, et al. Multi-ancestry genome-wide association study of 21,000 cases and 95,000 controls identifies new risk loci for atopic dermatitis. Nat Genet. 2015;47(12):1449.

34. Li K, Oh WJ, Park KY, Kim KH, Seo SJ. FLG mutations in the East Asian atopic dermatitis patients: genetic and clinical implication. Exp Dermatol. 2016;25(10):816–8.

35. Margolis DJ, Apter AJ, Gupta J, Hoffstad O, Papadopoulos M, Campbell LE, et al. The persistence of atopic dermatitis and filaggrin (FLG) mutations in a US longitudinal cohort. J Allergy Clin Immunol. 2012;130(4):912–7.

36. Margolis DJ, Gupta J, Apter AJ, Ganguly T, Hoffstad O, Papadopoulos M, et al. Filaggrin-2 variation is associated with more persistent atopic dermatitis in African Americans. J Allergy Clin Immunol. 2014;133(3):784–9.

37. Kaufman BP, Guttman-Yassky E, Alexis AF. Atopic dermatitis in diverse racial and ethnic groups—variations in epidemiology, genetics, clinical presentation and treatment. Exp Dermatol. 2018;27(4):340–57.

38. Bolognia J, Jorizzo JL, Schaffer JV. Dermatology. 3rd ed. Philadelphia: Elsevier Saunders; 2012.

39. Xu F, Yan S, Zheng Q, Li F, Chai W, Wu M, et al. Residential risk factors for atopic dermatitis in 3- to 6-year old children: a cross-sectional study in Shanghai, China. Int J Environ Res Public Health. 2016;13(6):537.

40. Horimukai K, Morita K, Narita M, Kondo M, Kitazawa H, Nozaki M, et al. Application of moisturizer to neonates prevents development of atopic dermatitis. J Allergy Clin Immunol. 2014;134(4):824–30.e6.

41. Sasaki T, Furusyo N, Shiohama A, Takeuchi S, Nakahara T, Uchi H, et al. Filaggrin loss-of-function mutations are not a predisposing factor for atopic dermatitis in an Ishigaki Island under subtropical climate. J Dermatol Sci. 2014;76(1):10–5.

42. Noda S, Suárez-Fariñas M, Ungar B, Kim SJ, de Guzman Strong C, Xu H, et al. The Asian atopic dermatitis phenotype combines features of atopic dermatitis and psoriasis with increased TH17 polarization. J Allergy Clin Immunol. 2015;136(5):1254–64.

43. Spergel JM, Paller AS. Atopic dermatitis and the atopic march. J Allergy Clin Immunol. 2003;112(6 Suppl):S118–27.

44. Syed ZU, Hamzavi IH. Photomedicine and phototherapy considerations for patients with skin of color. Photodermatol Photoimmunol Photomed. 2011;27(1):10–6.

45. Love PB. Inflammatory disorders. In: Vashi NA, Maibach HI, editors. Dermatoanthropology of ethnic skin and hair. Cham: Springer International Publishing; 2017. p. 129–41.

46. Hon KL, Tsang YC, Lee VW, Pong NH, Ha G, Lee ST, et al. Efficacy of sodium hypochlorite (bleach) baths to reduce Staphylococcus aureus colonization in childhood onset moderate-to-severe eczema: a randomized, placebo-controlled cross-over trial. J Dermatolog Treat. 2016;27(2):156–62.

47. Huang JT, Abrams M, Tlougan B, Rademaker A, Paller AS. Treatment of Staphylococcus aureus colonization in atopic dermatitis decreases disease severity. Pediatrics. 2009;123(5):e808–14.

48. Clark GW, Pope SM, Jaboori KA. Diagnosis and treatment of seborrheic dermatitis. Am Fam Physician. 2015;91(3):185–90.

49. Ostlere LS, Taylor CR, Harris DW, Rustin MH, Wright S, Johnson M. Skin surface lipids in HIV-positive patients with and without seborrheic dermatitis. Int J Dermatol. 1996;35(4):276–9.

50. Taylor SC. Treatments for skin of color. Edinburgh: Saunders/Elsevier; 2011. Available from: http://www.clinicalkey.com/dura/browse/bookChapter/3-s2.0-C20090395422; http://www.clinicalkey.com.au/dura/browse/bookChapter/3-s2.0-C20090395422; http://site.ebrary.com/id/10493316; http://search.ebscohost.com/login.aspx?direct=true&scope=site&db=nlebk&db=nlabk&AN=444950; http://www.myilibrary.com?id=754895; https://www.clinicalkey.com.au/dura/browse/bookChapter/3-s2.0-C20090395422; http://ezsecureaccess.balamand.edu.lb/login?url=https://www.clinicalkey.com/dura/browse/bookChapter/3-s2.0-C20090395422; https://nls.ldls.org.uk/welcome.html?ark:/81055/vdc_1000 52715963.0x000001.

51. Friedmann DP, Mishra V, Batty T. Progressive facial papules in an African-American patient: an atypical presentation of seborrheic dermatitis. J Clin Aesthet Dermatol. 2018;11(7):44–5.

52. Wannanukul S, Chiabunkana J. Comparative study of 2% ketoconazole cream and 1% hydrocortisone cream in the treatment of infantile seborrheic dermatitis. J Med Assoc Thail = Chotmaihet thangphaet. 2004;87(Suppl 2):S68–71.

53. Rodney IJ, Onwudiwe OC, Callender VD, Halder RM. Hair and scalp disorders in ethnic populations. J Drugs Dermatol: JDD. 2013;12(4):420–7.

54. Milani M, Antonio Di Molfetta S, Gramazio R, Fiorella C, Frisario C, Fuzio E, et al. Efficacy of betamethasone valerate 0.1% thermophobic foam in seborrhoeic dermatitis of the scalp: an open-label, multicentre, prospective trial on 180 patients. Curr Med Res Opin. 2003;19(4):342–5.

55. High WA, Pandya AG. Pilot trial of 1% pimecrolimus cream in the treatment of seborrheic dermatitis in African American adults with associated hypopigmentation. J Am Acad Dermatol. 2006;54(6):1083–8.

56. Stratigos JD, Antoniou C, Katsambas A, Bohler K, Fritsch P, Schmolz A, et al. Ketoconazole 2% cream versus hydrocortisone 1% cream in the treatment of seborrheic dermatitis. A double-blind comparative study. J Am Acad Dermatol. 1988;19(5 Pt 1):850–3.

57. Drenkard C, Parker S, Aspey LD, Gordon C, Helmick CG, Bao G, et al. Racial disparities in the incidence of primary chronic cutaneous lupus erythematosus in the Southeastern United States: the Georgia Lupus Registry. Arthritis Care Res. 2019;71(1):95–103.

58. Hopkinson ND, Doherty M, Powell RJ. Clinical features and race-specific incidence/prevalence rates of systemic lupus erythematosus in a geographically complete cohort of patients. Ann Rheum Dis. 1994;53(10):675–80.

59. Jarrett P, Thornley S, Scragg R. Ethnic differences in the epidemiology of cutaneous lupus erythematosus in New Zealand. Lupus. 2016;25(13):1497–502.

60. Rees F, Doherty M, Grainge M, Davenport G, Lanyon P, Zhang W. The incidence and prevalence of systemic lupus erythematosus in the UK, 1999–2012. Ann Rheum Dis. 2016;75(1):136–41.

61. Moser KL, Kelly JA, Lessard CJ, Harley JB. Recent insights into the genetic basis of systemic lupus erythematosus. Genes Immun. 2009;10(5):373–9.

62. Singh B, Walter S, Callaghan DJ, Paek J, Lam C. Autoimmune and connective tissue disease in skin of color. In: Vashi NA, Maibach HI, editors. Dermatoanthropology of ethnic skin and hair. Cham: Springer International Publishing; 2017. p. 161–95.

63. Schultz HY, Dutz JP, Furukawa F, Goodfield MJ, Kuhn A, Lee LA, et al. From pathogenesis, epidemiology, and genetics to definitions, diagnosis, and treatments of cutaneous lupus erythematosus and dermatomyositis: a report from the 3rd International Conference on Cutaneous Lupus Erythematosus (ICCLE) 2013. J Invest Dermatol. 2015;135(1):7–12.

64. Molomo EM, Bouckaert M, Khammissa RA, Motswaledi HM, Lemmer J, Feller L. Discoid lupus erythematosus-related squamous cell carcinoma of the lip in an HIV-seropositive black male. J Cancer Res Ther. 2015;11(4):1036.

65. Fernandes MS, Girisha BS, Viswanathan N, Sripathi H, Noronha TM. Discoid lupus erythematosus with squamous cell carcinoma: a case report and review of the literature in Indian patients. Lupus. 2015;24(14):1562–6.

66. Pons-Estel GJ, Aspey LD, Bao G, Pons-Estel BA, Wojdyla D, Saurit V, et al. Early discoid lupus erythematosus protects against renal disease in patients with systemic lupus erythematosus: longitudinal data from a large Latin American cohort. Lupus. 2017;26(1):73–83.

67. Lowe GC, Henderson CL, Grau RH, Hansen CB, Sontheimer RD. A systematic review of drug-induced subacute cutaneous lupus erythematosus. Br J Dermatol. 2011;164(3):465–72.

68. Magro CM, Crowson AN. The cutaneous pathology associated with seropositivity for antibodies to SSA (Ro): a clinicopathologic study of 23 adult patients

without subacute cutaneous lupus erythematosus. Am J Dermatopathol. 1999;21(2):129–37.

69. Lee A, Batra P, Furer V, Cheung W, Wang N, Franks A Jr. Rowell syndrome (systemic lupus erythematosus + erythema multiforme). Dermatol Online J. 2009;15(8):1.

70. Petit A, Dadzie OE. Multisystemic diseases and ethnicity: a focus on lupus erythematosus, systemic sclerosis, sarcoidosis and Behcet disease. Br J Dermatol. 2013;169(Suppl 3):1–10.

71. Hochberg MC. Updating the American College of Rheumatology revised criteria for the classification of systemic lupus erythematosus. Arthritis Rheum. 1997;40(9):1725.

72. Alarcon GS, Friedman AW, Straaton KV, Moulds JM, Lisse J, Bastian HM, et al. Systemic lupus erythematosus in three ethnic groups: III. A comparison of characteristics early in the natural history of the LUMINA cohort. LUpus in MInority populations: NAture vs. Nurture. Lupus. 1999;8(3):197–209.

73. Uribe AG, McGwin G Jr, Reveille JD, Alarcon GS. What have we learned from a 10-year experience with the LUMINA (Lupus in Minorities; Nature vs. nurture) cohort? Where are we heading? Autoimmun Rev. 2004;3(4):321–9.

74. Lim SS, Drenkard C. Epidemiology of lupus: an update. Curr Opin Rheumatol. 2015;27(5):427–32.

75. Patel M, Clarke AM, Bruce IN, Symmons DP. The prevalence and incidence of biopsy-proven lupus nephritis in the UK: evidence of an ethnic gradient. Arthritis Rheum. 2006;54(9):2963–9.

76. Agbai ON, Buster K, Sanchez M, Hernandez C, Kundu RV, Chiu M, et al. Skin cancer and photoprotection in people of color: a review and recommendations for physicians and the public. J Am Acad Dermatol. 2014;70(4):748–62.

77. Avgerinou G, Papafragkaki DK, Nasiopoulou A, Arapaki A, Katsambas A, Stavropoulos PG. Effectiveness of topical calcineurin inhibitors as monotherapy or in combination with hydroxychloroquine in cutaneous lupus erythematosus. J Eur Acad Dermatol Venereol: JEADV. 2012;26(6):762–7.

78. Abdulaziz N, Shah AR, McCune WJ. Hydroxychloroquine: balancing the need to maintain therapeutic levels with ocular safety: an update. Curr Opin Rheumatol. 2018;30(3):249–55.

79. Pons-Estel GJ, Catoggio LJ, Cardiel MH, Bonfa E, Caeiro F, Sato E, et al. Lupus in Latin-American patients: lessons from the GLADEL cohort. Lupus. 2015;24(6):536–45.

80. Tayer-Shifman OE, Rosen CF, Wakani L, Touma Z. Novel biological therapeutic approaches to cutaneous lupus erythematosus. Expert Opin Biol Ther. 2018;18(10):1041–7.

81. BENLYSTA [package insert]. Research Triangle Park: GlaxoSmithKline; 2018.

82. Kuhn A, Landmann A, Wenzel J. Advances in the treatment of cutaneous lupus erythematosus. Lupus. 2016;25(8):830–7.

83. Selva-O'Callaghan A, Pinal-Fernandez I, Trallero-Araguas E, Milisenda JC, Grau-Junyent JM, Mammen AL. Classification and management of adult inflammatory myopathies. Lancet Neurol. 2018;17(9):816–28.

84. Wolstencroft PW, Fiorentino DF. Dermatomyositis clinical and pathological phenotypes associated with myositis-specific autoantibodies. Curr Rheumatol Rep. 2018;20(5):28.

85. Werth VP, Callen JP, Ang G, Sullivan KE. Associations of tumor necrosis factor alpha and HLA polymorphisms with adult dermatomyositis: implications for a unique pathogenesis. J Invest Dermatol. 2002;119(3):617–20.

86. Hill CL, Zhang Y, Sigurgeirsson B, Pukkala E, Mellemkjaer L, Airio A, et al. Frequency of specific cancer types in dermatomyositis and polymyositis: a population-based study. Lancet. 2001;357(9250):96–100.

87. Peng JC, Sheen TS, Hsu MM. Nasopharyngeal carcinoma with dermatomyositis. Analysis of 12 cases. Arch Otolaryngol Head Neck Surg. 1995;121(11):1298–301.

88. Tersiguel AC, Longueville C, Beltan E, Vincent T, Tressieres B, Cordel N. Prevalence of cancer in the Afro-Caribbean population presenting dermatomyositis and anti-synthetase syndrome: a preliminary study conducted at Pointe-a-Pitre University Hospital, 2000–2012. Ann Dermatol Venereol. 2014;141(10):575–80.

89. Femia AN, Vleugels RA, Callen JP. Cutaneous dermatomyositis: an updated review of treatment options and internal associations. Am J Clin Dermatol. 2013;14(4):291–313.

90. Jorizzo JL. Dermatomyositis: practical aspects. Arch Dermatol. 2002;138(1):114–6.

91. Srivastava P, Dwivedi S, Misra R. Myositis-specific and myositis-associated autoantibodies in Indian patients with inflammatory myositis. Rheumatol Int. 2016;36(7):935–43.

92. Kang EH, Nakashima R, Mimori T, Kim J, Lee YJ, Lee EB, et al. Myositis autoantibodies in Korean patients with inflammatory myositis: anti-140-kDa polypeptide antibody is primarily associated with rapidly progressive interstitial lung disease independent of clinically amyopathic dermatomyositis. BMC Musculoskelet Disord. 2010;11:223.

93. Pinal-Fernandez I, Casal-Dominguez M, Huapaya JA, Albayda J, Paik JJ, Johnson C, et al. A longitudinal cohort study of the anti-synthetase syndrome: increased severity of interstitial lung disease in black patients and patients with anti-PL7 and anti-PL12 autoantibodies. Rheumatology (Oxford, England). 2017;56(6):999–1007.

94. Callen JP, Wortmann RL. Dermatomyositis. Clin Dermatol. 2006;24(5):363–73.

95. Vencovsky J, Jarosova K, Machacek S, Studynkova J, Kafkova J, Bartunkova J, et al. Cyclosporine A versus methotrexate in the treatment of poly-

myositis and dermatomyositis. Scand J Rheumatol. 2000;29(2):95–102.

96. Morganroth PA, Kreider ME, Werth VP. Mycophenolate mofetil for interstitial lung disease in dermatomyositis. Arthritis Care Res. 2010;62(10):1496–501.

97. Barnes H, Holland AE, Westall GP, Goh NS, Glaspole IN. Cyclophosphamide for connective tissue disease-associated interstitial lung disease. Cochrane Database Syst Rev. 2018;1:Cd010908.

98. Hollar CB, Jorizzo JL. Topical tacrolimus 0.1% ointment for refractory skin disease in dermatomyositis: a pilot study. J Dermatolog Treat. 2004;15(1):35–9.

99. Ang G, Werth VP. Combination antimalarials in the treatment of cutaneous dermatomyositis: a retrospective study. Arch Dermatol. 2005;141(7): 855–9.

100. Kurtzman DB, Wright NA, Lin J, et al. Tofacitinib citrate for refractory cutaneous dermatomyositis: an alternative treatment. JAMA Dermatol. 2016;152(8):944–5.

101. Gutierrez A Jr, Wetter DA. Calcinosis cutis in autoimmune connective tissue diseases. Dermatol Ther. 2012;25(2):195–206.

102. Welborn MC, Gottschalk H, Bindra R. Juvenile dermatomyositis: a case of calcinosis cutis of the elbow and review of the literature. J Pediatr Orthop. 2015;35(5):e43–6.

103. Leitenberger JJ, Cayce RL, Haley RW, Adams-Huet B, Bergstresser PR, Jacobe HT. Distinct autoimmune syndromes in morphea: a review of 245 adult and pediatric cases. Arch Dermatol. 2009;145(5):545–50.

104. Zwischenberger BA, Jacobe HT. A systematic review of morphea treatments and therapeutic algorithm. J Am Acad Dermatol. 2011;65(5):925–41.

105. Jacobe HT, Cayce R, Nguyen J. UVA1 phototherapy is effective in darker skin: a review of 101 patients of Fitzpatrick skin types I–V. Br J Dermatol. 2008;159(3):691–6.

106. Kroft EBM, Groeneveld TJ, Seyger MMB, Jong EMGJ. Efficacy of topical tacrolimus 0.1% in active plaque morphea. Am J Clin Dermatol. 2009;10(3):181–7.

107. Campione E, Paternò EJ, Diluvio L, Orlandi A, Bianchi L, Chimenti S. Localized morphea treated with imiquimod 5% and dermoscopic assessment of effectiveness. J Dermatol Treat. 2009;20(1):10–3.

108. Silver RM, Bogatkevich G, Tourkina E, Nietert PJ, Hoffman S. Racial differences between blacks and whites with systemic sclerosis. Curr Opin Rheumatol. 2012;24(6):642–8.

109. Gelber AC, Manno RL, Shah AA, Woods A, Le EN, Boin F, et al. Race and association with disease manifestations and mortality in scleroderma: a 20-year experience at the Johns Hopkins Scleroderma Center and review of the literature. Medicine. 2013;92(4):191–205.

110. Satoh M, Krzyszczak ME, Li Y, Ceribelli A, Ross SJ, Chan EK, et al. Frequent coexistence of anti-topoisomerase I and anti-U1RNP autoantibodies in African American patients associated with mild skin involvement: a retrospective clinical study. Arthritis Res Ther. 2011;13(3):R73.

111. Blanco I, Mathai S, Shafiq M, Boyce D, Kolb TM, Chami H, et al. Severity of systemic sclerosis-associated pulmonary arterial hypertension in African Americans. Medicine. 2014;93(5):177–85.

112. Steen V, Domsic RT, Lucas M, Fertig N, Medsger TA Jr. A clinical and serologic comparison of African American and Caucasian patients with systemic sclerosis. Arthritis Rheum. 2012;64(9):2986–94.

113. Reveille JD, Fischbach M, McNearney T, Friedman AW, Aguilar MB, Lisse J, et al. Systemic sclerosis in 3 US ethnic groups: a comparison of clinical, sociodemographic, serologic, and immunogenetic determinants. Semin Arthritis Rheum. 2001;30(5):332–46.

114. Wang J, Assassi S, Guo G, Tu W, Wu W, Yang L, et al. Clinical and serological features of systemic sclerosis in a Chinese cohort. Clin Rheumatol. 2013;32(5):617–21.

115. Pope JE. New classification criteria for systemic sclerosis (scleroderma). Rheum Dis Clin N Am. 2015;41(3):383–98.

116. Fett N. Scleroderma: nomenclature, etiology, pathogenesis, prognosis, and treatments: facts and controversies. Clin Dermatol. 2013;31(4):432–7.

117. Sinnathurai P, Schrieber L. Treatment of Raynaud phenomenon in systemic sclerosis. Intern Med J. 2013;43(5):476–83.

118. Chung L, Shapiro L, Fiorentino D, Baron M, Shanahan J, Sule S, et al. MQX-503, a novel formulation of nitroglycerin, improves the severity of Raynaud's phenomenon: a randomized, controlled trial. Arthritis Rheum. 2009;60(3):870–7.

119. Derk CT, Grace E, Shenin M, Naik M, Schulz S, Xiong W. A prospective open-label study of mycophenolate mofetil for the treatment of diffuse systemic sclerosis. Rheumatology. 2009;48(12):1595–9.

Inflammatory Disorders: Psoriasis, Lichen Planus, Pityriasis Rosea, and Sarcoidosis

Callie R. Mitchell and Porcia B. Love

Psoriasis

Psoriasis vulgaris is a chronic, multifactorial, hyperproliferative skin disease. Arthritis may be associated with skin disease in approximately 30% of patients. Psoriasis appears to be most prevalent in northern European populations and is thought to be observed less frequently in patients with skin of color [1]. A population-based study in the United States in 2005 showed that although psoriasis is less common in African Americans than in Caucasians, it is not rare and carries a substantial burden in both groups. In this study, the prevalence of psoriasis was 2.5% in Caucasians and 1.3% in African Americans. African Americans had an approximately 52% reduction in the prevalence of psoriasis compared with Caucasians [2]. In another cross-sectional study using National Health and Nutrition Examination Survey data from 2009 to 2010, the psoriasis prevalence was highest in Caucasians at 3.6%, followed by African Americans (1.9%),

Hispanics (1.6%), and others (1.4%) [3]. The psoriasis prevalence is estimated to be approximately 0.3% in Asians (18).

Pathophysiology

The pathophysiology of psoriasis involves genetic and immune-mediated factors leading to immune dysregulation and hyperproliferation of epidermal keratinocytes with increased epidermal cell turnover. Triggers include infectious episodes (i.e., staphylococcus, streptococcus, HIV), traumatic insult (i.e., surgery), alcohol, or medications (beta-blockers, steroid withdrawal, lithium, antimalarials) [4]. Once triggered, there appears to be substantial leukocyte recruitment to the dermis and epidermis resulting in the characteristic psoriatic plaques [5]. The major inflammatory cells are activated T cells that induce changes in keratinocytes, vascular endothelial cells, and other inflammatory cells. The antigen HLA-Cw6 has the strongest association with psoriasis and correlates with early age at onset and a positive family history [6]. HLA-Cw6 is found in approximately 50–80% of Caucasian psoriatic patients [7]. However, in one study, only 17–18% of Chinese [8] and Taiwanese [9] psoriatic patients, respectively, were found to have the HLA Cw6 allele. Outcome-based studies often suggest that patients with more severe psoriasis have an increased risk of major cardiovascular

C. R. Mitchell
River Region Dermatology and Laser,
Montgomery, AL, USA

P. B. Love (✉)
River Region Dermatology and Laser,
Montgomery, AL, USA

University of Alabama School of Medicine, River
Region Dermatology and Laser,
Montgomery, AL, USA
e-mail: plove@rrdermatologylaser.com

© Springer Nature Switzerland AG 2021
B. S. Li, H. I. Maibach (eds.), *Ethnic Skin and Hair and Other Cultural Considerations*, Updates in
Clinical Dermatology, https://doi.org/10.1007/978-3-030-64830-5_8

events independent of traditional risk factors [10]. The onset or worsening of psoriasis with weight gain and/or improvement with weight loss has also been observed [11].

Clinical Manifestations

Psoriasis presents similarly across skin types. Psoriasis is characterized by erythematous, well-demarcated plaques with silvery scale (Fig. 8.1a, b). Lesions are most commonly found on the elbows, knees, scalp, umbilicus, and intergluteal folds. The palms and soles may contain sterile

pustules and thick scale. External trauma (rubbing, scratching, surgery) may lead to the Koebner phenomenon [5]. In darker skin, the distribution is similar; however, plaques may be violaceous with gray scale, and erythema is sometimes difficult to identify (Fig. 8.1c). Psoriasis has two peak age ranges; early onset occurs in the second decade, and late onset peaks between the ages of 50 and 60 [12].

Guttate psoriasis is characterized by the rapid onset of red, salmon-colored papules and plaques that may be covered with fine silvery scale. In darker skin, violaceous and gray colors predominate. Guttate psoriasis most commonly occurs in

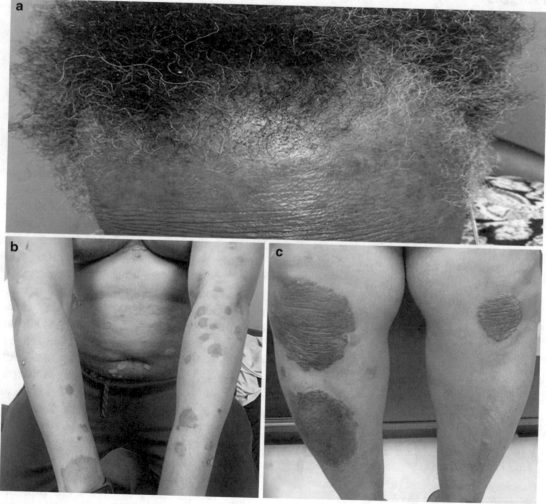

Fig. 8.1 Psoriasis. Erythematous, well-demarcated plaques with silvery scale are noted on the scalp (**a**) and arms (**b**). In darker skin, the distribution is similar; how-ever, plaques are often brown or violaceous, and erythema is sometimes difficult to appreciate (**c**)

young patients and is often associated with viral or streptococcal pharyngitis. Pustular psoriasis is characterized by groups of sterile pustules at the periphery of stable plaques. Pustular psoriasis may occur as a primary manifestation of palmoplantar psoriasis and can be confused with dyshidrotic eczema. Generalized psoriasis, a potentially fatal disorder, is characterized by large sheets of pustules on a fiery red base. It is seen in patients with extensive psoriasis who have been treated with systemic or intensive and prolonged topical corticosteroids. Patients often have systemic symptoms (fever, chills, or peripheral leukocytosis). Erythrodermic psoriasis is characterized by generalized redness, scaling, and warmth of the skin. Body temperature is often erratic, and patients are severely ill, secondary to sudden withdrawal of long-term steroids [12].

Psoriasiform nail findings include nail pitting (most common finding), leukonychia, longitudinal grooves and ridges, the oil drop sign, and subungual hyperkeratosis. Psoriatic arthritis, affecting approximately 10–30% of those with skin disease, produces stiffness, pain, and progressive joint damage, usually in the hands and feet [12].

Treatment

Treatment for psoriasis is similar across ethnicities. Mild to moderate psoriasis is treated with topical corticosteroids, vitamin D derivatives, retinoids, anthralin, and tar-based formulations. For psoriasis that is nonresponsive to topical treatments and for moderate to severe psoriasis, systemic treatment is often needed. Options include systemic retinoids, methotrexate, cyclosporine, and apremilast [13]. Many of the systemic therapies for psoriasis manipulate the function of the immune system and expose the patient to the risk of severe infections while blunting the body's response. In these patients, findings suggestive of minor infections must be taken seriously, and the risk versus the benefit of continuing the drug in the face of the infection must be weighed [13].

Biologic immune-modifying agents have revolutionized psoriasis therapy. Several are now available and block TNF-alpha, IL 12/23, and IL 17, all inflammatory cytokines involved in psoriasis pathogenesis. The risks of these biologic agents include infections, tuberculosis reactivation, and hematologic malignancies [14]. Therefore, the benefit of using these medications must be weighed against the side effects while selecting appropriate patients for treatment. Phototherapy may also be used to treat moderate to severe plaque psoriasis. There is a risk of increased pigmentation (tanning) and post-inflammatory hyperpigmentation in skin of color. Various ultraviolet light treatments are used, with UVB being the most common, although psoralen + UVB (PUVA) is still used [15]. The 308-nm excimer laser is also an effective and safe modality for localized plaques of psoriasis, with good results achieved in a relatively short time [16].

Lichen Planus

Lichen planus is an autoimmune inflammatory mucocutaneous condition that can affect the scalp, oral mucosa, skin, and nails. Lichen planus can be found in approximately 1% of adults [1]. There is no overt racial predisposition, and women develop the condition more than men. Two-thirds develop the disease between 30 and 60 years old; however, lichen planus can occur at any age [17, 18]. Oral lichen planus is found in 50–70% of cutaneous lichen planus, and cutaneous lichen planus is found in 10–20% of oral lichen planus. One-fourth have solely mucosal involvement [18].

Pathogenesis

Lichen planus is a T cell-mediated autoimmune process against basal keratinocytes. Caspase 3 is often elevated in cutaneous and oral lesions, and it is suspected that apoptosis of basal keratinocytes as mediated by cytotoxic T cells is involved [19]. Five percent of hepatitis C patients have lichen planus. Medications that may cause lichen planus include beta-blockers, ACE inhibitors,

NSAIDs, antimalarials, quinidine, hydrochloro-thiazide, gold, and penicillamine. Autoimmune liver disease, myasthenia gravis, and ulcerative colitis may also be associated with lichen planus [18]. There is a higher prevalence of serum auto-antibodies in Chinese patients with oral lichen planus [20] and a strong correlation between the presence of hepatitis C and lichen planus in the Japanese. In one study, long-standing hepatitis C virus infection, hypoalbuminemia, and smoking were significant risk factors for the presence of oral lichen planus in patients [21]. In oral lichen planus, prolonged exposure to amalgam fillings has also been implicated. Many have regression of disease with removal of the metal [22].

Clinical Features

Cutaneous lichen planus is characterized by small, polygonal, violaceous, flat-topped papules that coalesce into plaques (Fig. 8.2). The surface is often shiny with a network of fine lines, also known as Wickham's striae. The Koebner phenomenon is commonly seen. Lesions often involve the flexor surfaces of the wrists and forearms, the dorsal surfaces of the hands, and the anterior aspect of the lower legs. In skin of color, the classic purple color may be black, gray, brown, or violaceous. If exacerbation occurs, it usually takes 2–16 weeks for maximal spread

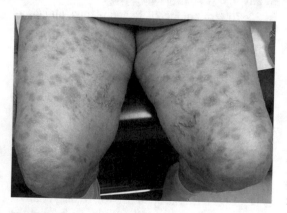

Fig. 8.2 Lichen planus. Polygonal, violaceous, flat-topped papules that coalesce into plaques with Wickham's striae are noted on the thighs

to occur. Lesions are intensely pruritic, often out of proportion to the amount of disease [18]. There are numerous variants of lichen planus (Table 8.1).

Lichen planus actinicus, also known as actinic lichen planus, is a photodistributed variant of lichen planus more common in darker-skinned individuals from subtropical climates and individuals of Middle Eastern, African, and Asian descent [18, 23]. Sun exposure is a triggering factor. The lateral aspect of the forehead is the most common involved area. It has an earlier age of onset and a longer course. There is a female predominance. Pruritus, scaling, nail involvement, and the Koebner phenomenon are often present [18, 24]. Lichen planus pigmentosus is another variant that is more common in Latin Americans and darker skin. Asymptomatic dark brown macules or patches in sun-exposed areas and flexural folds are observed (Fig. 8.3).

Treatment

Lichen planus is often self-limiting with lesions resolving after 1 year in most patients; however, treatment is often indicated to prevent post-inflammatory hyperpigmentation. Topical corticosteroids are first-line treatment. For lesions refractory to topical treatment or lesions that are more hyperkeratotic, intralesional or systemic corticosteroids may be indicated. Additional therapy for lesions that are refractory to topical treatment and are steroid sparing include acitretin, dapsone, methotrexate, hydroxychloroquine, cyclosporine, thalidomide, low molecular weight heparin, mycophenolate mofetil, and metronidazole. Narrowband UVB phototherapy may also be used [25]. It is important to check for exacerbating factors (e.g., medications and infections). Treatment of oral lichen planus is often more difficult and includes topical, intralesional, or systemic steroids, topical immunomodulators, retinoids, cyclosporine, griseofulvin, antimalarials, and methotrexate [22]. Removal of a contact allergen is also often indicated.

Table 8.1 Variants of lichen planus

Variants	Characteristics	Notes
Acute lichen planus	Eruptive lesions that occur most often on the trunk	
Annular lichen planus	Lesions with central inactivity or involution	Occurs in about 10% of patients
Atrophic lichen planus	Resolving lesions that are classically found on the lower leg	
Bullous lichen planus	Lesions that exhibit blisters within long-standing plaques	
Hypertrophic lichen planus	Lesions that present with thick hyperkeratotic plaques	Risk of squamous cell carcinoma, more common in Blacks
Lichen nitidus	Presents as tiny skin-colored or hypopigmented papules involving the trunk or extremities	Most common in children
Lichen planopilaris	Follicular variant that can result in scarring alopecia of the scalp	
Lichen planus actinicus	Photodistributed variant	More common in darker-skinned individuals from subtropical climates and individuals of Middle Eastern, African, and Asian descent
Lichen planus pemphigoides	Manifests as bullae in previously uninvolved skin of patients with LP	Circulating IgG autoantibodies against BPAG2 (type XVII collagen)
Lichen planus pigmentosus	Asymptomatic dark brown macules or patches in sun-exposed areas and flexural folds are found	More common in Latin Americans and darker skin
Linear lichen planus	Linear lesions that occur spontaneously along the lines of Blaschko	
Lichen planus-lupus erythematosus overlap syndrome	Patients with characteristics of both lichen planus and lupus erythematosus	
Nail lichen planus	Nail thinning, ridging, fissuring, pterygium formation	
Oral lichen planus	White, reticular lacy patches on the buccal mucosa	More common in women; occurs in ~50–75% of patients; risk of squamous cell carcinoma
Ulcerative lichen planus	Consists of bullae and permanent loss of toenails	

Adapted from [18]

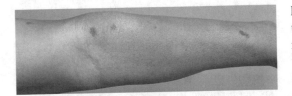

Fig. 8.3 Lichen planus pigmentosus. Dark brown macules and patches found on the arms

Pityriasis Rosea

Pityriasis rosea is a common, self-limiting, papulosquamous eruption that most often occurs in healthy children and young adults. The eruption usually lasts 6–8 weeks. Although there is no racial predilection for pityriasis rosea, patients with skin of color seem to have a more widespread distribution [26]. It has been noted to present atypically in Indian adolescent patients [27].

Pathophysiology

The exact cause of pityriasis rosea remains unknown. The eruption seems to be more prevalent during the spring and fall. A viral etiology has been suspected to induce pityriasis rosea due to its occasional prodromal symptoms, a low rate of recurrence, and correlation with the changing of seasons. Oxidative stress may also play a role [28]. Human herpes viruses HHV 6 and HHV 7 have also been implicated [29]. A higher incidence of pityriasis rosea is noted among patients with decreased immunity (i.e., pregnant women and bone marrow transplant recipients). Pityriasis rosea during pregnancy may be associated with premature delivery and miscarriage, especially when it develops within the first 15 weeks of gestation [30].

Clinical Presentation

Pityriasis rosea typically presents with a solitary "herald patch" with a well-circumscribed border and collarette of scale on the back (Fig. 8.4) [28]. The herald patch may be absent in 10–15% of cases, especially in drug-induced pityriasis rosea. Within 2 weeks, a generalized truncal exanthem characterized by papules and patches occurs along the Langer lines in a Christmas tree distribution. The eruption most commonly occurs on the chest, abdomen, and back; the palms and soles are spared. Pruritus may occur. Patients with lighter skin tones portray pale pink lesions; the lesions are less noticeable on patients with

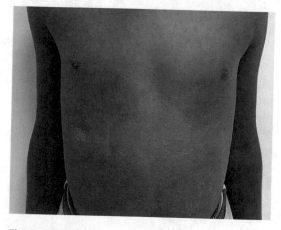

Fig. 8.4 Pityriasis rosea. Generalized papulosquamous eruption on trunk. Note "herald patch" on the right upper abdomen

darker skin. Approximately 5–10% of patients may have a prodrome of fever, chills, fatigue, headache, and lymphadenopathy. The eruption can last as long as 6–8 weeks [31].

Several atypical presentations of pityriasis rosea may occur. Papular pityriasis rosea tends to be more common in African Americans. African American patients may experience a more widespread distribution of lesions than Caucasian patients, and there is a higher risk of lymphadenopathy and scalp and face involvement [26, 32]. Patients with skin of color may have post-inflammatory hyperpigmentation that lasts for months. Pityriasis rosea usually will remain on the trunk; however, approximately 10–15% of patients may have oral lesions, such as ulcers, punctate hemorrhages, and petechiae. The majority of patients with oral lesions are patients with skin of color [33]. Pityriasis rosea is often known as the "great mimicker"; tinea corporis, tinea versicolor, atopic dermatitis, psoriasis, and syphilis are often included in the differential diagnosis.

Treatment

Pityriasis rosea is a self-limiting condition; however, topical steroids may help with pruritus and speed up resolution. Informational handouts and reassurance should be provided to the patient and/or their parents [34]. Patients with pityriasis rosea may require antihistamines to help with pruritus. Narrowband UVB phototherapy may also help severe cases of pruritus [35]. Hot water, fragrances, and harsh soaps can cause the eruption to worsen. Systemic steroids are generally not indicated, but they may help with severe disease with pruritus or vesicles. Although acyclovir has been shown to be ineffective against HHV6 and HHV7, some evidence suggests that acyclovir may be useful in the treatment of pityriasis rosea [36]. Patients with skin of color tend to have a high risk of post-inflammatory pigmentation, and topical treatments for dyschromia should be used after the eruption heals.

Sarcoidosis

Sarcoidosis is a multisystem, granulomatous, and inflammatory disease that, depending on the organ involved, has different clinical presentations, with varying degrees severity. The most common organs involved include the lungs, lymph nodes, and skin, with the skin being involved in 20–35% of cases [37]. The most common symptoms of systemic sarcoidosis are low-grade fever, weight loss, cough, dyspnea, chronic fatigue, arthralgia, and lymphadenopathy. Several studies have documented the higher incidence of sarcoidosis in African Americans compared to Caucasians [38]. In a population-based study conducted in the United States, Rybicki et al. found the age-adjusted incidence in African Americans to be 35.5/100,000 compared to 10.9/100,000 in Caucasians [39]. Sarcoidosis has also been found to occur at an earlier age and have a more severe course in African Americans compared to Caucasians [37]. In addition, Black patients are more likely to have cutaneous involvement than Caucasians [40]. The incidence of sarcoidosis may also be higher in other skin of color populations [41]. In a retrospective survey of Caucasian, Black West Indian/African, and Indo-Pakistan Asian patients treated at South London hospitals, the incidence of sarcoidosis was similar in Blacks and Asians, and these two groups had more widespread extrathoracic disease compared to Caucasians [42].

Pathophysiology

No causative agent has been identified for sarcoidosis; however, T cells play a central role in the disease [43], and both tumor necrosis factor (TNF) and receptors [44] are increased in patients with the disease. There are reports that genetically predisposed individuals who are exposed to different mycobacterial, viral, and other environmental antigens are susceptible to developing the disease, and this may initiate the immunologic cascade that produces the noncaseating granulomas most commonly found in the lung, skin, heart, and liver [45]. Recent genetic epidemiology studies from the Black Women's Health Study support the role of the BTNL2 gene and the 5q31 locus in the etiology of sarcoidosis, and also demonstrate that African ancestry is associated with disease risk [46].

Clinical Presentation

Cutaneous sarcoidosis may present as a part of systemic disease but may also only involve the skin. Skin involvement manifests with a wide variety of morphologies. Table 8.2 highlights the different morphologic types of cutaneous sarcoidosis.

Some of the more common lesions presenting in patients with skin of color include the maculopapular (Fig. 8.5), lupus pernio (Fig. 8.6), plaque, nodular ulcerative, and hypopigmented (Fig. 8.7) forms of sarcoidosis. Maculopapular sarcoidosis is the most common lesion seen in cutaneous sarcoidosis, especially in Black women [41]. Lupus pernio is usually more common in Black women with long-standing systemic disease [41]. Sarcoidosis is often called the "great imitator" because it can present with almost any morphology. Scarring alopecia and nail dystrophy may also occur.

The lungs are affected in nearly all cases (90%) of sarcoidosis and are characterized by granulomatous involvement of the interstitium, alveoli, blood vessels, and bronchioles. A third to half of all patients experience dyspnea, dry cough, and chest pain. Bilateral hilar adenopathy is the most common diagnostic radiographic finding. Overall, Blacks tend to have more severe lung disease as compared with Caucasians on presentation, a higher likelihood of progressive pulmonary dysfunction, and a poorer long-term prognosis [39, 41].

Table 8.2 Morphologic subtypes of cutaneous sarcoidosis

Subtype	Clinical features	Characteristics
Maculopapular sarcoidosis	Reddish brown macules and papules involving the cheeks, periorbital area, and nasolabial folds. Lesions may resolve without scarring	Most common manifestation of cutaneous sarcoidosis, especially in Black women. Commonly associated with hilar lymphadenopathy, acute uveitis, and parotid enlargement [40]
Lupus pernio	Red and violaceous, indurated papules, plaques, and nodules that usually affect the nose, lips, cheeks, and ears. Nasal ulceration and septal perforation may occur	More common in Black women [40]. Higher frequency of pulmonary and ocular disease
Plaque sarcoidosis	Annular, erythematous, brown, or violaceous, infiltrated plaques that may be atrophic or scaly. Angiolupoid plaques may have large telangiectasias. Plaques may heal with scarring and alopecia	Patients usually have more chronic and severe systemic involvement [45]
Subcutaneous nodular sarcoidosis (Darier-Roussy)	Nontender, firm, skin-colored, or violaceous mobile subcutaneous nodules commonly found on the trunk or extremities. Usually appear in the early stages of the disease. Nodules may resolve spontaneously	Usually associated with less severe systemic disease [45]
Scar-associated sarcoidosis	Scars from previous trauma, surgery, venipuncture, or tattoo may become infiltrated with sarcoidosis and show a red or violaceous color. These lesions may be tender	May appear early in the disease or parallel chronic systemic findings [45]
Erythema nodosum	Tender, erythematous subcutaneous nodules on the extremities (most commonly anterior tibias)	Associated with a good prognosis and spontaneous resolution of the disease. More common in Scandinavian women [45]
Lofgren syndrome	Triad of erythema nodosum, polyarthritis, and hilar adenopathy. Anterior uveitis, fever, ankle periarthritis, arthralgias, and pulmonary involvement	Acute syndrome with excellent prognosis [45]

Treatment

The goal of therapy is to alleviate symptoms by minimizing the inflammatory process. Treatment is selected based on the type of lesion, the cosmetic disfigurement, and the symptoms [37]. In general, patients presenting with cutaneous disease in the setting of systemic involvement benefit from being treated systemically. In cases where disease is localized to the skin, ultrapotent topical steroids or intralesional steroid injections are first-line treatments. Intralesional injections are most appropriate for papule or plaque sarcoidal lesions and aid in suppressing granuloma formation. Steroid-sparing topical agents such as the topical immunomodulators, topical tacrolimus and pimecrolimus, can be alternated with topical steroids to decrease the risk of steroid-induced skin atrophy or hypopigmentation.

Patients with severely scarring sarcoidosis, lesions refractory to local treatment, or those experiencing cutaneous and systemic involvement may require systemic corticosteroids. Minocycline or doxycycline may also be used as first-line treatment [47]. Widespread, cutaneous disease (especially lupus pernio, mucosal, and nail disease) may require oral corticosteroids or antimalarial agents, such as hydroxychloroquine or chloroquine. Antimalarial agents halt

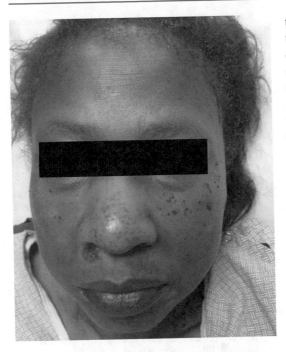

Fig. 8.5 Maculopapular sarcoidosis. Multiple red to violaceous macules are noted on the nose. Scattered violaceous papules coalescing into a thin plaque were noted on the upper cutaneous lip

the body's inflammatory response by preventing the antigen presentation necessary for the process of granuloma formation. Given the potential for ocular toxicity with antimalarial agents, patients should be followed by an ophthalmologist with an eye examination every 6–12 months to monitor for the development of corneal deposits and retinopathy. Patients of African, Mediterranean, or Southeastern Asian descent should be screened for glucose-6-phosphate-dehydrogenase deficiency before prescribing antimalarial medication to avoid precipitating a hemolytic episode [41, 48].

Recalcitrant disease may require the addition of methotrexate, azathioprine, or mycophenolate mofetil. Tumor necrosis factor (TNF) plays an important role in both formation and maintenance of the sarcoidal granulomas, and the TNF-alpha inhibitors, infliximab and adalimumab, have been used successfully in some patients with sarcoidosis [49]. However, it is important to note that there have been cases of TNF-alpha inhibitor-induced sarcoidosis [50].

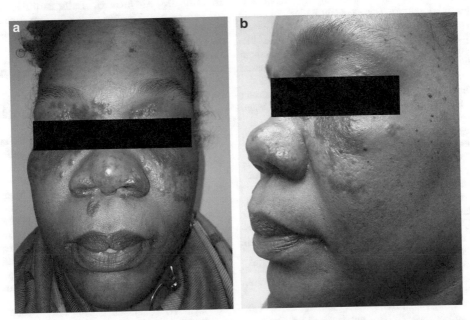

Fig. 8.6 (a, b) Lupus pernio. Multiple disfiguring violaceous papules and plaques are noted on the periorbital, malar cheeks, upper cutaneous lip, and bilateral nasal rims

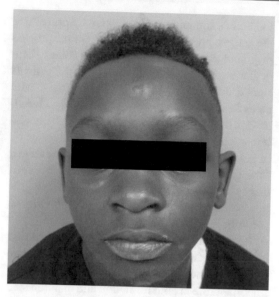

Fig. 8.7 Hypopigmented sarcoid. Scattered hypopigmented subcutaneous nodules are noted on the forehead, cheeks, and chin

References

1. Love PB. Inflammatory disorders. In: Vashi NA, Maibach HI, editors. Dermatoanthropology of ethnic skin and hair. Cham: Springer; 2017.
2. Gelfand JM, Stern RS, Nijsten T, Feldman SR, Thomas J, Kist J, et al. The prevalence of psoriasis in African Americans: results from a population-based study. J Am Acad Dermatol. 2005;52(1):23–6.
3. Rachakonda TD, Schupp CW, Armstrong AW. Psoriasis prevalence among adults in the United States. J Am Acad Dermatol. 2014;70(3):512–6.
4. Krueger JG, Bowcock A. Psoriasis pathophysiology: current concepts of pathogenesis. Ann Rheum Dis. 2005;64(Suppl 2):ii30–6.
5. Shah NJ. Psoriasis. In: Love PB, editor. Clinical cases in skin of color. Cham: Springer; 2016. p. 73–80.
6. Ikaheimo I, Tiilikainen A, Karvonen J, Silvennoinen-Kassinen S. HLA risk haplotype Cw6,DR7,DQA1*0201 and HLA-Cw6 with reference to the clinical picture of psoriasis vulgaris. Arch Dermatol Res. 1996;288(7):363–5.
7. Wuepper KD, Coulter SN, Haberman A. Psoriasis vulgaris: a genetic approach. J Invest Dermatol. 1990;95(5 Suppl):2S–4S.
8. Cao K, Song FJ, Li HG, Xu SY, Liu ZH, Su XH, et al. Association between HLA antigens and families with psoriasis vulgaris. Chin Med J. 1993;106(2):132–5.
9. Tsai TF, Hu CY, Tsai WL, Chu CY, Lin SJ, Liaw SH, et al. HLA-Cw6 specificity and polymorphic residues are associated with susceptibility among Chinese psoriatics in Taiwan. Arch Dermatol Res. 2002;294(5):214–20.
10. Parisi R, Rutter MK, Lunt M, Young HS, Symmons DP, Griffiths CE, et al. Psoriasis and the risk of major cardiovascular events: cohort study using the clinical practice research datalink. J Invest Dermatol. 2015;135(9):2189–97.
11. Correia B, Torres T. Obesity: a key component of psoriasis. Acta Biomed. 2015;86(2):121–9.
12. Geng A, Zeikus PS, McDonald CJ. Psoriasis. In: Kelly AP, editor. Dermatology for skin of color. New York: McGraw-Hill; 2009. p. 139–46.
13. Menter A, Korman NJ, Elmets CA, Feldman SR, Gelfand JM, Gordon KB, et al. Guidelines of care for the management of psoriasis and psoriatic arthritis: section 4. Guidelines of care for the management and treatment of psoriasis with traditional systemic agents. J Am Acad Dermatol. 2009;61(3):451–85.
14. Menter A, Gottlieb A, Feldman SR, Van Voorhees AS, Leonardi CL, Gordon KB, et al. Guidelines of care for the management of psoriasis and psoriatic arthritis: section 1. Overview of psoriasis and guidelines of care for the treatment of psoriasis with biologics. J Am Acad Dermatol. 2008;58(5):826–50.
15. Menter A, Korman NJ, Elmets CA, Feldman SR, Gelfand JM, Gordon KB, et al. Guidelines of care for the management of psoriasis and psoriatic arthritis: section 5. Guidelines of care for the treatment of psoriasis with phototherapy and photochemotherapy. J Am Acad Dermatol. 2010;62(1):114–35.
16. Hadi SM, Al-Quran H, de Sa Earp AP, Hadi AS, Lebwohl M. The use of the 308-nm excimer laser for the treatment of psoriasis. Photomed Laser Surg. 2010;28(5):693–5.
17. Balasubramaniam P, Ogboli M, Moss C. Lichen planus in children: review of 26 cases. Clin Exp Dermatol. 2008;33(4):457–9.
18. Bridges K. Lichen planus. In: Kelly AP, editor. Dermatology for skin of color. New York: McGraw Hill; 2009. p. 152–7.
19. Abdel-Latif AM, Abuel-Ela HA, El-Shourbagy SH. Increased caspase-3 and altered expression of apoptosis-associated proteins, Bcl-2 and Bax in lichen planus. Clin Exp Dermatol. 2009;34(3):390–5.
20. Chang JY, Chiang CP, Hsiao CK, Sun A. Significantly higher frequencies of presence of serum autoantibodies in Chinese patients with oral lichen planus. J Oral Pathol Med. 2009;38(1):48–54.
21. Nagao Y, Sata M. A retrospective case-control study of hepatitis C virus infection and oral lichen planus in Japan: association study with mutations in the core and NS5A region of hepatitis C virus. BMC Gastroenterol. 2012;12:31.
22. Goyal AKR, Planus L. In: Love PBKR, editor. Clinical cases in skin of color. Cham: Springer; 2016. p. 91–101.
23. Sharma VK, Sahni K, Wadhwani AR. Photodermatoses in pigmented skin. Photochem Photobiol Sci. 2013;12(1):65–77.

24. Meads SB, Kunishige J, Ramos-Caro FA, Hassanein AM. Lichen planus actinicus. Cutis. 2003;72(5):377–81.

25. Taylor S. Treatments for skin of color. St. Louis: Saunders/Elsevier; 2011.

26. Zawar V. Pityriasis amiantacea-like eruptions in scalp: a novel manifestation of pityriasis rosea in a child. Int J Trichol. 2010;2(2):113–5.

27. Drago F, Ciccarese G, Thanasi H, Agnoletti AF, Cozzani E, Parodi A. Facial involvement in pityriasis rosea: differences among Caucasian and dark-skinned patients. G Ital Dermatol Venereol. 2016;151(5):571–2.

28. Emre S, Akoglu G, Metin A, Demirseren DD, Isikoglu S, Oztekin A, et al. The oxidant and antioxidant status in Pityriasis Rosea. Indian J Dermatol. 2016;61(1):118.

29. Neoh CY, Tan AW, Mohamed K, Sun YJ, Tan SH. Characterization of the inflammatory cell infiltrate in herald patches and fully developed eruptions of pityriasis rosea. Clin Exp Dermatol. 2010;35(3):300–4.

30. Drago F, Ciccarese G, Herzum A, Rebora A, Parodi A. Pityriasis Rosea during pregnancy: major and minor alarming signs. Dermatology. 2018;234(1–2):31–6.

31. Drago F, Broccolo F, Agnoletti A, Drago F, Rebora A, Parodi A. Pityriasis rosea and pityriasis rosea-like eruptions. J Am Acad Dermatol. 2014;70(1):196.

32. Amer A, Fischer H, Li X. The natural history of pityriasis rosea in black American children: how correct is the "classic" description? Arch Pediatr Adolesc Med. 2007;161(5):503–6.

33. Alzahrani NA, AlJasser MI. Geographic tonguelike presentation in a child with pityriasis rosea: case report and review of oral manifestations of pityriasis rosea. Pediatr Dermatol. 2018;35(2):e124–e7.

34. Villalon-Gomez JM. Pityriasis rosea: diagnosis and treatment. Am Fam Physician. 2018;97(1):38–44.

35. Jairath V, Mohan M, Jindal N, Gogna P, Syrty C, Monnappa PM, et al. Narrowband UVB phototherapy in pityriasis rosea. Indian Dermatol Online J. 2015;6(5):326–9.

36. Drago F, Vecchio F, Rebora A. Use of high-dose acyclovir in pityriasis rosea. J Am Acad Dermatol. 2006;54(1):82–5.

37. Haimovic A, Sanchez M, Judson MA, Prystowsky S. Sarcoidosis: a comprehensive review and update for the dermatologist: part I. Cutaneous disease. J Am Acad Dermatol. 2012;66(5):699. e1–18; quiz 717-8.

38. Wheat CM, Love PB. Sarcoidosis. In: Love PB, editor. Clinical cases in skin of color. 2nd ed. Cham: Springer; 2016.

39. Rybicki BA, Major M, Popovich J Jr, Maliarik MJ, Iannuzzi MC. Racial differences in sarcoidosis incidence: a 5-year study in a health maintenance organization. Am J Epidemiol. 1997;145(3):234–41.

40. Guss L, Ghazarian S, Daya N, Sarcoidosis in African Americans OG. Austin. J Dermatol. 2014;1(6):1028.

41. Heath CR, David J, Taylor SC. Sarcoidosis: are there differences in your skin of color patients? J Am Acad Dermatol. 2012;66(1):121. e1-14.

42. Edmondstone WM, Wilson AG. Sarcoidosis in Caucasians, blacks and Asians in London. Br J Dis Chest. 1985;79(1):27–36.

43. Facco M, Cabrelle A, Teramo A, Olivieri V, Gnoato M, Teolato S, et al. Sarcoidosis is a Th1/Th17 multisystem disorder. Thorax. 2011;66(2):144–50.

44. Yee AM, Pochapin MB. Treatment of complicated sarcoidosis with infliximab anti-tumor necrosis factor-alpha therapy. Ann Intern Med. 2001;135(1):27–31.

45. McKinley-Grant L, Warnick M, Singh S. Cutaneous manifestations of systemic diseases. In: Kelly A, Taylor S, editors. Dermatology for skin of color. New York: McGraw-Hill; 2009.

46. Cozier Y, Ruiz-Narvaez E, McKinnon C, Berman J, Rosenberg L, Palmer J. Replication of genetic loci for sarcoidosis in US black women: data from the Black Women's Health Study. Hum Genet. 2013;132(7):803–10.

47. Bachelez H, Senet P, Cadranel J, Kaoukhov A, Dubertret L. The use of tetracyclines for the treatment of sarcoidosis. Arch Dermatol. 2001;137(1):69–73.

48. Jones E, Callen JP. Hydroxychloroquine is effective therapy for control of cutaneous sarcoidal granulomas. J Am Acad Dermatol. 1990;23(3 Pt 1):487–9.

49. Crommelin HA, Vorselaars AD, van Moorsel CH, Korenromp IH, Deneer VH, Grutters JC. Anti-TNF therapeutics for the treatment of sarcoidosis. Immunotherapy. 2014;6(10):1127–43.

50. Scailteux LM, Guedes C, Polard E, Perdriger A. Sarcoidosis after adalimumab treatment in inflammatory rheumatic diseases: a report of two cases and literature review. Presse Med. 2015;44(1):4–10.

Pigmentary Disorders

Loren Krueger and Nada Elbuluk

Disorders of Hyperpigmentation
(See Table 9.1)

Melasma

Melasma is a common disorder of acquired hyperpigmentation with an estimated prevalence of 1% in the general population [1]. It is thought to occur more commonly in women and in those with darker skin types. The most frequently reported age of onset is in the second and third decades of life [2]. Over 60% of those affected endorse a positive family history of the disorder [3].

Melasma is multifactorial with many suggested aggravating factors, including light exposure. More specifically, ultraviolet and visible light have been found to lead to hyperpigmentation via secretion of stem cell factor (SCF), which is the ligand for c-kit, the tyrosine kinase receptor which controls proliferation of melanocytes. This may explain the presence of mast cells in lesional skin as mast cells also express

L. Krueger
The Ronald O. Perelman Department of
Dermatology, New York University,
New York, NY, USA
e-mail: Loren.krueger@nyumc.org

N. Elbuluk (✉)
Department of Dermatology, University of Southern
California, Keck School of Medicine,
Los Angeles, CA, USA

c-kit tyrosine kinase receptors [4]. Additionally, Wnt signaling-related proteins may be increased in skin with melasma [5]. Changes suggestive of solar elastosis are increasingly identified in skin with melisma, and these dermal changes may play a role in its development [6]. Increased angiogenesis and vascular endothelial growth factor (VEGF) have also been noted, and although the implications are unclear, melanocytes have been found to express VEGF receptors [7]. Moreover, hormonal exposures including pregnancy and oral contraceptives are also thought to trigger or worsen the condition. Although the exact roles of estrogens, progesterone, and antiandrogens are unclear, it is well established that melanocytes express estrogen receptors and these receptors have a role in melanogenesis [8].

Clinically, melasma is characterized by symmetric, light to dark brown macules and patches in sun-exposed areas, often in a reticular pattern. Patterns of distribution include *centrofacial*, involving the forehead, cheeks, upper lip, and chin; *malar*, involving the cheeks; and *mandibular*, involving the mandibular jawline (Fig. 9.1) [2]. Extrafacial forms of melasma have also been described, occurring most commonly on the arms (95%), forearms, chest, and back [9]. On dermoscopy, a brown pseudo-network pattern that spares follicular openings has been described, in addition to brown dots, granules, and arcuate structures [10, 11]. Wood's lamp examination will accentuate epidermal forms of melasma [2].

© Springer Nature Switzerland AG 2021
B. S. Li, H. I. Maibach (eds.), *Ethnic Skin and Hair and Other Cultural Considerations*, Updates in
Clinical Dermatology, https://doi.org/10.1007/978-3-030-64830-5_9

Table 9.1 Disorders of pigmentation

Hyperpigmentation	Hypopigmentation	Depigmentation
Melasma	Tinea versicolor	Vitiligo
Exogenous ochronosis	Progressive macular hypomelanosis	Chemical leukoderma
Erythema dyschromicum perstans	Leprosy	Oculocutaneous albinism
Lichen planus pigmentosus	Nevus depigmentosus	Piebaldism
Confluent and reticulated papillomatosis	Idiopathic guttate hypomelanosis	Waardenburg syndrome
Prurigo pigmentosa	Pityriasis alba	Onchocerciasis
Post-inflammatory hyperpigmentation	Sarcoidosis	Pinta
Genetic disorders	Hypopigmented mycosis fungoides	
Systemic disorders		
Drug-induced/exogenous hyperpigmentation		
Lichen amyloidosis		
Maturational dyschromia		
Acanthosis nigricans		
Pigmented contact dermatitis		

Histopathology has shown epidermal, dermal, and mixed forms of melasma. The affected skin may demonstrate increased melanin in all epidermal layers. It is unclear whether the number of melanocytes is increased in lesional skin; however, lesional melanocytes demonstrate increased number of organelles including melanosomes suggesting amplified activity [6, 12]. Dermal melanophages are present in dermal forms of melasma [4].

Although the clinical presentation alone typically suffices for diagnosing melasma, the differential diagnosis is broad. Lentigines develop in sun-exposed areas, however, are typically more discreet macules and are not always symmetric. Nevus of Ota and Hori's nevus can present similarly to melasma; however, these conditions tend to be less reticulated, have a predominant blue/gray hue, and are stable following their development (Fig. 9.2). Maturational dyschromia may present with gray/brown patches on the cheeks and temples. Exogenous ochronosis, which can be found in the same distribution, can occur as a result of long-term treatment of melasma with lightening agents. This condition tends to be darker brown to black, can present with fine caviar-like papules in later stages, and does not respond to melasma treatments. PIH is also on the differential but requires history of antecedent inflammation in the area.

Exogenous Ochronosis

Exogenous ochronosis (EO) develops in the setting of chronic, continuous use of skin-lightening agents that contain hydroquinone, resorcinol, and/or phenolic compounds [13]. The prevalence of EO is underreported but is likely higher in African and Asian countries than in the USA [14, 15]. The exact mechanism remains unclear; however, it has been proposed that hydroquinone inhibits the enzyme homogentisic acid oxidase, leading to the precipitation of ochre pigment from accumulated homogentisic acid [16].

Establishing the diagnosis of EO can be challenging. Clinically, EO presents with dark brown/black macules and patches, typically symmetrically in sun-exposed areas. However, EO can occur anywhere the precipitating agent is applied. The development of colloid milia, described as *caviar-like* fine papules, helps to distinguish this condition from melasma (Fig. 9.3a). Atrophy and hypopigmentation may also be seen in EO [17]. One severity classification scheme describes disease progression with *grade 1*, initial macular pigmentation; *grade 2*, macular stippling and fine papules; *grade 3*, dark deposits and papules; and *grade 4*, the development of colloid milia [18]. On dermoscopy, dense, dark brown/black globules and curvilinear (wormlike) structures have been identified. These structures obliterate fol-

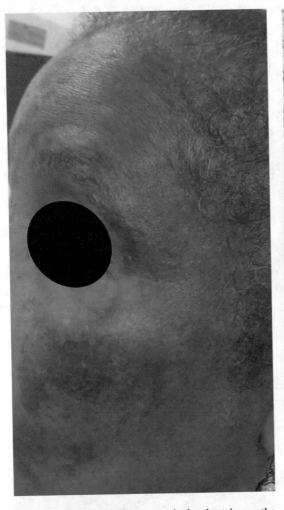

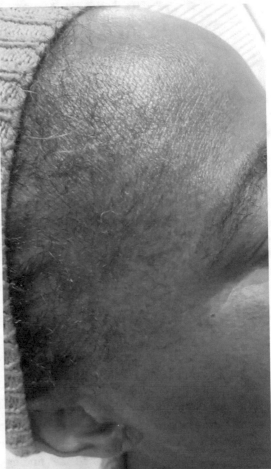

Fig. 9.2 Nevus of Ota: Confluent blue-gray patch on the temple and forehead since birth

Fig. 9.1 Melasma: Dark brown reticulated patches on the forehead, temples, and cheeks

licular openings, which distinguishes this from melasma dermoscopically [19].

Histopathology demonstrates yellow-brown pigment deposits in the dermis, which are thought to correspond to the globules seen on dermoscopy (Fig. 9.3b).

The clinical differential diagnosis includes melasma as well as the conditions discussed in this chapter as the differential for melasma. Distinguishing between EO and melasma is imperative in guiding appropriate and effective treatment.

Erythema Dyschromicum Perstans

Erythema dyschromicum perstans (EDP), also known as ashy dermatosis, is an uncommon pigmentary disorder that was first described by Ramirez in El Salvador [20]. The disease occurs most commonly in Caucasian and Hispanic children and young adults, although it has been described in older adults as well. The etiology remains unclear.

Clinically, EDP presents with symmetric blue-gray macules and patches predominantly on the

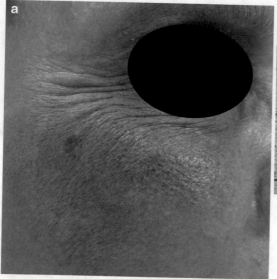

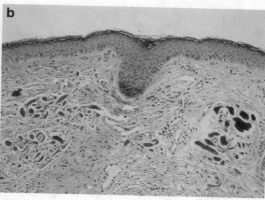

Fig. 9.3 (**a**) Exogenous ochronosis: Brown ill-defined patch on malar cheek consisting of "caviar-like" fine papules. (**b**) Exogenous ochronosis: Yellow-brown deposits in the dermis (H&E, 20×). (Photo courtesy of Drs. Lu Chen and Shane Meehan from NYU – The Ronald O. Perelman Department of Dermatology)

trunk and non-photoexposed sites. It can become confluent and extensive with patches reaching up to 5 cm or larger in size. Evolving macules and patches may have an erythematous, sometimes raised border in the early inflammatory phase; one retrospective review identified this finding in 17% of patients [21]. On dermoscopy, blue/gray-hued small, homogenous dots are appreciated [22].

On histopathology, pigment incontinence with dermal melanophages is most commonly seen. The active, erythematous border features lymphocytic inflammation at the dermoepidermal junction and vacuolization of the basal layer (Fig. 9.4) [21].

The differential diagnosis includes lichen planus pigmentosus, confluent and reticulated papillomatosis, multifocal fixed drug eruption, post-inflammatory hyperpigmentation, and drug-induced causes of hyperpigmentation. EDP can be most difficult to distinguish from lichen planus pigmentosus; however, age, distribution, and deeper blue/gray hue can help in distinguishing the two conditions [23].

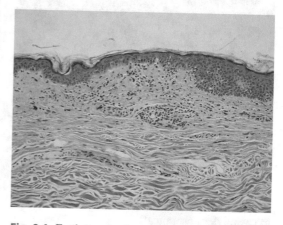

Fig. 9.4 Erythema dyschromicum perstans: Superficial perivascular lymphohistiocytic infiltrates with vacuolization of the basal layer and scattered dermal melanophages (H&E, 20×). (Photo courtesy of Drs. Lu Chen and Shane Meehan from NYU – The Ronald O. Perelman Department of Dermatology)

Lichen Planus Pigmentosus

Lichen planus pigmentosus (LPP) is a disorder of hyperpigmentation that occurs more commonly in patients with skin types III–V. The prevalence is unknown, but literature suggests the disease may not be uncommon, especially in patients of Indian, African, and Latin American descent [24, 25]. It can co-occur with lichen planus in a percentage of patients. In a study of 40 Indian patients with LPP, over 30% of the patients had an additional form of lichen planus; however, other studies have not consistently confirmed such a strong coexistence [23, 26]. LPP is also increasingly recognized in a subset of patients with skin of color with frontal fibrosing alopecia, a patterned form of lichen planopilaris [25].

LPP presents with brown to blue/gray macules and patches most commonly on the head and neck and other photoexposed sites (Fig. 9.5). When involving the face, the forehead, temples, and preauricular cheeks are commonly involved [23]. Involvement of axillary and intertriginous areas can be seen, which suggests non-sun-exposed areas could also be affected [23]. One study describes the clinical patterns as *diffuse*, seen in 77.4% of patients, *reticular* in 9.7%, *blotchy* in 7.3%, and *perifollicular* in 5.6% [24]. Few descriptive studies on the use of dermoscopy in LPP have suggested a role in helping to establish the diagnosis. Pseudonetwork, dots, and globules are described, with patterned deposition of dots and globules [27, 28]. Dots and globules can be uniformly distributed and appear in circles or in a linear pattern [27, 28]. Pruritus has been reported in up to 85% of patients and may reflect disease activity [29].

On histopathology, LPP demonstrates a band-like lymphohistiocytic infiltrate with melanophages in the upper dermis indicative of pigment incontinence. In later stages, the epidermis may appear atrophic with scattered necrotic keratinocytes [30].

The differential diagnosis is broad and when involving the face should include melasma, pigmented contact dermatitis, and post-inflammatory hyperpigmentation. Truncal predominance may suggest EDP over LPP, although both commonly occur on the neck. As LPP can be associated with other forms of lichen planus, thorough evaluation for additional findings on the scalp, mucous membranes, and nails is prudent.

Confluent and Reticulated Papillomatosis

Confluent and reticulated papillomatosis of Gougerot and Carteaud, or CARP, is an acquired disorder of keratinization. Although most cases are sporadic, there does appear to be a familial variant [31]. The cause of the disorder has been debated. Some have theorized that *Malassezia furfur* or *Dietzia papillomatosis* infection may play a role [32]. Endocrinologic imbalance has also been suggested due to its association with obesity and insulin resistance [32]. Roles for UV light, amyloid, and keratin 16 have also been suggested [33]. Epidemiologic information is varied but suggests a younger age of onset with an average between 19 and 21 years of age [34, 35]. There is no clear racial or gender predilection [34].

CARP is characterized by brown to gray macules and flat-topped papules that coalesce centrally with a reticular appearance periph-

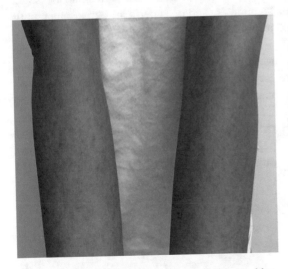

Fig. 9.5 Lichen planus pigmentosus: Brown to blue-gray, ill-defined macules and patches on the extensor and ventral forearms

erally. Lesions appear to have scale or hyper-keratosis. The central chest and upper trunk are common sites of involvement. The eruption is typically asymptomatic, although pruritus has been reported [36, 37]. On dermoscopy, white scales are seen, with either a background "sulci and gyri" pattern or a "cobblestone" appearance [36, 38].

Histopathology demonstrates hyperkerato-sis and papillomatosis with heavily pigmented bulbous rete ridges; a sparse perivascular lym-phohistiocytic infiltrate may also be appreciated (Fig. 9.6) [34]. This constellation of findings may be seen in benign neoplasms including sebor-rheic keratoses and epidermal nevi, and therefore clinical information should be provided.

The diagnosis of CARP can typically be made through a combination of patient age, chest/trun-cal distribution, and reticular pattern. The differ-ential diagnosis for CARP includes acanthosis nigricans, tinea versicolor, prurigo pigmentosa in resolution phase, and post-inflammatory hyper-pigmentation. Although the hyperkeratosis seen in CARP may resemble acanthosis nigricans, the latter tends to appear primarily on the neck and intertriginous areas. Tinea versicolor and CARP both occur commonly on the chest and back but can be distinguished by potassium hydroxide (KOH) examination.

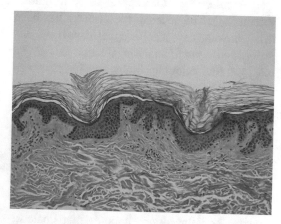

Fig. 9.6 Confluent and reticulated papillomatosis: Hyperkeratosis and papillomatosis with bulbous rete ridges (H&E, 20×). (Photo courtesy of Drs. Lu Chen and Shane Meehan from NYU – The Ronald O. Perelman Department of Dermatology)

Prurigo Pigmentosa

Prurigo pigmentosa (PP) was originally described in Japanese patients by Nagashima [39]. The eti-ology remains unknown. There appears to be a predominance in females and young adults [39]. Since its initial description, it has been reported in patients from Korea, the Middle East, and the USA [40, 41]. Case reports suggest a correlation with pregnancy as well as ketotic diet [42–44].

Prurigo pigmentosa presents with recurrent crops of intensely pruritic, erythematous papules that are initially urticarial and then progress to a vesicular morphology [45]. Lesions become crusted or scaly and heal with brown macules that coalesce into reticulated pigmentation [46].

The histopathologic findings are variable; however, they likely reflect the clinical stage of the lesions in PP. Early lesions demonstrate superficial perivascular infiltrate with neutro-phils. Papillary dermal edema and epidermal exocytosis and/or spongiosis may also be appre-ciated at this stage. More developed lesions may demonstrate spongiosis with balloon degenera-tion, necrotic keratinocytes, and clusters of neu-trophils. There is a dense mixed dermal infiltrate. Older lesions demonstrate parakeratosis, slight spongiosis, and/or superficial perivascular infil-trate with melanophages [46].

The differential diagnosis varies based on the stage of the PP lesions. Erythematous, inflamma-tory papules may resemble lesions of atopic der-matitis, urticaria, dermatitis herpetiformis, and linear IgA dermatosis. Reticulated hyperpigmen-tation may resemble confluent and reticulated papillomatosis, acanthosis nigricans, lichen pla-nus pigmentosus, Dowling-Degos disease, and post-inflammatory hyperpigmentation [45].

Post-inflammatory Hyperpigmentation

Post-inflammatory hyperpigmentation (PIH) results after injury to the skin, which can be endogenous from conditions including inflam-matory dermatoses or exogenous from external trauma. PIH is more common in patients with skin of color [47]. The propensity to develop PIH following cutaneous injury has been proposed to be secondary to one's *individual chromatic tendency* or the likelihood for an individual's melanocytes to respond with increased, decreased, or stable melanin production following inflammation [48]. In PIH, melanocytes respond to inflammation and/or trauma with increased melanin production and transfer to keratinocytes. Melanin may also drop from the epidermis following injury resulting in melanophages [47, 49]. A linear variant of post-inflammatory hyperpigmentation may be seen following various conditions including Rhus dermatitis, phytophotodermatosis, koebnerization of certain inflammatory conditions, flagellate hyperpigmentation, and trauma.

The clinical history is especially important in establishing the diagnosis. Clinical examination reveals brown, blue, or gray-hued macules or patches at sites of previous inflammation or trauma.

Histopathology will demonstrate increased epidermal melanin and/or dermal melanophages. Fontana-Masson may be used to stain melanin. The findings may be similar to those seen in post-inflammatory hypopigmentation, and clinicopathologic correlation is required [47].

The differential diagnosis of post-inflammatory hyperpigmentation varies based on location. For facial hyperpigmentation, melasma, pigmented contact dermatitis, and maturational dyschromia should all be considered. Additional conditions that could resemble more diffuse PIH include lichen planus pigmentosus, lichen amyloidosis (Fig. 9.7), and drug-induced hyperpigmentation.

Genetic Disorders of Hyperpigmentation

Dyskeratosis congenita (DKC) is characterized clinically by nail dystrophy, leukoplakia, and reticulated hyperpigmentation. Mutations on the DKC1 gene encoding the dyskerin protein, which is responsible for telomere maintenance, cause DKC. Although autosomal dominant and recessive forms exist, the most common form is X-linked recessive; therefore, 90% of those

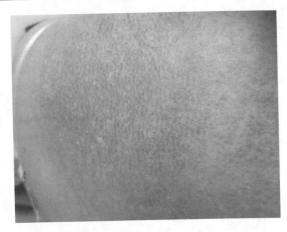

Fig. 9.7 Lichen amyloidosis: Light brown rippled patch on mid upper back

affected are male. Reticulated hyperpigmentation presents in the first decade of life on the neck, chest, and back. Histopathology of the reticular hyperpigmentation will demonstrate epidermal atrophy and melanophages in the superficial dermis. Degeneration of basal keratinocytes can also be seen [50]. Bone marrow failure is the major cause of mortality in these patients. The differential includes Fanconi's anemia, which can present with pigmentary changes in the setting of hematologic abnormalities and Naegeli-Franceschetti-Jadassohn syndrome [51].

Naegeli-Franceschetti-Jadassohn syndrome (NFJ syndrome) is caused by a mutation in keratin 14 with an autosomal dominant inheritance. One of the initial presenting signs is reticulated hyperpigmentation on the abdomen and periorificial skin. This hyperpigmentation usually fades following puberty. Histopathology of the hyperpigmentation will demonstrate melanophages in the superficial dermis. Onychodystrophy, dental anomalies, and hypoplastic dermatoglyphics may also be appreciated. Lack of hematologic abnormalities suggests against dyskeratosis congenita [52, 53].

Dowling-Degos disease (DDD) is a rare disorder caused by a mutation in keratin 5 which typically occurs after puberty. Inheritance is autosomal dominant. It is characterized by reticular hyperpigmentation of intertriginous and flexural sites. Comedo-like lesions can be appreciated in these areas as well. Histopathology of the hyperpigmentation demonstrates increased epidermal pigmentation of elongated rete ridges with thin suprapapillary plates, at times referred to as "antlers" [54]. Dermal melanophages may also be appreciated [55, 56]. The differential diagnosis includes acanthosis nigricans, reticulate acropigmentation of Kitamura (predominant on the hands and feet), and Galli-Galli disease, which is similar to DDD but with the addition of acantholysis [54].

Systemic Disorders

Addison's disease is an autoimmune endocrine disorder of primary adrenal insufficiency. Adrenal glands are unable to produce sufficient steroid hormones, which leads to increased adrenocorticotropic hormone levels that act on the melanocyte-stimulating hormone. This results in diffuse hyperpigmentation, with some accentuation noted at sun-exposed sites. The hair, nails, and mucosae may also be involved. Additional signs of Addison's disease include dehydration, hypoglycemia, weight loss, muscle aches, and weakness [57].

Hyperthyroidism may also cause localized or generalized hyperpigmentation. Additional cutaneous manifestations include skin thickening, pretibial myxedema, urticaria, and hair thinning. Serum thyroid-stimulating hormone level is the initial screening test [58].

Drug-Induced/Exogenous Hyperpigmentation

Flagellate erythema/hyperpigmentation presents with linear hyperpigmentation that can be pruritic. At times it is preceded by an erythematous or urticarial eruption. It has been associated with bleomycin, including intralesional forms, as well as raw shiitake mushroom ingestion, and dermatomyositis [59].

Heavy metals, including arsenic and silver, can also cause hyperpigmentation. Elevation in arsenic levels, due to consumption of contaminated well water, can lead to cutaneous changes

over time. Skin hyperpigmentation may present before skin hyperkeratosis in the setting of arsenicosis [60]. The hyperpigmentation is often in sun-protected areas with a typical description of diffuse hyperpigmentation with overlying "raindrop" hypopigmentation. Hyperkeratosis of the palms and soles and keratinocytic skin cancers are also seen [61]. Hyperpigmentation is also seen as a side effect of silver ingestion, referred to as argyria. Blue-gray discoloration involves the skin, nails, and conjunctiva [62]. A localized cutaneous variant can also occur secondary to acupuncture, topical medications containing silver nitrate, and jewelry [63]. Histopathology demonstrates brown-black granules in the basement membrane and around eccrine coils (Fig. 9.8) [64].

Several medications can also cause hyperpigmentation (Table 9.2). Antimalarials including chloroquine and hydroxychloroquine, tetracyclines, and chemotherapeutic agents are common culprits in drug-induced hyperpigmentation. Of the tetracyclines, minocycline most commonly causes pigmentary changes that can be categorized into three types. Type I features blue-gray hyperpigmentation at sites of inflammation or trauma (including acne) on the face, and histopathology will demonstrate iron and melanin both within macrophages and extracellularly. Type II presents clinically with blue-gray hyperpigmen-

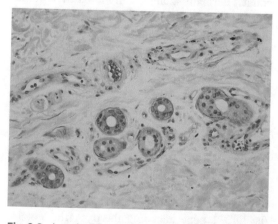

Fig. 9.8 Argyria: Blue-black granules near dermal elastic fibers and around the basement membrane of eccrine coils and blood vessels (H&E, 40×). (Photo courtesy of Drs. Lu Chen and Shane Meehan from NYU – The Ronald O. Perelman Department of Dermatology)

Table 9.2 Causes of drug-induced hyperpigmentation

Heavy metals	Antibiotics/antivirals	Antimalarials	Chemotherapeutics	Other
Arsenic	Tetracyclines	Chloroquine	Bisulfan	Amiodarone
Bismuth	Doxycycline	Hydroxychloroquine	Bleomycin	NSAIDs
Gold	Minocycline	Quinacrine	Cyclophosphamide	Oral contraceptives
Lead	Clofazimine		Doxorubicin	Amytriptiline
Silver	Zidovudine		Daunorubicin	Carotenoids
Mercury				

tation of the extremities (favoring shins), and histopathologic findings are similar to type I. Type III presents with a diffuse brown-gray pigmentation in sun-exposed areas with increased melanin and dermal melanophages present on histopathology. Whereas types I and II fade gradually with time, type III persists and can be disfiguring for patients [64, 65].

Disorders of Hypopigmentation and Depigmentation (See Table 9.1)

Tinea Versicolor

Tinea versicolor (TV), also known as pityriasis versicolor, is a common and ubiquitous disorder that can cause hypopigmentation. It is unclear whether a racial predilection exists; however, the disease may be more easily recognized in darker skin types [66, 67]. TV has a higher prevalence in men, presumably due to increased sebaceous activity. The disease is also more common in adolescence and young adulthood, suggesting a role for hormonal changes [68]. Immunosuppression and corticosteroid overuse may also increase the risk for development of TV [68, 69]. TV is caused by the yeast *Malassezia*, commensal, lipophilic yeasts that can colonize healthy skin [70]. *Malassezia* species *M. globosa* has been isolated most commonly in cases of TV; however, *M. sympodialis* and *M. furfur* have also been isolated [70]. Hypopigmentation results from both the yeast's production of dicarboxylic acid that inhibits tyrosinase and to the accumulation of "lipid-like" material in the stratum corneum blocking ultraviolet penetration [69, 71].

On clinical examination, TV presents with 3–5 mm round or oval-shaped macules that may

coalesce (Fig. 9.9a) [69]. Overlying scale is a classic feature and can be evaluated with potassium hydroxide preparation. Lesions most commonly appear on the upper trunk, neck, face, and intertriginous areas. The macules may be hypopigmented, hyperpigmented, or salmon colored [72]. Lesions may be asymptomatic or pruritic. Histopathology demonstrates hyphae and spores in the stratum corneum with variable superficial perivascular lymphohistiocytic infiltrate (Fig. 9.9b) [73].

The differential diagnosis includes progressive macular hypomelanosis, idiopathic guttate hypomelanosis, pityriasis alba, hypopigmented mycosis fungoides, and post-inflammatory hypopigmentation. When hyperpigmented, CARP and post-inflammatory hyperpigmentation should also be considered.

Progressive Macular Hypomelanosis

Progressive macular hypomelanosis (PMH) is a condition of hypopigmentation that predominantly affects the trunk. The disorder was previously known as *cutis trunci variata*, *creole dyschromia*, *progressive macular confluent hypomelanosis*, and *idiopathic multiple large-macule hypomelanosis* [74–76]. PMH occurs more commonly in women and young adults. One epidemiologic study from Brazil found the average age of onset to be 20 years old and 79% of those affected were women [77]. The disorder is likely more common in patients with darker skin types. Although the etiology of the disorder is not fully elucidated, it has been linked to *Propionibacterium acnes*. *P. acnes* has been isolated and cultured from lesional skin, and it is proposed that some strains (strain III) may pro-

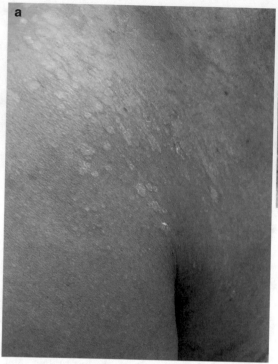

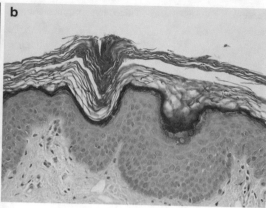

Fig. 9.9 (**a**) Tinea versicolor: Round, coalescing hypopigmented macules with overlying scale on the anterior shoulder. (**b**) Tinea versicolor. Innumerable hyphae and spores in the stratum corneum (H&E, 40×). (Photo courtesy of Drs. Lu Chen and Shane Meehan from NYU – The Ronald O. Perelman Department of Dermatology)

duce a factor capable of altering pigmentation [78, 79]. No association with acneiform lesions has been identified [75].

Progressive macular hypomelanosis manifests with ill-defined, round, hypopigmented macules that coalesce into patches typically on the trunk. Extremity and facial lesions are uncommon. The lesions are non-scaly and asymptomatic. Wood's lamp can help confirm the diagnosis of PMH through demonstration of punctate orange-red fluorescence around follicles [80].

Histopathology demonstrates decreased epidermal melanin, with some reports suggesting mild lymphocytic papillary dermal infiltrate [75, 81]. There does not appear to be a decrease in melanocyte density in lesional skin [81]. However, electron microscopy reveals a decrease in mature melanosomes (decrease in type IV) and an increase in smaller melanosomes (smaller types II–IV) [81].

PMH is commonly mistaken for tinea versicolor, and potassium hydroxide preparation can be useful to distinguish these two entities. Pityriasis alba should also be considered in this age group, although this more commonly involves the face than trunk. Additional diagnoses to consider in the differential include leprosy, pinta, and hypopigmented mycosis fungoides.

Leprosy

Leprosy, or Hansen's disease, has diverse clinical presentations determined by the host's immune response to the infectious bacillus, *Mycobacterium leprae*. Although disease incidence has decreased, leprosy is still seen in regions of Central and South America as well as Africa and Asia.

Initial infection manifests in a macular morphology. Depending on the host's immunity, these lesions can then progress toward tuberculoid, lepromatous, or indeterminate forms. Hypopigmented macules, patches, and plaques suggest indeterminate or tuberculoid forms of leprosy; however, they have also been described in the lepromatous form [82, 83]. Annular lesions with central hypopigmentation and a slightly elevated border can be seen; this border represents an ideal location for histologic sampling. Close assessment for alopecia and hypoesthesia within these lesions is critical for diagnosis.

Histopathology is diagnostic and will reveal foamy macrophages with variable number of acid-fast bacilli. It has also been reported to have focal areas of decreased epidermal melanin [82].

The differential diagnosis is broad and includes pinta, hypopigmented mycosis fungoides, pityriasis lichenoides chronica, pityriasis alba, post-inflammatory hypopigmentation, and the hypopigmented variant of sarcoidosis.

Nevus Depigmentosus

Nevus depigmentosus (ND), or nevus achromicus, is a hypopigmented dermatologic condition that typically develops by 3 years of age. It is commonly grouped with disorders of hypopigmentation which occur along the lines of Blaschko [84]. ND is not inherited [85]. The condition's name is misleading as it is hypopigmented and not depigmented. ND does not change or progress; however, the development of lentigines and melanocytic nevi within ND has been reported [86, 87]. A developmental defect of melanocytes, perhaps involving the transfer of melanosomes to keratinocytes, is thought to cause ND [88]. Coupe proposed diagnostic criteria for ND which include (1) presence at birth or early in life, (2) stable distribution without progression, (3) no change in texture or sensation of the area, and (4) lack of hyperpigmented border around the lesion [89].

ND appears most commonly on the trunk in either a segmental or isolated pattern [90]. Multiple lesions have been described in some patients [90]. The lesion is well circumscribed with clearly demarcated borders and does not blanch with pressure.

Multiple studies have reproduced similar histopathologic findings of ND showing a decreased density of epidermal melanin [85, 90]. However, data conflict as to whether melanocyte number is decreased in lesional skin [85, 90, 91].

The differential diagnosis includes segmental vitiligo, which would demonstrate depigmentation with complete loss of melanocytes. Nevus anemicus is nearly indistinguishable clinically, but diascopy can distinguish between the two, as it will blanch the surrounding skin of nevus anemicus but not ND.

Idiopathic Guttate Hypomelanosis

Idiopathic guttate hypomelanosis (IGH) is a common, acquired disorder of hypopigmentation seen in older patients. Factors including genetic predisposition, normal aging, and ultraviolet light exposure are associated with its development and progression [92]. Several studies have demonstrated a high prevalence of IGH, with one epidemiologic study finding it present in over 80% of patients age >40 years [93]. The development of IGH in the setting of either ultraviolet-A or narrowband ultraviolet-B therapy suggests a pathogenic role for exposure to light [94]. Additionally, IGH has been identified in association with other signs of photoaging, including solar lentigines [93].

On physical examination, sharply demarcated, 2–5 mm "ivory-white" macules favor the extensor extremities, although they also occur on the trunk and rarely the face [92, 93]. In one study, the average number of IGH macules per patient was 13 [93]. Three distinct morphologies of the presentation of IGH have been described: (1) hypopigmented macule on sun-damaged skin, (2) white, well-demarcated macule on either sun-exposed or sun-protected skin, and (3) well-demarcated lesion with keratotic crust, frequently with a "scalloped" border [95]. Newly described dermoscopic findings suggest a "cloudy" pattern or overlapping white macules that lead to varying intensity of the white color [96]. Borders of the macules are described as "amoeboid," "petaloid," "feathery," or indistinct (Fig. 9.10) [97].

Histopathology demonstrates hyperkeratosis and acanthosis of the stratum corneum as well as

Fig. 9.10 Idiopathic guttate hypomelanosis: Dermoscopic image of sharply demarcated white macules with "scalloped" or "petaloid" borders. (Dermlite DL200)

flattening of the rete ridges with variable epidermal atrophy. Epidermal melanin and melanocyte density are also both decreased [98].

The differential diagnosis includes progressive macular hypomelanosis, hypopigmented mycosis fungoides, pityriasis alba, post-inflammatory hypopigmentation, vitiligo, and tinea versicolor [92].

Pityriasis Alba

Pityriasis alba is (PA) a common disorder in children and adolescents, especially those with atopic diathesis. In fact, PA is considered one of the minor forms of atopic dermatitis [99–101]. It is one of the leading dermatologic conditions seen in children, with reported prevalence over 8% [102]. The disorder is more frequently recognized in patients with darker skin types and after summer following tanning of normal skin [103]. Excessive bathing and hot water temperatures may increase risk [103].

Pityriasis alba presents with ill-defined, hypopigmented patches (average of 0.6–6 cm) typically on the face [99, 103]. The lesions can initially be erythematous, and in some cases peripheral erythema and/or scaling is appreciated [104]. Lesions are usually asymptomatic;

however, pruritus has been reported. The clinical course is difficult to predict and can include relapses, remission, and spontaneous resolution [104].

Histopathology of pityriasis alba demonstrates spongiosis, hyperkeratosis, and acanthosis. Superficial lymphocytic infiltrate may also be appreciated. Hair follicles demonstrate plugging as well as associated atrophic sebaceous glands [105]. Epidermal melanin is decreased, and studies are mixed as to whether melanocyte density is decreased or preserved [105, 106].

The differential diagnosis includes vitiligo, tinea versicolor, nevus depigmentosus, nevus anemicus, and post-inflammatory hypopigmentation. Pityriasis lichenoides chronica and hypopigmented mycosis fungoides should also be considered. Concomitant additional cutaneous manifestations of atopic dermatitis support the diagnosis of pityriasis alba.

Sarcoidosis

Sarcoidosis is a complex, multi-organ granulomatous disease with a myriad of cutaneous presentations. Rates of sarcoidosis are elevated in African Americans, especially women, with worse disease severity and mortality [107]. It is prudent to evaluate patients with cutaneous sarcoidosis for systemic involvement, as systemic disease is seen in 25–82% [108, 109]. Cutaneous manifestations are widely varied and include macules, papules, plaques, infiltration of scars or tattoos, nodules, ulceration, and hypopigmentation [109]. Forms including subcutaneous nodules and lupus pernio are more likely to portend systemic involvement [109, 110]. Various syndromes can occur which also include sarcoidosis with a constellation of other signs and symptoms such as Lofgren syndrome and Darier-Roussy [111].

Hypopigmented patches and plaques may be seen in sarcoidosis; this form is more commonly seen in patients with darker skin types [112]. The lesions are most commonly seen on the extremities, although they have also been described on the face and neck [113]. Lesions may be palpable or indurated [114].

The histopathologic hallmark of cutaneous sarcoidosis is the presence of naked granulomas on histopathology. However, it is important to note that hypopigmented forms may not feature pathognomonic granulomas [113, 114]. Case series suggest that hypopigmented macular or patch-like lesions without induration are less likely to reveal sarcoidal granulomas on histopathology; therefore, sampling should be directed at palpable areas [114, 115].

The differential diagnosis includes post-inflammatory hypopigmentation, pityriasis alba, hypopigmented mycosis fungoides, and pityriasis lichenoides chronica. Clinicopathologic correlation should inform the need for systemic evaluation. Thorough history and review of systems with special attention to the pulmonary system is prudent, along with consideration of chest radiograph [116].

Hypopigmented Mycosis Fungoides

Hypopigmented mycosis fungoides is a rare subtype of cutaneous T-cell lymphoma that is more commonly seen in patients with skin of color. Although the disease has a mean age between 30 and 40, it has been described in children and adolescents as well [117]. There does not appear to be a gender predilection [117]. The vast majority of patients are either stage IA or IB at initial diagnosis [117, 118]. Hypopigmented mycosis fungoides has a particularly indolent course, rarely advancing beyond patch stages [119]. Disease recurrence is common, and albeit rare, disease progression and large-cell transformation can occur [120].

Clinically, hypopigmented mycosis fungoides favors sun-protected areas, similar to other forms of cutaneous T-cell lymphoma. Hypopigmented macules and patches are present on the trunk, buttocks, and/or extremities [117]. Erythema, scale, and atrophy are also seen [121]. The lesions are asymptomatic. Examination with Wood's lamp does not reveal fluorescence.

Repeat biopsies may be needed to establish the diagnosis. Findings include superficial perivascular lymphocytic infiltrate and epi-dermotropic atypical lymphocytes with large, hyperchromatic, cerebriform nuclei. CD8+ cells predominate, although CD4+ cells may also be seen [119]. Loss of CD7 is noted in hypopigmented mycosis fungoides [119].

It is prudent to consider hypopigmented mycosis fungoides in the differential for hypopigmented patches as diagnosis is frequently delayed due to misdiagnosis; one epidemiologic study suggests an average delay in diagnosis of 5 years [117]. The differential diagnosis includes pityriasis lichenoides chronica, cutaneous sarcoidosis, and post-inflammatory hypopigmentation. Consider also pityriasis alba, especially in children and adolescents.

Vitiligo

Vitiligo is a complex, multifactorial disorder that can have devastating psychosocial effects. It is the most common depigmenting disorder with an estimated prevalence of 0.5–1% of the world's population [122]. Indian studies have suggested a prevalence as high as 8.8% [123]. Men and women are affected at equal rates [124, 125]. Peak incidence is in the second and third decades of life [125]. HLA-DR4 and HLA-A2 have strong evidence supporting their roles as genetic risk factors in vitiligo [126, 127]. Non-MHC gene associations include CTLA4 and PTPN22 [128, 129]. Genome-wide association studies continue to identify genetic loci which contribute as risk factors for vitiligo, with more studies needed in those of non-European backgrounds [130]. Monozygotic twin studies suggest concordance of 23%, so although heritability plays a role, other factors contribute to the pathogenesis of vitiligo [131]. The exact pathophysiology of vitiligo is still not fully known and is considered multifactorial with genetic, cytotoxic, neurohumoral, environmental, and autoimmune causes [132, 133]. The onset of vitiligo may varies and is often related to internal or external stress to the body. These can include pregnancy, trauma, and psychosocial stressors [134, 135].

Vitiligo is characterized by well-defined, depigmented macules and patches (Fig. 9.11a).

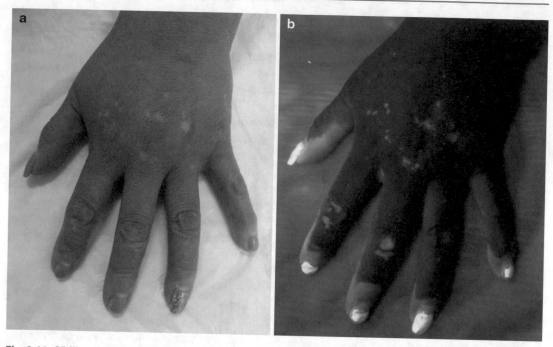

Fig. 9.11 Vitiligo: (**a**) Depigmented macules and patches on the dorsal hand. (**b**) Fluorescence of depigmented skin in vitiligo with Wood's lamp

Wood's lamp examination reveals bright fluorescence of the depigmented areas (Fig. 9.11b) [136]. Vitiligo is classified based on extent and distribution. The two main categories are segmental and nonsegmental vitiligo. The latter can be further subdivided into localized, generalized, or universal forms. Universal forms are particularly challenging to treat with near complete depigmentation (>80% body surface area) [137]. Segmental vitiligo manifests as a rapidly progressive depigmented unilateral patch that eventually stabilizes [137, 138]. It is important for providers to recognize signs of active disease activity including confetti-like depigmentation, trichome coloration, inflammatory lesions (elevated, erythematous borders), and koebnerization. Repigmentation in vitiligo begins as brown macules surrounding follicles, which can expand into larger brown macules and patches (Fig. 9.12). Dermoscopy has been utilized in the assessment of disease activity with *starburst*, *comet tail*, and *micro-Koebner's* patterns signifying disease progression [139].

Histopathology will demonstrate decreased epidermal melanin; however, immunohistochemical staining is needed to establish the diagnosis.

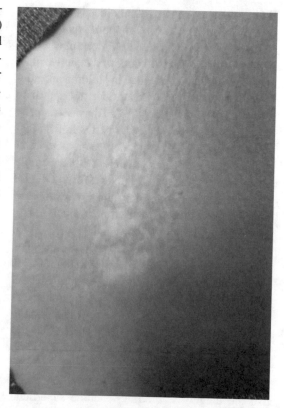

Fig. 9.12 Repigmenting vitiligo: Perifollicular brown macules within a depigmented patch

Studies suggest melanocytes are near-completely or completely absent in vitiligo lesions [140, 141]. A CD8+ -predominant lymphocytic infiltrate may be present at the dermoepidermal junction in early or evolving lesions [138].

Vitiligo has been found in association with additional autoimmune conditions, most commonly thyroid disease (hypothyroid>hyperthyroid) in over 19% [131]. Rheumatoid arthritis, alopecia areata, inflammatory bowel disease, and other autoimmune and inflammatory diseases have also been found to be associated with vitiligo [131, 142].

The differential diagnosis is broad and includes chemical leukoderma as well as genetic causes of depigmentation. Trauma, burns, and post-inflammatory hypopigmentation can mimic vitiligo. Pityriasis alba, hypopigmented sarcoidosis, pityriasis lichenoides chronica, and hypopigmented mycosis fungoides should also be considered. Nevus depigmentosus may also be considered in the differential of segmental vitiligo.

Chemical Leukoderma

Chemical leukoderma is an acquired disorder of hypo- or depigmentation resulting from exposure to a melanotoxic agent. Common agents include phenols and sulfhydryls. The ability of these agents to cause skin lightening is capitalized as phenolic agents hydroquinone and monobenzyl ether of hydroquinone, which can be used in the treatment of melasma and vitiligo, respectively.

Clinical findings are varied and not distinctive; however, confetti-like distribution of small macules is suggestive. In the setting of hand and upper extremity involvement, one should consider occupational exposures as this has been seen in janitors and those exposed more frequently to chemicals from cleaning products. In those with a facial distribution of leukoderma, cosmetic products including makeups and hair dyes should be considered (Fig. 9.13) [143]. Associated pruritus can be seen [144] (Table 9.3).

Histopathologic findings in chemical leukoderma are very similar to those in vitiligo.

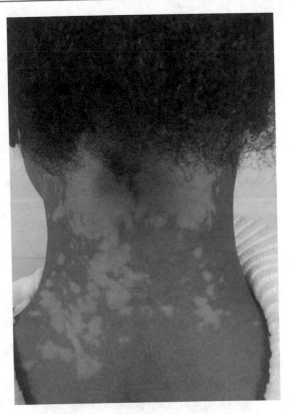

Fig. 9.13 Chemical leukoderma: Hypopigmented and depigmented macules and patches on the posterior neck

Table 9.3 Causes of chemical leukoderma

Causes of chemical leukoderma
Phenol derivatives
Catechol derivatives
P-phenylenediamine
Chemical agents: hair dyes, deodorants, perfumes, detergents, rubber, makeup, insecticides
Occupational exposures
Acrylates

Melanocytes are dramatically decreased or absent. However, chemical leukoderma will lack the lymphocytic infiltrate seen in vitiligo [143].

Considerations for the differential diagnosis include vitiligo and the conditions discussed in this chapter as part of the differential for vitiligo. With cessation of the causative agent, chemical leukoderma tends to have a good prognosis [144].

Genetic Disorders of Hypo-/Depigmentation

Oculocutaneous albinism (OCA) is a group of hereditary disorders with multiple subtypes, OCA1–OCA7. Most forms have an autosomal recessive inheritance pattern. Prevalence is estimated to be as high as 1:17000, with OCA2 as the most common subtype [145]. The disorder results in diffuse loss of pigmentation resulting from a partial or total loss of melanin. OCA has both ocular and cutaneous manifestations. Ocular manifestations include photophobia, nystagmus, and strabismus, and reduction in visual acuity can be seen. The lack of protective melanin in skin predisposes these patients to keratinocytic carcinomas [145].

Piebaldism is caused by mutations in the KIT proto-oncogene. It has an autosomal dominant inheritance. Patients present from birth with depigmented patches, typically toward the central face and body. These lesions remain stable. The more severe form may present with the white forelock or frontal scalp poliosis [146].

Waardenburg syndrome is a rare genetic disorder caused by mutations in genes encoding various transcription factors including *SOX10*, *MITF*, *PAX3*, and *SNAI2*. Four subtypes have been described, and clinical features help to distinguish these subtypes. Clinical features include central white forelock, dystopia canthorum (widening of the distance between the inner canthi), deafness, and heterochromia irides.

The differential diagnosis for these genetic disorders includes all three genetic conditions discussed as well as vitiligo and leukoderma. Associated manifestations of each syndrome can help in distinguishing them from each other [146, 147].

Conclusion

Pigmentary disorders are common yet disfiguring skin conditions that affect millions of people around the world. These disorders are especially prevalent in patients with skin of color. Although there can be overlap in the presentations of these disorders, greater understanding of the clinical and histopathologic features of each condition can help in attaining the proper diagnosis and determining appropriate treatment options.

References

1. Ogbechie-Godec OA, Elbuluk N. Melasma: an up-to-date comprehensive review. Dermatol Ther. 2017;7(3):305–18.
2. Achar A, Rathi SK. Melasma: a clinico-epidemiological study of 312 cases. Indian J Dermatol. 2011;56(4):380–2.
3. Handel AC, Lima PB, Tonolli VM, Miot LD, Miot HA. Risk factors for facial melasma in women: a case-control study. Br J Dermatol. 2014;171(3):588–94.
4. Hernández-Barrera R, Torres-Alvarez B, Castanedo-Cazares JP, Oros-Ovalle C, Moncada B. Solar elastosis and presence of mast cells as key features in the pathogenesis of melasma. Clin Exp Dermatol. 2008;33(3):305–8.
5. Kim JY, Lee TR, Lee AY. Reduced WIF-1 expression stimulates skin hyperpigmentation in patients with melasma. J Invest Dermatol. 2013;133(1):191–200.
6. Kang WH, Yoon KH, Lee E-S, Kim J, Lee KB, Yim H, et al. Melasma: histopathological characteristics in 56 Korean patients. Br J Dermatol. 2002;146(2):228–37.
7. Kim EH, Kim YC, Lee E-S, Kang HY. The vascular characteristics of melasma. J Dermatol Sci. 2007;46(2):111–6.
8. Lee AY. Recent progress in melasma pathogenesis. Pigment Cell Melanoma Res. 2015;28(6):648–60.
9. Ritter CG, Fiss DVC, Borges da Costa JAT, de Carvalho RR, Bauermann G, Cestari TF. Extra-facial melasma: clinical, histopathological, and immunohistochemical case-control study. J Eur Acad Dermatol Venereol. 2013;27(9):1088–94.
10. Sonthalia S, Jha AK, Langar S. Dermoscopy of melasma. Indian Dermatol Online J. 2017;8(6):525–6.
11. Yalamanchili R, Shastry V, Betkerur J. Clinico-epidemiological study and quality of life assessment in melasma. Indian J Dermatol. 2015;60(5):519.
12. Grimes PE, Yamada N, Bhawan J. Light microscopic, immunohistochemical, and ultrastructural alterations in patients with melasma. Am J Dermatopathol. 2005;27(2):96–101.
13. Findlay GH, Morrison JG, Simson IW. Exogenous ochronosis and pigmented colloid milium from hydroquinone bleaching creams. Br J Dermatol. 1975;93(6):613–22.
14. Simmons BJ, Griffith RD, Bray FN, Falto-Aizpurua LA, Nouri K. Exogenous ochronosis: a comprehensive review of the diagnosis, epidemiology, causes, and treatments. Am J Clin Dermatol. 2015;16(3):205–12.

15. Zawar V, Chuh A. Exogenous ochronosis in Asians. Int J Dermatol. 2010;49(1):101; author reply.

16. Penneys NS. Ochronosislike pigmentation from hydroquinone bleaching creams. Arch Dermatol. 1985;121(10):1239–40.

17. Dogliotti M, Leibowitz M. Granulomatous ochronosis – a cosmetic-induced skin disorder in Blacks. S Afr Med J (Suid-Afrikaanse tydskrif vir geneeskunde). 1979;56(19):757–60.

18. Hardwick N, Van Gelder LW, Van der Merwe CA, Van der Merwe MP. Exogenous ochronosis: an epidemiological study. Br J Dermatol. 1989;120(2):229–38.

19. Khunger N, Kandhari R. Dermoscopic criteria for differentiating exogenous ochronosis from melasma. Indian J Dermatol Venereol Leprol. 2013;79(6):819–21.

20. Ramirez C. Los cenicientos: problema clinica. Memoraia del Primer Congresso Centroamericano de Dermatologica, San Salvador. 1957:122–30.

21. Chang SE, Kim HW, Shin JM, Lee JH, Na JI, Roh MR, et al. Clinical and histological aspect of erythema dyschromicum perstans in Korea: a review of 68 cases. J Dermatol. 2015;42(11):1053–7.

22. Errichetti E, Angione V, Stinco G. Dermoscopy in assisting the recognition of ashy dermatosis. JAAD Case Rep. 2017;3(6):482–4.

23. Kumarasinghe SPW, Pandya A, Chandran V, Rodrigues M, Dlova NC, Kang HY, et al. A global consensus statement on ashy dermatosis, erythema dyschromicum perstans, lichen planus pigmentosus, idiopathic eruptive macular pigmentation, and Riehl's melanosis. Int J Dermatol. 2019;58(3):263–72.

24. Kanwar AJ, Dogra S, Handa S, Parsad D, Radotra BD. A study of 124 Indian patients with lichen planus pigmentosus. Clin Exp Dermatol. 2003;28(5):481–5.

25. Dlova NC. Frontal fibrosing alopecia and lichen planus pigmentosus: is there a link? Br J Dermatol. 2013;168(2):439–42.

26. Bhutani LK, Bedi TR, Pandhi RK, Nayak NC. Lichen planus pigmentosus. Dermatologica. 1974;149(1):43–50.

27. Pirmez R, Duque-Estrada B, Donati A, Campos-do-Carmo G, Valente NS, Romiti R, et al. Clinical and dermoscopic features of lichen planus pigmentosus in 37 patients with frontal fibrosing alopecia. Br J Dermatol. 2016;175(6):1387–90.

28. Sharma VK, Gupta V, Pahadiya P, Vedi KK, Arava S, Ramam M. Dermoscopy and patch testing in patients with lichen planus pigmentosus on face: a cross-sectional observational study in fifty Indian patients. Indian J Dermatol Venereol Leprol. 2017;83(6):656–62.

29. Muthu SK, Narang T, Saikia UN, Kanwar AJ, Parsad D, Dogra S. Low-dose oral isotretinoin therapy in lichen planus pigmentosus: an open-label non-randomized prospective pilot study. Int J Dermatol. 2016;55(9):1048–54.

30. Al-Mutairi N, El-Khalawany M. Clinicopathological characteristics of lichen planus pigmentosus and its response to tacrolimus ointment: an open label, non-randomized, prospective study. J Eur Acad Dermatol Venereol: JEADV. 2010;24(5):535–40.

31. Henderson Berg M-H, Pehr K. Familial confluent and reticulated papillomatosis in 2 kindreds including 3 generations. J Cutan Med Surg. 2018;22(3):330–2.

32. Le C, Bedocs PM. Confluent and reticulated papillomatosis. Treasure Island: StatPearls Publishing LLC; 2018.

33. Lim JH, Tey HL, Chong WS. Confluent and reticulated papillomatosis: diagnostic and treatment challenges. Clin Cosmet Investig Dermatol. 2016;9:217–23.

34. Lee MP, Stiller MJ, McClain SA, Shupack JL, Cohen DE. Confluent and reticulated papillomatosis: response to high-dose oral isotretinoin therapy and reassessment of epidemiologic data. J Am Acad Dermatol. 1994;31(2, Part 2):327–31.

35. Hamilton D, Tavafoghi V, Shafer JC, et al. Confluent and reticulated papillomatosis of Gougerot and Carteaud. J Am Acad Dermatol. 1980;2:401–10.

36. Errichetti E, Maione V, Stinco G. Dermatoscopy of confluent and reticulated papillomatosis (Gougerot-Carteaud syndrome). JDDG: J Dtsch Dermatol Ges. 2017;15(8):836–8.

37. Davis MD, Weenig RH, Camilleri MJ. Confluent and reticulate papillomatosis (Gougerot-Carteaud syndrome): a minocycline-responsive dermatosis without evidence for yeast in pathogenesis. A study of 39 patients and a proposal of diagnostic criteria. Br J Dermatol. 2006;154(2):287–93.

38. Bernardes Filho F, Quaresma MV, Rezende FC, Kac BK, Nery JA, Azulay-Abulafia L. Confluent and reticulate papillomatosis of Gougerot-Carteaud and obesity: dermoscopic findings. An Bras Dermatol. 2014;89(3):507–9.

39. Nagashima M. Prurigo pigmentosa--clinical observations of our 14 cases. J Dermatol. 1978;5(2):61–7.

40. Kim JK, Chung WK, Chang SE, Ko JY, Lee JH, Won CH, et al. Prurigo pigmentosa: clinicopathological study and analysis of 50 cases in Korea. J Dermatol. 2012;39(11):891–7.

41. Whang T, Kirkorian AY, Krishtul A, Phelps R, Shim-Chang H. Prurigo pigmentosa: report of two cases in the United States and review of the literature. Dermatol Online J. 2011;17(12):2.

42. Leone L, Colato C, Girolomoni G. Prurigo pigmentosa in a pregnant woman. Int J Gynaecol Obstet. 2007;98(3):261–2.

43. Hanami Y, Yamamoto T. Bullous prurigo pigmentosa in a pregnant woman with hyperemesis gravidarum. J Dermatol. 2015;42(4):436–7.

44. Choi JR, Kim JK, Won CH, Lee MW, Oh ES, Chang S. Prurigo pigmentosa treated with Jessner's peel and irradiation with an 830-nm light-emitting diode. J Dermatol. 2012;39(5):493–6.

45. Beutler BD, Cohen PR, Lee RA. Prurigo pigmentosa: literature review. Am J Clin Dermatol. 2015;16(6):533–43.

46. Satter E, Rozelle C, Sperling L. Prurigo pigmentosa: an under-recognized inflammatory dermatosis characterized by an evolution of distinctive clinicopathological features. J Cutan Pathol. 2016;43(10):809–14.

47. Silpa-archa N, Kohli I, Chaowattanapanit S, Lim HW, Hamzavi I. Postinflammatory hyperpigmentation: a comprehensive overview. J Am Acad Dermatol. 2017;77(4):591–605.

48. Ruiz-Maldonado R, Orozco-Covarrubias ML. Postinflammatory hypopigmentation and hyperpigmentation. Semin Cutan Med Surg. 1997;16(1): 36–43.

49. Nordlund JJ. Postinflammatory hyperpigmentation. Dermatol Clin. 1988;6(2):185–92.

50. Güngör Ş, Erdemir AV, Göncü EK, Gürel MS, Özekinci S. A case of dyskeratosis congenita with dermoscopic and reflectance confocal microscopic features. J Am Acad Dermatol. 2015;73(1):e11–e3.

51. Garofola C, Gross GP. Dyskeratosis congenita. Treasure Island: StatPearls Publishing LLC; 2018.

52. Papini M. Natural history of the Naegeli-Franceschetti-Jadassohn syndrome. J Am Acad Dermatol. 1994;31(5 Pt 1):830.

53. Itin PH, Burger B. Spontaneous fading of reticular pigmentation in Naegeli-Franceschetti-Jadassohn syndrome. Dermatology. 2010;221(2):135–6.

54. CCEA. Dowling-Degos disease: classic clinical and histopathological presentation. An Bras Dermatol. 2011;86(5):979–82.

55. Rice AS, Cook C. Dowling Degos disease. Treasure Island: StatPearls Publishing LLC; 2018.

56. Kim YC, Davis MD, Schanbacher CF, Su WP. Dowling-Degos disease (reticulate pigmented anomaly of the flexures): a clinical and histopathologic study of 6 cases. J Am Acad Dermatol. 1999;40(3):462–7.

57. Patel LM, Lambert PJ, Gagna CE, Maghari A, Lambert WC. Cutaneous signs of systemic disease. Clin Dermatol. 2011;29(5):511–22.

58. Pokhrel B, Bhusal K. Graves disease. Treasure Island: StatPearls Publishing LLC; 2018.

59. Bhushan P, Manjul P, Baliyan V. Flagellate dermatoses. Indian J Dermatol Venereol Leprol. 2014;80(2):149–52.

60. Yajima I, Ahsan N, Akhand AA, Al Hossain MA, Yoshinaga M, Ohgami N, et al. Arsenic levels in cutaneous appendicular organs are correlated with digitally evaluated hyperpigmented skin of the forehead but not the sole in Bangladesh residents. J Expo Sci Environ Epidemiol. 2018;28(1):64–8.

61. Sengupta S, Das N, Datta P. Pathogenesis, clinical features and pathology of chronic arsenicosis. Indian J Dermatol Venereol Leprol. 2008;74(6):559–70.

62. Raychaudhuri SP, Raychaudhuri S. The blue nails of argyria. Int J Dermatol. 2014;53(9):e400–e1.

63. Beutler BD, Lee RA, Cohen PR. Localized cutaneous argyria: report of two patients and literature review. Dermatol Online J. 2016;22(11).

64. Granstein RD, Sober AJ. Drug- and heavy metal-induced hyperpigmentation. J Am Acad Dermatol. 1981;5(1):1–18.

65. Geria AN, Tajirian AL, Kihiczak G, Schwartz RA. Minocycline-induced skin pigmentation: an update. Acta Dermatovenerol Croat: ADC. 2009;17(2):123–6.

66. Berry M, Khachemoune A. Extensive tinea versicolor mimicking Pityriasis rubra pilaris. J Drugs Dermatol: JDD. 2009;8(5):490–1.

67. Child, Fuller, Higgins, Vivier D. A study of the spectrum of skin disease occurring in a black population in south-east London. Br J Dermatol. 1999;141(3):512–7.

68. Rao G, Kuruvilla M, Kumar P, Vinod V. Clinico-epidermiological studies on tinea versicolor. Indian J Dermatol Venereol Leprol. 2002;68(4):208–9.

69. Kallini JR, Riaz F, Khachemoune A. Tinea versicolor in dark-skinned individuals. Int J Dermatol. 2014;53(2):137–41.

70. Prohic A, Jovovic Sadikovic T, Krupalija-Fazlic M, Kuskunovic-Vlahovljak S. Malassezia species in healthy skin and in dermatological conditions. Int J Dermatol. 2016;55(5):494–504.

71. Borgers M, Cauwenbergh G, Van De Ven M-A, Hernanz AP, Degreef H. Pityriasis versicolor and pityrosporum ovale. Int J Dermatol. 1987;26(9):586–9.

72. Ajaykrishnan, Thappa DM. Morphological and pigmentary variations of tinea versicolor in South Indian patients. Indian J Dermatol. 2003;48(02):83–6.

73. Zhou H, Tang XH, De Han J, Chen M-K. Dermoscopy as an ancillary tool for the diagnosis of pityriasis versicolor. J Am Acad Dermatol. 2015;73(6):e205–e6.

74. Lesueur A, Garcia-Granel V, Helenon R, Cales-Quist D. Progressive macular confluent hypomelanosis in mixed ethnic melanodermic subjects: an epidemiologic study of 511 patients. Ann Dermatol Venereol. 1994;121(12):880–3.

75. Westerhof W, Relyveld GN, Kingswijk MM, de Man P, Menke HE. Propionibacterium acnes and the pathogenesis of progressive macular hypomelanosis. Arch Dermatol. 2004;140(2):210–4.

76. Guillet G, Helenon R, Gauthier Y, Surleve-Bazeille JE, Plantin P, Sassolas B. Progressive macular hypomelanosis of the trunk: primary acquired hypopigmentation. J Cutan Pathol. 1988;15(5):286–9.

77. Duarte I, Nina BID, Gordiano MC, Buense R, Lazzarini R. Hipomelanose macular progressiva: estudo epidemiológico e resposta terapêutica à fototerapia. An Bras Dermatol. 2010;85:621–4.

78. Cavalcanti SM, de Franca ER, Lins AK, Magalhaes M, de Alencar ER, Magalhaes V. Investigation of Propionibacterium acnes in progressive macular hypomelanosis using real-time PCR and culture. Int J Dermatol. 2011;50(11):1347–52.

79. Barnard E, Liu J, Yankova E, Cavalcanti SM, Magalhaes M, Li H, et al. Strains of the

Propionibacterium acnes type III lineage are associated with the skin condition progressive macular hypomelanosis. Sci Rep. 2016;6:31968.

80. Pflederer RT, Wuennenberg JP, Foote C, Aires D, Rajpara A. Use of Wood's lamp to diagnose progressive macular hypomelanosis. J Am Acad Dermatol. 2017;77(4):e99–e100.

81. Wu X-G, Xu A-E, Song X-Z, Zheng J-H, Wang P, Shen H. Clinical, pathologic, and ultrastructural studies of progressive macular hypomelanosis. Int J Dermatol. 2010;49(10):1127–32.

82. Tomimori-Yamashita J, Maeda SM, Sunderkotter C, Kaminsky SK, Michalany NS, Rotta O, et al. Leukomelanodermic leprosy. Int J Dermatol. 2002;41(8):513–5.

83. Massone C, Cavalchini A, Clapasson A, Nunzi E. Hypopigmented macules: leprosy, atopy or pityriasis versicolor? Giornale italiano di dermatologia e venereologia: organo ufficiale. Societa italiana di dermatologia e sifilografia. 2010;145(6):779–82.

84. Nehal KS, PeBenito R, Orlow SJ. Analysis of 54 cases of hypopigmentation and hyperpigmentation along the lines of blaschko. Arch Dermatol. 1996;132(10):1167–70.

85. Lee H-S, Chun Y-S, Hann S-K. Nevus depigmentosus: clinical features and histopathologic characteristics in 67 patients. J Am Acad Dermatol. 1999;40(1):21–6.

86. Oiso N, Kawara S, Kawada A. Acquired melanocytic naevus in naevus depigmentosus. Clin Exp Dermatol. 2009;34(7):e311–e2.

87. Zhang W, Chen H, Sun J. Development of lentigines within nevus depigmentosus. J Dermatol. 2012;39(11):928–30.

88. Bolognia JL, Pawelek JM. Biology of hypopigmentation. J Am Acad Dermatol. 1988;19(2 Pt 1):217–55.

89. Coupe RL. Unilateral systematized achromic naevus. Dermatologica. 1967;134(1):19–35.

90. Kim SK, Kang HY, Lee E-S, Kim YC. Clinical and histopathologic characteristics of nevus depigmentosus. J Am Acad Dermatol. 2006;55(3):423–8.

91. Jimbow K, Fitzpatrick TB, Szabo G, Hori Y. Congenital circumscribed hypomelanosis: a characterization based on Electron microscopic study of tuberous sclerosis, nevus depigmentosus, and piebaldism. J Investig Dermatol. 1975;64(1):50–62.

92. Juntongjin P, Laosakul K. Idiopathic guttate hypomelanosis: a review of its etiology, pathogenesis, findings, and treatments. Am J Clin Dermatol. 2016;17(4):403–11.

93. Shin MK, Jeong KH, Oh IH, Choe BK, Lee MH. Clinical features of idiopathic guttate hypomelanosis in 646 subjects and association with other aspects of photoaging. Int J Dermatol. 2011;50(7):798–805.

94. Friedland R, David M, Feinmesser M, Fenig-Nakar S, Hodak E. Idiopathic guttate hypomelanosis-like lesions in patients with mycosis fungoides: a new adverse effect of phototherapy. J Eur Acad Dermatol Venereol: JEADV. 2010;24(9):1026–30.

95. Kumarasinghe SP. 3–5 second cryotherapy is effective in idiopathic guttate hypomelanosis. J Dermatol. 2004;31(5):437–9.

96. Errichetti E, Stinco G. Dermoscopy of idiopathic guttate hypomelanosis. J Dermatol. 2015;42(11):1118–9.

97. Ankad BS, Beergouder SL. Dermoscopic evaluation of idiopathic guttate hypomelanosis: a preliminary observation. Indian Dermatol Online J. 2015;6(3):164–7.

98. Kim SK, Kim EH, Kang HY, Lee ES, Sohn S, Kim YC. Comprehensive understanding of idiopathic guttate hypomelanosis: clinical and histopathological correlation. Int J Dermatol. 2010;49(2): 162–6.

99. Watkins DB. Pityriasis alba: a form of atopic dermatitis: a preliminary report. Arch Dermatol. 1961;83(6):915–9.

100. Wahab MA, Rahman MH, Khondker L, Hawlader AR, Ali A, Hafiz MA, et al. Minor criteria for atopic dermatitis in children. Mymensingh Med J: MMJ. 2011;20(3):419–24.

101. Hanifin JM, Rajka G. Diagnostic features of atopic dermatitis. Acta Derm Venereol (Stockh) Suppl. 1980;92:44–7.

102. Dogra S, Kumar B. Epidemiology of skin diseases in school children: a study from northern India. Pediatr Dermatol. 2003;20(6):470–3.

103. Blessmann Weber M, Sponchiado de Ávila L, Albaneze R, Magalhães de Oliveira O, Sudhaus B, Ferreira Cestari T. Pityriasis alba: a study of pathogenic factors. J Eur Acad Dermatol Venereol. 2002;16(5):463–8.

104. Miazek N, Michalek I, Pawlowska-Kisiel M, Olszewska M, Rudnicka L. Pityriasis alba--common disease, enigmatic entity: up-to-date review of the literature. Pediatr Dermatol. 2015;32(6):786–91.

105. Vargas-Ocampo F. Pityriasis alba: a histologic study. Int J Dermatol. 1993;32(12):870–3.

106. In SI, Yi SW, Kang HY, Lee ES, Sohn S, Kim YC. Clinical and histopathological characteristics of pityriasis alba. Clin Exp Dermatol. 2009;34(5):591–7.

107. Gerke AK, Judson MA, Cozier YC, Culver DA, Koth LL. Disease burden and variability in sarcoidosis. Ann Am Thorac Soc. 2017;14(Supplement_6):S421–s8.

108. García-Colmenero L, Sánchez-Schmidt JM, Barranco C, Pujol RM. The natural history of cutaneous sarcoidosis. Clinical spectrum and histological analysis of 40 cases. Int J Dermatol. 2019;58(2):178–84.

109. Ahmed I, Harshad SR. Subcutaneous sarcoidosis: is it a specific subset of cutaneous sarcoidosis frequently associated with systemic disease? J Am Acad Dermatol. 2006;54(1):55–60.

110. Spiteri MA, Matthey F, Gordon T, Carstairs LS, James DG. Lupus pernio: a clinico-radiological study of thirty-five cases. Br J Dermatol. 1985;112(3):315–22.

111. Brown F, Tanner LS. Lofgren syndrome. Treasure Island: StatPearls Publishing LLC; 2018.

112. Fernandez-Faith E, McDonnell J. Cutaneous sarcoidosis: differential diagnosis. Clin Dermatol. 2007;25(3):276–87.

113. Alexis JB. Sarcoidosis presenting as cutaneous hypopigmentation with repeatedly negative skin biopsies. Int J Dermatol. 1994;33(1):44–5.

114. Hall RS, Floro JF, King LE Jr. Hypopigmented lesions in sarcoidosis. J Am Acad Dermatol. 1984;11(6):1163–4.

115. Hubler WR Jr. Hypomelanotic canopy of sarcoidosis. Cutis. 1977;19(1):86–8.

116. Wanat KA, Rosenbach M. Cutaneous sarcoidosis. Clin Chest Med. 2015;36(4):685–702.

117. Amorim GM, Niemeyer-Corbellini JP, Quintella DC, Cuzzi T, Ramos-e-Silva M. Hypopigmented mycosis fungoides: a 20-case retrospective series. Int J Dermatol. 2018;57(3):306–12.

118. Virmani P, Levin L, Myskowski PL, Flores E, Marchetti MA, Lucas AS, et al. Clinical outcome and prognosis of young patients with mycosis fungoides. Pediatr Dermatol. 2017;34(5):547–53.

119. Rodney IJ, Kindred C, Angra K, Qutub ON, Villanueva AR, Halder RM. Hypopigmented mycosis fungoides: a retrospective clinicohistopathologic study. J Eur Acad Dermatol Venereol: JEADV. 2017;31(5):808–14.

120. Pradhan D, Jedrych JJ, Ho J, Akilov OE. Hypopigmented mycosis fungoides with large cell transformation in a child. Pediatr Dermatol. 2017;34(5):e260–e4.

121. Youssef R, Mahgoub D, Zeid OA, Abdel-Halim DM, El-Hawary M, Hussein MF, et al. Hypopigmented interface T-cell dyscrasia and hypopigmented mycosis fungoides: a comparative study. Am J Dermatopathol. 2018;40(10):727–35.

122. Taieb A, Picardo M. The definition and assessment of vitiligo: a consensus report of the Vitiligo European Task Force. Pigment Cell Res. 2007;20(1):27–35.

123. Dwivedi M, Laddha NC, Shajil EM, Shah BJ, Begum R. The ACE gene I/D polymorphism is not associated with generalized vitiligo susceptibility in Gujarat population. Pigment Cell Melanoma Res. 2008;21(3):407–8.

124. Dogra S, Parsad D, Handa S, Kanwar AJ. Late onset vitiligo: a study of 182 patients. Int J Dermatol. 2005;44(3):193–6.

125. Onunu AN, Kubeyinje EP. Vitiligo in the Nigerian African: a study of 351 patients in Benin City, Nigeria. Int J Dermatol. 2003;42(10):800–2.

126. Foley LM, Lowe NJ, Misheloff E, Tiwari JL. Association of HLA-DR4 with vitiligo. J Am Acad Dermatol. 1983;8(1):39–40.

127. Liu JB, Li M, Chen H, Zhong SQ, Yang S, Du WD, et al. Association of vitiligo with HLA-A2: a meta-analysis. J Eur Acad Dermatol Venereol: JEADV. 2007;21(2):205–13.

128. Kemp EH, Ajjan RA, Waterman EA, Gawkrodger DJ, Cork MJ, Watson PF, Weetman AP. Analysis of a microsatellite polymorphism of the cytotoxic T-lymphocyte antigen-4 gene in patients with vitiligo. Br J Dermatol. 1999;140(1):73–8.

129. Cantón I, Akhtar S, Gavalas NG, Gawkrodger DJ, Blomhoff A, Watson PF, et al. A single-nucleotide polymorphism in the gene encoding lymphoid protein tyrosine phosphatase (PTPN22) confers susceptibility to generalised vitiligo. Genes Immun. 2005;6:584.

130. Spritz RA, Andersen GH. Genetics of vitiligo. Dermatol Clin. 2017;35(2):245–55.

131. Alkhateeb A, Fain PR, Thody A, Bennett DC, Spritz RA. Epidemiology of vitiligo and associated autoimmune diseases in Caucasian probands and their families. Pigment Cell Res. 2003;16(3):208–14.

132. Alikhan A, Felsten LM, Daly M, Petronic-Rosic V. Vitiligo: a comprehensive overview Part I. Introduction, epidemiology, quality of life, diagnosis, differential diagnosis, associations, histopathology, etiology, and work-up. J Am Acad Dermatol. 2011;65(3):473–91.

133. Dillon AB, Sideris A, Hadi A, Elbuluk N. Advances in vitiligo: an update on medical and surgical treatments. J Clin Aesthet Dermatol. 2017;10(1):15–28.

134. Mason CP, Gawkrodger DJ. Vitiligo presentation in adults. Clin Exp Dermatol. 2005;30(4):344–5.

135. Manolache L, Benea V. Stress in patients with alopecia areata and vitiligo. J Eur Acad Dermatol Venereol. 2007;21(7):921–8.

136. Asawanonda P, Taylor CR. Wood's light in dermatology. Int J Dermatol. 1999;38(11):801–7.

137. Ezzedine K, Lim HW, Suzuki T, Katayama I, Hamzavi I, Lan CCE, et al. Revised classification/nomenclature of vitiligo and related issues: the vitiligo global issues consensus conference. Pigment Cell Melanoma Res. 2012;25(3):E1–E13.

138. Rodrigues M, Ezzedine K, Hamzavi I, Pandya AG, Harris JE. New discoveries in the pathogenesis and classification of vitiligo. J Am Acad Dermatol. 2017;77(1):1–13.

139. Kumar Jha A, Sonthalia S, Lallas A, Chaudhary RKP. Dermoscopy in vitiligo: diagnosis and beyond. Int J Dermatol. 2018;57(1):50–4.

140. Seleit I, Bakry OA, Abdou AG, Dawoud NM. Immunohistochemical study of melanocyte-melanocyte stem cell lineage in vitiligo; a clue to interfollicular melanocyte stem cell reservoir. Ultrastruct Pathol. 2014;38(3):186–98.

141. Kim YC, Kim YJ, Kang HY, Sohn S, Lee ES. Histopathologic features in vitiligo. Am J Dermatopathol. 2008;30(2):112–6.

142. Sheth VM, Guo Y, Qureshi AA. Comorbidities associated with vitiligo: a ten-year retrospective study. Dermatology. 2013;227(4):311–5.

143. Bonamonte D, Vestita M, Romita P, Filoni A, Foti C, Angelini G. Chemical leukoderma. Dermatitis. 2016;27(3):90–9.

144. Ghosh S, Mukhopadhyay S. Chemical leucoderma: a clinico-aetiological study of 864 cases in the perspective of a developing country. Br J Dermatol. 2009;160(1):40–7.

145. Federico JR, Krishnamurthy K. Albinism. Treasure Island: StatPearls Publishing LLC; 2018.

146. Oiso N, Fukai K, Kawada A, Suzuki T. Piebaldism. J Dermatol. 2013;40(5):330–5.

147. Que SK, Weston G, Suchecki J, Ricketts J. Pigmentary disorders of the eyes and skin. Clin Dermatol. 2015;33(2):147–58.

Management of Pigmentary Disorders

10

Lauren C. Payne, Kamaria Nelson, and Valerie D. Callender

Post-inflammatory Hypopigmentation

Post-inflammatory hypopigmentation (PIH) is an acquired consequence of prior skin inflammation, trauma, or exposure to an outside agent that leads to partial or complete loss of pigmentation in the skin. The extent of pigment loss directly correlates with the severity of the inciting process. Though PIH occurs in both sexes and all ethnicities, some individuals are more susceptible to developing PIH than others. It is also more clinically appreciable in dark-skinned individuals. PIH lesions present as hypopigmented macules or patches on virtually any area of the skin from the head to toe in an area of prior skin affliction (Fig. 10.1). Associated overlying epidermal and surface change may or may not be

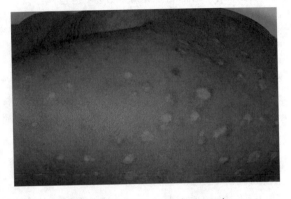

Fig. 10.1 Post-inflammatory hypopigmentation

present, dependent upon depth of involvement of the inciting event.

The specific cause of acquired PIH as a result of skin injury remains to be completely elucidated; however, it is suspected that susceptibility is genetically predetermined in an autosomal dominant fashion with some individuals possessing melanocytes that are more at risk of damage due to stressful events and inflammation [1]. It is hypothesized that PIH occurs mainly due to inhibition of melanogenesis; however, in some conditions, direct destruction of melanocytes leading to permanent hypo- or depigmented lesions can also occur.

There are many underlying skin conditions that result in PIH. These categories include inflammatory skin diseases such as atopic dermatitis, pityriasis alba, psoriasis, sarcoidosis, lichen striatus,

L. C. Payne (✉)
Veteran Affairs Medical Center, Howard University Hospital, George Washington University, Department of Dermatology, Washington, DC, USA
e-mail: lauren.payne@cmmpmed.org

K. Nelson
George Washington University, Medical Faculty Associates, Department of Dermatology, Washington, DC, USA

V. D. Callender
Howard University College of Medicine, Department of Dermatology, Washington, DC, USA

Callender Dermatology & Cosmetic Center, Glenn Dale, MD, USA

© Springer Nature Switzerland AG 2021
B. S. Li, H. I. Maibach (eds.), *Ethnic Skin and Hair and Other Cultural Considerations*, Updates in Clinical Dermatology, https://doi.org/10.1007/978-3-030-64830-5_10

and pityriasis lichenoides chronica. Cutaneous infections such as secondary syphilis, tuberculosis, leprosy, tinea versicolor, and mycobacteria can also cause lesions of hypopigmentation. Connective tissue disorders like Lichen Sclerosus et. Atrophicus (LS&A) and scleroderma can also present with hypopigmented skin areas. Along with inflammatory skin disease and infection, prior physical trauma can cause PIH lesions, including exposure to various chemicals such as phenols, corticosteroids, monobenzyl ether of hydroquinone (MBEH), and chemical peels, as well as physical trauma through accidental injury, cryotherapy, dermabrasion, and lasers [2–4].

Investigation of hypopigmented lesions to distinguish PIH lesions secondary to injury/trauma or chemical exposure from other more serious diseases or infections that lead to hypopigmentation is vital. Clinical examination should include evaluation of the area with a Wood's lamp to distinguish PIH from depigmented fluorescent lesions of vitiligo, coppery orange fluorescent lesions of progressive macular hypomelanosis, and yellowish fluorescence seen in tinea versicolor. Histopathologic evaluation is also important to rule out underlying conditions that can present with hypopigmented lesions such as lupus, mycosis fungoides (MF), and sarcoidosis that have distinguishing path findings. Histology of PIH lesions is nonspecific and can include a mild to severe lymphohistiocytic infiltrate, reduction in dermal melanin, and scattered melanophages.

Regarding treatment of PIH, it is important to first identify the underlying culprit. Once that has been treated, hypopigmentation will most often gradually resolve on its own over time. Preparations containing both a topical steroid and tar have been reported to aid in repigmentation of PIH lesions, with the steroid addressing residual inflammation and tar inducing melanin production [5, 6]. Topical calcineurin inhibitors have also been reported to treat PIH associated with seborrheic dermatitis in one open label, pilot trial. Pimecrolimus 1% cream was applied to affected areas twice daily for 16 weeks leading to improvement of PIH [7]. Ultraviolet light exposure can also aid in repigmentation of PIH

lesions; however, it can also enhance contrast with the surrounding skin as that often also becomes tanned through the same light exposure. Topical 0.1–0.5% 8-methoxypsoralen, coal tar, or anthralin in combination with UVA exposure has been reported to improve PIH. 8-methoxypsoralen compounded in Aquaphor is applied to the affected areas of PIH for 20–30 min, followed by exposure of these areas to UVA light at an initial dose of 0.2–0.5 J/cm^2 1–3 times weekly. The dose is increased by 0.2–0.5 J/cm^2 weekly until improvement is noted, and then the dose is maintained [8, 9]. Reports of improvement in PIH with the 308 nm excimer laser have also been noted to induce pigmentation in hypopigmented scars, with a reported response of 60–70% after 9 weeks of treatments twice weekly. Maintenance treatments will likely be needed every 1–4 months to maintain pigmentation. For extensive cases of PIH, NB-UVB has also been shown to lead to repigmentation of hypopigmented lesions, especially in cases of vitiligo [10]. Cosmetic makeup, self-tanning products, and tattooing may be alternative camouflage options available for some patients. Surgical grafting of tissue or cells can also be considered in vitiligo lesions.

Hypopigmented Mycosis Fungoides

Mycosis fungoides is the most common type of primary cutaneous T cell lymphoma, accounting for up to 60% of all cases [11]. It mainly affects the skin, with minimal systemic involvement until advanced stages. The mean age of onset in most cases is during the fifth decade, with various clinical presentations, including patches, plaques, granulomatous, folliculotropic, and ichthyosiform lesions [12, 13].

One additional subtype, hypopigmented mycosis fungoides (HMF), is a unique variant in that it differs from the other types of cutaneous T cell lymphoma in several ways. First, hypopigmented MF usually presents in the younger population, for which the average age of onset is in the second to third decade of life [14]. It most commonly presents as asymptomatic hypopig-

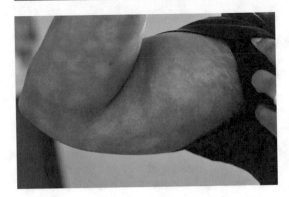

Fig. 10.2 Hypopigmented mycosis fungoides

mented to slightly scaly patches and plaques mainly localized to the proximal lower body (i.e., buttocks, upper thighs) and trunk (Fig. 10.2). Occasional involvement of the face and upper extremities can occur [15, 16].

Histopathologic findings of HMF include focal parakeratosis, minimal to absent spongiosis, with a lymphocytic infiltrate in the upper dermis with epidermotropism. Pautrier microabscesses are rare. The malignant cell population in HMF is mainly composed of clonal CD8 T cells, which differs from the CD4 T cells most commonly found in classic MF. It is suspected that these neoplastic cells attack and destroy melanocytes leading to their destruction and decreased melanogenesis, contributing to the hypopigmentation of the affected areas (HMF [17, 18]).

Along with a skin biopsy to confirm the diagnosis, patients with HFM should also be evaluated with a complete blood count and peripheral blood smear to identify the presence of Sezary cells, as well as T cell clonal population using flow cytometry.

Since HMF is typically skin limited, treatment is mainly targeted toward the skin only. Limited skin involvement (<10% BSA) can be treated with topical steroids and calcineurin inhibitors, nitrogen mustard, bexarotene, mechlorethamine, and carmustine. For more advanced cases with >10% BSA involvement, combination treatment is often recommended including both topical medications and phototherapy (both UVA and NB-UVB) [19–23]. In one study, more patients

reported preference for NB-UVB phototherapy over UVA for treatment of Stage 1A disease, and this is often the preferred treatment for clinicians as well, due to lower side effect profile [24].

Pityriasis Alba

Pityriasis alba (p alba) is a common benign skin condition presenting with round or oval slightly scaly hypopigmented patches most commonly found on the face (especially cheeks) and upper trunk of children and adolescents, ranging from 3 to 16 years old [25–27] (Fig. 10.3). Occasionally, patients may report of mild pruritis, but most times, lesions are asymptomatic. There is no known racial predilection of p alba; however, lesions are more appreciable in patients with darker skin types and can also be accentuated with UV exposure during the summer months.

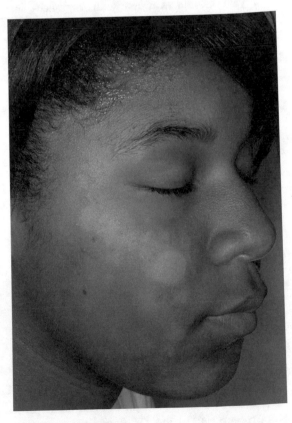

Fig. 10.3 Pityriasis alba

Oftentimes, patients also report a history of atopic dermatitis. Pigmentation of the lesions will spontaneously return over time, usually within 1 year.

Histopathologic findings of p alba include hyperkeratosis, parakeratosis, acanthosis, and spongiosis, with a mild perivascular infiltrate. The hypopigmentation is due to reduced melanin in the basal layer with decreased number of active melanocytes, as well as decreased number and size of melanosomes. The number of total melanocytes, however, is not decreased [28–30]. It is important to rule out underlying causes of hypopigmentation patches in children including tinea versicolor, vitiligo, seborrheic dermatitis, hypopigmented mycosis fungoides, and nevus depigmentosus. This can be done via evaluation of lesions with a Wood's lamp, KOH prep, and skin biopsy.

Treatment of p alba is not required as it most commonly spontaneously resolves over time on its own, though often taking several months to up to 1 year. Gentle skin care with fragrance- and dye-free products should be encouraged. Low-potency topical steroids, calcineurin inhibitors, and topical vitamin D analogs such as calcitriol can be used to reduce associated erythema or pruritis and accelerate repigmentation of the area [31, 32]. The excimer 308 nm laser can also be used for isolated areas to promote repigmentation [33]. Sunscreen should also be applied to the affected and surrounding area to minimize risk of sunburn and decrease darkening of the surrounding skin.

Tinea Versicolor

Tinea versicolor (TV) is a common superficial dermatophyte infection caused by fungi from the *Malassezia* genus. The most common species causing the condition is *M. globosa* followed *M. furfur*. *Malassezia* is commonly found on the skin but becomes pathogenic when it is converted from the yeast to the mycelial form [34]. Worldwide prevalence is 1–4% in temperate climates and 30–40% in tropical areas [35]. Recurrence rate of the TV after discontinuation of treatments can be up to 80% in the first 2 years

[36]. There is no known gender or racial predilection; however, the condition might be more visible in darker-skinned individuals. The classic clinical presentation is annular and oval-shaped hypo-/hyperpigmented and even pink scaly plaques occurring most commonly on the trunk, neck, upper arms, and occasionally the face (Fig. 10.4). Often these lesions are asymptomatic; however, patients may also report of mild pruritis [37]. Patients also report that the conditions recur and are most pruritic with heat and moist conditions.

The hypopigmentation that commonly occurs in TV is due to inhibition of tyrosinase by dicarboxylic acid, which is produced by *Malassezia*. In addition, it is also hypothesized that the fungus damages melanocytes and causes accumulation of material in the stratum corneum which blocks ultraviolet light [38]. The hypopigmentation may persist for several months even after the fungus has been cleared.

Malassezia is usually eradicated by T cells in immunocompetent individuals; however, certain environmental conditions support its overgrowth including heat and humidity, as well as the use of oily topical preparations, and genetic predisposition [39].

Diagnosis of TV is most often made clinically due to its classic presentation; however, a KOH preparation of scaling from an active lesion can also reveal fungal elements in the stratum corneum, often referred to as "spaghetti and meatballs." Wood's lamp evaluation can also reveal a bright yellow or gold fluorescence of TV lesions.

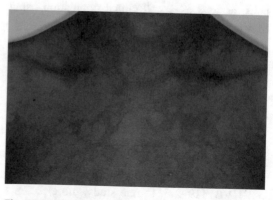

Fig. 10.4 Tinea versicolor

Treatment of tinea versicolor most commonly includes topical antifungal and non-antifungal shampoos and creams. Nonspecific antifungals include selenium sulfide, salicylic acid, zinc pyrithione, and ciclopirox in various preparations including shampoos, lotions, foams, and creams. Direct antifungal creams and shampoos are also used including clotrimazole, ketoconazole, and terbinafine applied daily to twice daily for up to 14 days with up to 80% clearance [37]. In certain recalcitrant cases, oral antifungals might be indicated, including fluconazole and itraconazole. Standard itraconazole dosing is 200 mg per day for 7 days with 80% clearance [40]. Fluconazole dosed at 300 mg/week × 2 weeks leads to 97% cure rate [39]. Pramiconazole is a new oral antifungal that is currently being investigated as a future TV treatment [41]. Prophylactic treatment with weekly or monthly use of a topical or oral antifungals might also be beneficial in patients who often have recurrent episodes of TV. Several case reports have noted a possible role of NB-UVB phototherapy in TV treatment [42].

Progressive Macular Hypomelanosis

Progressive macular hypomelanosis (PMH) is an [...] of hypopigmentation. It classi[...] [...]ymptomatic hypopigmented [...]atches on the trunk and [...]ccasional involvement [...] Fig. 10.5). There is

usually no preceding identifiable skin condition in areas of involvement [44]. Pathogenesis of PMH has not been definitively elucidated; however, multiple studies report a causal relationship between the Type III strain of *Propionibacterium acnes*, a Gram-positive anaerobic rod, and the development of PMH. Prior studies have shown that biopsies from PMH hypopigmented skin revealed *P. acnes* in pilosebaceous ducts, which were absent in non-lesional skin. Lesional skin also revealed coppery-orange/red fluorescence, indicating the presence of P. *acnes* [45]. The hypopigmentation within the lesions is thought to be due to both a decrease in melanin production and change in melanosome distribution (favoring aggregated or clustered melanosomes instead of the usually single dispersed pattern), both leading to a decrease in epidermal melanin and subsequent hypopigmentation.

Histologic examination of PMH often reveals normal skin, with only very mild decrease in epidermal melanin pigment. PMH is a diagnosis of exclusion after other conditions with similar presentations have been ruled out, including tinea versicolor, mycosis fungoides, seborrheic dermatitis, pityriasis alba, and leprosy. Wood's lamp evaluation can also reveal coral red fluorescence of PMH lesions [44].

Given the presence of *P. acne* bacteria in lesional skin, suggested treatment of PMH often incudes antibacterial medications, including benzoyl peroxide and clindamycin, with various improvements reported, ranging from 30% to 80% over 8–12 months, with no recurrence or relapse up to 2 years after [45]. Spontaneous resolution has also been reported in some cases, usually taking at least 1 year. Other reported successful treatments of PMH include NB-UVB phototherapy with response rate of up to 50–90% of patients having up to 90% repigmentation. The typical protocol is NB-UVB phototherapy twice weekly for at least 3 months to note improvement [...]. In multiple studies, an initial response t[...] [...]ent is seen after an average of six tre[...] [...] sessions. Maximum repigmentation t[...] [...]ally occurs after 22 sessions. If no improve[...] is noted after 3–6 months, the treatment s[...] be considered a failure and discontinue[...]

mechanism of action for NB-UVB treatment is thought to be due to both a stimulated release of inflammatory markers that help to eradicate *P. acnes* and stimulating residual melanocytes to increase melanin production [47]. Along with phototherapy and antibiotics as treatment for PMH, one case report noted a patient's PMH responding and resolving with low-dose isotretinoin 10 mg/day after 1 month of treatment, which remained clear at 10 months follow-up. The potential mechanism for isotretinoin's treatment of PMH is through its inhibitory effect on sebum production and reduced *P. acnes* colonization, leading to repigmentation [48]. In most cases of PMH, patients are treated with a combination of treatments, including both topical antibiotics and phototherapy for maximum benefit.

Idiopathic Guttate Hypomelanosis

Idiopathic guttate hypomelanosis (IGH) is a benign dermatosis characterized by scattered hypopigmented round to oval macules often identified on the extremities of older individuals with up to 80% of patients over the age of 40 [49, 50] (Fig. 10.6). Lesions are usually asymptomatic and have no overlying surface changes. There is no racial predilection; however, lesions are often more noticeable in darker skin types. The pathogenesis of IGH is unknown, but it is thought to be due to a combination of both genetic and environmental factors. Sun exposure has often been reported as a causative factor; however, this has

not been fully elucidated. Genetics has also been identified as a contributing factor, as reports have shown IGH lesions in patients with a positive family history [51]. Repeated trauma has also been proposed as a precipitating cause of IGH lesions, explaining common areas of involvement including the anterior tibia which are often subject to accidental external trauma.

The underlying mechanism behind the hypopigmentation in IGH lesions may be due to a slight reduction in the overall total number of melanocytes. Other findings in IGH lesions might also include decreased tyrosinase activity, decreased number of melanosomes, or abnormal keratinocyte uptake of melanosomes [52]. There may also be a mild mononuclear inflammatory infiltrate in some lesion samples. Diagnosis of IGH is most commonly made via clinical observation alone; however, if a biopsy is conducted, it will likely reveal hyperkeratosis, an atrophic epidermis, flattened rete ridges, and a decrease in the number of active melanocytes in the basal layer of the epidermis and decreased melanin production [51].

Given that lesions of IGH are asymptomatic and benign, no treatment is necessary. However, because it is thought that sunlight is a contributing factor, sunscreen and sun protection with physical barriers are important. Other reported treatments to improve IGH lesions have in[...] cryotherapy, topical calcineurin inhibitor[...] cal retinoids, as well as excimer laser [...] Fractional CO_2 laser and dermabrasion [...] been reported as potential treatment[...] lesions with variable results [56]. [...] Wambier demonstrated repigment[...] lesions after microinfusing 5-fluo[...] lesions using tattoo equipment [5[...]

Vitiligo

Vitiligo is an autoimmune [...] acterized by the appeara[...] lesions on the skin and [...] It is suggested that 0.5–[...] tion is affected by vitil[...] lished predilection for [...]

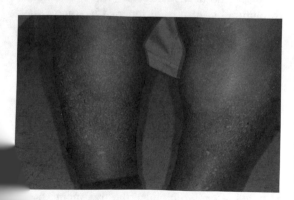

10.6 Idiopathic guttate hypomelanosis

Regarding age, almost 50% of cases affect the adolescent population before the age of 20 [60]. Vitiligo classically presents with depigmented macules and patches on the skin and mucosal surfaces, with occasional involvement of hair follicles (Fig. 10.7). Factors that have been reported to induce vitiligo lesions include trauma (known as the Koebner phenomenon), stress, sunburn, and pregnancy [61–63]. Chemicals such as 4-tert-butylphenol, rhododendrol, and various hair dyes, which all contain phenol that acts as a tyrosinase inhibitor, can also induce vitiligo-like lesions [64, 65].

The appearance of vitiligo patterns can be classified into localized, segmental, and universal. Localized lesions present as isolated, small depigmented patches that often appear in a symmetric distribution. Acrofacial pattern is a sub type of localized vitiligo where the lesions are mainly confined to the head, hands, and feet. "Lip tip" vitiligo is another localized subtype that involves only the distal fingers, toes, and facial orifices. Segmental vitiligo is a rapidly progressive condition in which a unilateral often linear depigmented patch occurs quickly (often over 6 months) and is associated with rapid leukotrichia (loss of hair pigment), which is a hallmark finding. It most often stabilizes earlier than other types of vitiligo; however, it is a very rare subtype. Segmental vitiligo is less responsive to treatment, and this is thought to be due to involvement of the hair follicles, which leads to a lack of melanocyte repository available for repigmentation. Universal vitiligo is a term reserved

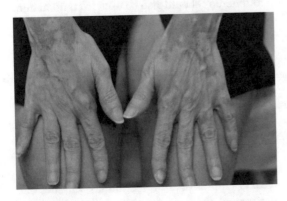

Fig. 10.7 Vitiligo

for near-complete or complete depigmentation of the skin of greater than 80% body surface area [66, 67].

The pathogenesis of vitiligo is thought to be one of autoimmunity that targets melanocytes for destruction. It has been reported that melanocytes are more susceptible to stress-induced injury because they produce large amounts of the protein melanin which can activate a stress pathway and lead to the production of reactive oxygen species. This in turn leads to the release of inflammatory cells including CD8 T cells that release IFN-gamma and induce the release of CXCL10 and its receptor CXCR3 to recruit additional T cells to attack melanocytes [68–70]. Prior studies have reported vitiligo as inherited in a polygenic pattern, meaning that multiple alleles are involved in the melanocyte's increased susceptibility to injury leading to the condition.

Vitiligo has been associated with various other autoimmune diseases in both the affected patient and their first-degree relatives. Some of these conditions include autoimmune thyroiditis, Type 1 diabetes mellitus, pernicious anemia, rheumatoid arthritis, and lupus [71, 72]. There are also several conditions that present with both vitiligo lesions and changes in the eyes and ears (which also contain melanocytes). Vogt-Koyanagi-Harada syndrome presents with depigmented skin lesions and leukotrichia, as well as ear pain, vertigo, hearing loss, meningitis, and symptomatic uveitis which can lead to blindness [73]. Alezzandrini syndrome often shows similar clinical findings; however, the skin findings typically present with segmental vitiligo [74].

Diagnosis of vitiligo can often be made clinically; however, thorough evaluation of vitiligo lesions is also important. This includes examination with a Wood's lamp exam which will commonly fluoresce with vitiligo lesions as well as a skin biopsy. The biopsy will often show loss of basal melanocytes in the center of the lesion with a possible inflammation with CD4 and CD8 T cells at the border of an active lesion (even without active erythema on clinical exam) [75].

Treatment of vitiligo should focus on two goals: stopping progression of depigmentation and repigmentation of existing lesions.

Identifying active disease is vital, as halting the progression is time sensitive to minimize the extent of disease involvement. There are three findings that should raise suspicion of active disease. These include Koebner phenomenon, inflammatory lesions (i.e., erythematous), and confetti-like lesions. Treatment options of vitiligo include topical medications, phototherapy, surgical interventions, as well as immunomodulation and camouflage [76].

Initial treatment of localized vitiligo includes potent topical steroids and calcineurin inhibitors applied to the affected areas twice daily. In combination, these medications have been shown to be effective in halting inflammation and inducing repigmentation while providing an intermittent break from chronic topical steroid use. In cases where BSA involvement is 5–10% or greater, topical treatment should be combined with phototherapy for maximum results. Vitamin D analogs such as calcipotriene, when combined with phototherapy, may also expedite repigmentation and reduce overall required treatment with phototherapy; however, no studies have shown improvement in repigmentation when calcipotriene is used as a single agent [76].

Phototherapies that have been shown to stabilize disease progression and lead to repigmentation include NB-UVB, PUVA, PUVA plus psoralen, BB-UVB, and excimer. Phototherapy induces apoptosis of T cells in active lesions as well as concomitantly stimulating active melanocytes in perilesional skin and hair follicles, which can lead to repigmentation of the depigmented areas [77]. Response rates for both PUVA and NB-UVB range from 40% to up to 75% with better responses reported in patients with new-onset lesions [78]. In the past, PUVA was the treatment of choice; however, in a review, PUVA was determined to be inferior to NB-UVB, even though PUVA causes more rapid repigmentation [78]. NB-UVB has been found to be more effective in stabilizing disease and causing repigmentation, with one report showing 75% maximum repigmentation rate with NB-UVB at 1 year. Patients are often started at a dose of 100–200 mJ two to three times weekly with the dose gradually increased 10–20% each week until the desired

light erythema is appreciated within vitiligo lesions. Once this occurs, the dose should be maintained until this erythema is no longer present. At that point, the dose should again be gradually increased [79–81]. The most responsive areas to phototherapy are often the face and neck, followed by the limbs and trunk. Acral areas show the lowest rates of repigmentation. Excimer 308 nm laser can also induce stability and repigmentation of vitiligo lesions; however, given the limited visual treatment field of the handheld laser, it is often reserved for localized cases when less than 10% BSA is involved. A lack of response to any of the treatments after 6 months indicates nonresponse and should be discontinued. In all types of phototherapy, patients should not apply any topical treatment immediately prior to treatment and should be adamant about sun protection with sunscreen and sun-protective clothing to minimize side effects from additive UV sunlight exposure.

In cases of rapidly progressive disease, oral minipulse steroid therapy is often used. One study reported that low-dose (5 or 7.5 mg) betamethasone or dexamethasone taken on two consecutive days each week for 3–6 months leads to halting of progression, with almost 90% of treated patients having stabilization of disease within 1–3 months [82, 83]. This is most often combined with phototherapy and topical treatment. Other immunosuppressive medications including methotrexate and cyclophosphamide have also been reported as effective treatments in stabilizing vitiligo in limited studies [84–87]. With the use of all immunosuppressive treatment, phototherapy should also be used in combination. Newer medications under current investigation to treat vitiligo include afamelanotide and JAK inhibitors including tofacitinib and ruxolitinib.

With all nonsurgical interventions for the treatment of vitiligo, it is important to be prepared for restarting treatment in the cases of relapse, which occurs in up to 40% of cases within the first year of stopping treatment. One study reported patients that had completed phototherapy treatment continued a maintenance regimen of twice weekly application of tacrolimus ointment to the treated areas on the head and neck. In this group, 96% of patients reported no relapse; however, 60% of patients using a placebo ointment experienced recurrence of lesions. Therefore, it has been suggested to continue a maintenance regimen of tacrolimus 0.1% ointment to the treated areas twice weekly to minimize the risk of relapse [88].

In addition to topical medications and phototherapy, several surgical treatment options are also available that can provide repigmentation of stable vitiligo lesions. A benefit of surgical intervention over nonsurgical intervention is that when repigmentation occurs in previously affected areas, relapse and recurrence of vitiligo in those areas are uncommon. Surgical options available today include minipunch grafts, suction epidermal grafting, and cellular grafting. These treatments should only be reserved for stable vitiligo cases. Stable vitiligo is defined as a patient without new or expanding lesions for a period of time from 6 months to 2 years. In addition, the patient should not have inflammatory, trichome, or confetti-like lesions, as these also indicate active disease. It is also important to be aware that certain areas are less responsive to surgical interventions, including over the joints (possibly due to repeated trauma and friction) and acrofacial areas, whereas head and neck recipient sites tend to portend the best outcomes.

Tissue grafts involve the transfer of non-affected pigmented tissue to a depigmented area. In contrast, cellular grafts are reserved for larger surface areas. These grafts are comprised of suspensions of donor site melanocytes and keratinocytes.

There are two types of tissue transplants: minipunch and epidermal suction grants. In performing minipunch graft transplants, 1–1.5 mm punch biopsies from an area of non-affected, pigmented skin are transferred into a prepared recipient, depigmented site. Though the technique is simple, potential complications include irregular surface changes and a risk of scarring and keloid formation at both the donor and recipient sites [89, 90]. Another tissue transfer technique is suction blister epidermal grafting. In this process, blister roofs are created from a normal skin with a suction tool and transferred to the affected skin

that has been pretreated with epidermal abrasion. This option has a lower risk of textural changes, scarring, or dyspigmentation; however, the risk of hemorrhagic blisters can be a concern [91].

The other type of surgical transplant in vitiligo is cellular grafting, also known as melanocyte keratinocyte transplant procedure. In most cases, noncultured cellular skin grafts are developed by creating a suspension of melanocytes and keratinocytes from a thin pigmented donor skin graft. The thin grafts are suspended in trypsin to allow separation and removal of the epidermis, which is then manually separated and centrifuged to create a liquid suspension. This product is then resuspended in lactated Ringer's and applied to a recipient depigmented site that has first been prepared with superficial abrasion to encourage absorption of the cellular product. Patients should be careful with the treated areas and remove the covered dressings 4–7 days after treatment [92]. This technique has positive results; however, there are disadvantages, which include the required equipment to create the cellular suspension, which can be costly. When comparing the overall efficacy of all three surgical treatments of vitiligo, noncultured cellular graft suspension has been shown to yield a more aesthetically appealing outcome; however, blister and punch grafts are easier techniques and require minimal extra-expensive equipment or tissue processing procedures.

In cases where vitiligo affects >50% BSA, some patients prefer to depigment the remaining pigmented skin to provide a more even physical appearance. Monobenzylether of hydroquinone (MBEH) is the only drug currently approved by the FDA for the treatment of vitiligo and is used to depigment the skin. Compounded MBEH at 20% concentration is applied to areas of pigmentation twice daily. This treatment often requires 4–12 months of application in order to obtain the desired effects of complete depigmentation. The most common side effect of MBEH is an irritant contact dermatitis. Strict sun exposure should be minimized to prevent perifollicular repigmentation from hair melanocyte reserves. Even after complete depigmented results are achieved, it will likely be necessary to touch up early-repigmenting areas with MBEH several times per week if necessary [93].

There are also several newer medications currently under current investigation for treatment of vitiligo including afamelanotide and JAK inhibitors such as tofacitinib and ruxolitinib. Afamelanotide is a synthetic analogue of alpha-melanocyte-stimulating hormone. One study used this synthetic hormone in conjunction with NB-UVB to treat vitiligo patients in a double blind, multicenter study. Those patients who received both treatments together reported repigmentation rates of almost 50% compared to 33% of patients only receiving NB-UVB phototherapy in the study. Commonly reported side effects associated with afamelanotide include nausea, itching, and generalized hyperpigmentation [94, 95]. Additional future studies need to be conducted to further elucidate this potential treatment option.

Tofacitinib and ruxolitinib are JAK inhibitors that are also currently being investigated as potential treatments for vitiligo. The mechanism behind JAK inhibitors affecting vitiligo is based on the known increase in interferon gamma-CXCL10 identified in vitiligo lesions. JAK inhibitors directly inhibit interferon signaling, allowing for melanocyte stabilization, survival, and increased melanin production, leading to repigmentation. One study reported that after oral ingestion of tofacitinib, which is a JAK1/3 inhibitor, the patient's serum CXCL10 level was lower than the initial value, possibly providing insight that JAK inhibitors affect vitiligo patients through inhibition of interferon gamma-CXCL10. This finding might be a way to quantitatively evaluate a patient's disease activity and response to treatment in the future. Topical forms of ruxolitinib in small studies have also begun to show promising results; however, additional replicative studies are necessary to validate results [96–99].

In addition to pharmacologic, phototherapy, and surgical interventions in vitiligo, several studies have hypothesized a potential role of various vitamin supplementation to improve repigmentation, including vitamin C, D, E, folate, B12, and zinc. This is thought to be due to their anti-oxidative properties which can decrease the effect of reactive oxygen species on their attack of melanocytes. These studies are continuing to be investigated [100].

Finally, discussing camouflage techniques with makeup, self-tanners, and possible permanent pigment tattooing should be discussed with patients [101, 102]. Various support groups for vitiligo patients exist, and it is important to provide education and support resources for all patients, as this disease can affect them not only physically but also psychologically [103–105].

Post-inflammatory Hyperpigmentation

Post-inflammatory hyperpigmentation (PIH) is an acquired pigmentary disorder that results after an inflammatory reaction such as acne vulgaris, psoriasis, atopic dermatitis, allergic or irritant contact dermatitis, trauma to the skin, or laser/light therapy [106–111]. It can present anywhere on the body, as it is a result of an existing inflammatory process or injury. Lesions appear as tan-brown to dark brown macules or patches, though they can even be a dark gray or blue-gray color when the inciting event occurs within dermis (Fig. 10.8) [110]. PIH is most common in Fitzpatrick skin types III–IV and is due to hyperreactive melanocytes known as hypermelanosis [106, 108, 110]. Melanocytes react to the initiating inflammatory process and become hypertrophic, secreting more melanin [109]. PIH can be divided into two categories: epidermal hypermelanosis and dermal hypermelanosis. The exact pathogenesis of epidermal hypermelanosis is not well understood but is thought to be due to melanocyte response to inflammatory markers, whereas dermal hypermelanosis occurs when melanophages accumulate at the site of injury and destroy basal keratinocytes [110]. The severity of PIH is determined by the degree of inflammation, patient's skin type, involvement of the dermo-epidermal junction, and the stability of melanocytes [111].

PIH is more common in darker skin types including African American, Hispanic/Latino, Asian, Native American, Pacific Islander, and

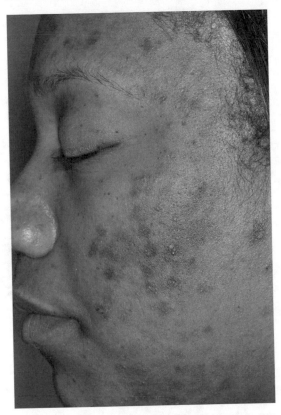

Fig. 10.8 Post-inflammatory hyperpigmentation

Middle Eastern and is the second most common diagnosis in African Americans [109, 112]. A clinical history and exam can usually support a diagnosis of PIH without need for further workup. Some physicians have found utility in the Wood's lamp which can be useful in determining the location of excess pigment. Wood's lamp can reveal if pigment is located in the epidermis or dermis, which is important when determining the best treatment option. New advances using polarized light photography, colorimetry, and diffuse reflectance spectroscopy (DRS) can assist in diagnosis by producing quantitative information about the affected areas [6]. Biopsy is rarely used but can give a definitive answer when there is question about the diagnosis. Histopathology will reveal superficial dermal melanophages and increased epidermal melanin without basal cell vacuolization [111].

There are many treatment options available for PIH which range from topical to systemic

to surgical therapies. The first steps in management include prevention and adequate management of the underlying skin disorder, proper sun protection, and behavior modification to encourage patients not to scratch affected areas. Photoprotection can prevent worsening of the hyperpigmentation, and patients should use a daily broad-spectrum sunscreen and wear protective clothing when possible [108, 110, 112].

Topical depigmenting agents are the first-line option for epidermal PIH and can be used as monotherapy or in combination with other agents [108, 109]. Common topical depigmenting agents include hydroquinone, azelaic acid, kojic acid, and retinoids. Hydroquinone is the gold standard for treating PIH and works by inhibiting tyrosinase. More specifically, it is a phenolic compound that blocks the conversion of dihydroxyphenyl-alanine (DOPA) to melanin [108, 110]. It is often used by mixing it with retinoids, corticosteroids, or antioxidants to obtain maximum results. It has been shown that hydroquinone 4% can be used twice daily for up to 6 months with good results [107]. Some adverse events reported include contact dermatitis, permanent leukoderma, and hypopigmentation of the unaffected skin also known as the "halo effect." One of the more concerning adverse events is exogenous ochronosis where homogentisic acid accumulates in the dermis causing permanent hyperpigmentation [110, 113]. Similar to hydroquinone, mequinol is a derivative of hydroquinone and is found to be less irritating than its counterpart. The exact pathway is unknown, but it is thought to also be a tyrosinase inhibitor [108].

Retinoids are effective in treating PIH through their skin-lightening effects. Retinoids are vitamin A derivatives and work through cell proliferation, differentiation, induction of apoptosis, and expression of anti-inflammatory properties. The most commonly seen side effect is mild to moderate irritation [106, 108].

Other topical agents with varying effects include azelaic acid, kojic acid, arbutin, niacinamide, vitamin C, and licorice root extract. Azelaic acid aids in depigmentation by tyrosinase inhibition along with selective antiproliferative mechanisms against hyperactive melanocytes [108]. Kojic acid is a fungal metabolite species found in *Penicillium*, *Aspergillum*, and *Acetobacter* and works as a tyrosinase inhibitor to aid in its skin-brightening effects [106, 108]. Arbutin is found naturally in bearberry, pear, cranberry, or blueberry leaves; it is derived from hydroquinone but has less side effects [108]. Niacinamide is the active form of vitamin B3 and works by decreasing melanosome transfer to keratinocytes. It has not been widely used in PIH, but studies show great promise due to its benefit in treating hyperpigmentation found in melasma. Vitamin C or ascorbic acid is a naturally occurring antioxidant that works in depigmentation by interacting with the active sites of tyrosinase and reducing dopaquinone oxidation which is an important product in the melanin synthesis pathway. Lastly, licorice root extract has anti-inflammatory and anti-tyrosinase activity with minimal side effects for the patient [104].

Chemical peels using glycolic acid or salicylic acid are effective in treating and reducing the appearance of PIH [99, 104]. Glycolic acid is a naturally occurring alpha-hydroxy acid found in sugar cane and works through epidermolysis. Salicylic acid is a beta-hydroxy acid found in willow tree bark that works by causing keratolysis. Both glycolic and salicylic acid have shown great safety and efficacy for PIH management [104]. Laser/light therapy has also shown utility in the treatment of PIH. A systemic review looking at the use of lasers for PIH therapy found that Q-switched Nd:YAG is the most effective laser in reducing the appearance of lesions [108]. Cosmetic camouflage can be used by patients to conceal pigmented lesions, improve appearance, and positively impact quality of life [104].

Melasma

Melasma is an acquired pigmentary disorder of unknown etiology. It classically presents with hyperpigmented brown to dark brown macules with "moth-eaten" or scalloped borders that are typically located on the face, mainly on the

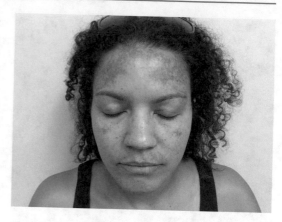

Fig. 10.9 Melasma

malar cheeks, centrofacial area, and mandibular areas (Fig. 10.9). Occasional involvement of the upper chest or extremities can be seen [114, 115]. Prior associations with exposure to ultraviolet radiation (UVR), increased estrogen levels, genetic predisposition, and phototoxic drugs [107, 113] have been theorized as underlying culprits or exacerbating factors. It is less commonly associated with ovarian dysfunction, thyroid disease, and liver disease [107]. UVR is known to worsen melasma, and increased exposure leads to the production of alpha-melanocyte-stimulating hormone (MSH), interleukin (IL)-1, and corticotrophin which stimulate melanin production [107]. However, visible light may also induce skin pigmentation of affected areas [116]. Estrogen is thought to induce melasma as it develops frequently during pregnancy, use of oral contraceptives (OCPs), and with hormone replacement therapy (HRT) [109]. The four different classifications of melasma are epidermal, dermal, mixed epidermal-dermal, and intermediate. Epidermal is attributed to increased melanin production in the epidermis and is the most common and easiest type to treat. Dermal is characterized by melanin-laden macrophages in the dermis and is the least responsive to treatment. Mixed epidermal-dermal is a combination of the two, and the intermediate type is more commonly found in darker skin types, Fitzpatrick skin types V–VI [113].

Melasma occurs predominately in women and can be seen in all ethnic groups; however, it is more common in Fitzpatrick skin types IV–VI. Exact prevalence is unknown but has been reported as 4–10% in Latin America and more specifically up to around 50% of women of Mexican descent of childbearing age [113, 114]. The true prevalence worldwide is not known yet [117]. Melasma can be diagnosed clinically and rarely requires a skin biopsy. Histopathology will show pigment accumulation in the epidermis, dermis, or both as well as melanin-laden macrophages [115]. The Melasma Area Severity Index (MASI) was created to evaluate the severity of melasma. Clinicians assess the forehead, malar cheeks, and chin for the presence of lesions and add up scores based on the area involved, darkness of the lesions, and homogeneity. The higher the score, the more severe the condition [113].

The goal for treatment of melasma is to slow the proliferation of melanocytes and to stop melanosome formation. Photoprotection is key to preventing worsening of dark lesions, and it is recommended for all patients to wear a broad-spectrum sunscreen. Discontinuation of OCPs or HRT may result in clearance of melasma since estrogen is thought to be involved in its presentation. Treatment of melasma in pregnancy is usually held until after delivery because of its increased resistance to treatment. Further, melasma may resolve after delivery of the baby [109].

Hydroquinone is the gold standard for treatment and can be used as monotherapy or combined with other lightening agents [113, 117]. Hydroquinone inhibits melanin production through the inhibition of tyrosinase, which is the rate-limiting step in melanin synthesis. In the United States, there is a triple combination cream that consists of 4% hydroquinone, 0.01% fluocinolone acetone, and 0.05% tretinoin and is often used for initial treatment for melasma. Patients should be made aware of the common side effects including skin atrophy and irritant reactions, and therefore the combination cream should be used for no longer than 6 months [109, 114]. Tretinoin reduces pigmentation by inhibiting tyrosinase and stops melanin production. Some side effects include mild irritation and increased pigmentation [109, 117]. Adapalene is a synthetic retinoid

that often causes less irritation than tretinoin and may be appropriate for long-term therapy. Azelaic and kojic acid have similar effects in inhibiting tyrosinase and have been shown to improve the appearance of melasma. Side effects include acneiform eruptions and mild irritation [109, 113]. Cysteamine is a newer topical agent that aids in treating hyperpigmentation through inhibition of tyrosinase and peroxidase in the melanin synthesis pathway. It has also been found to remove dopaquinone, bind and remove iron and copper, and increase glutathione, all which lead to the lightening of melasma [118]. Oligopeptides are a new class of tyrosinase inhibitors that are being studied for the treatment of melasma and may be a good alternative to hydroquinone due to its decreased side effects. Chemical peels with salicylic acid have also been found to be effective in management [114].

There have been some new research studies looking at the utility of laser/light therapy for the management of melasma, which have produced good results. Carbon dioxide fractional ablative lasers are ablative treatment that non-selectively destroys the epidermis. The laser is fractional so the amount of epidermal injury is decreased, and there is less risk of dyspigmentation. Quality-switched neodymium-doped yttrium aluminum garnet laser (Nd:YAG) targets melanin specifically and can be used with low, short pulses to reduce the side effect of hypopigmentation. 1550 nm fractional non-ablative laser has shown promise but is still being investigated for the treatment of melasma [114].

Tranexamic acid (TA) and methimazole are oral agents that may be useful in depigmenting lesions in melasma. Tranexamic acid works in hyperpigmentation by decreasing melanocyte-stimulating hormone; however, more studies are needed to evaluate the effectiveness. The major side effect associated with this therapy is the risk of deep venous thrombosis, so patients will need to be carefully screened before starting this treatment for a history or increased risk of thromboembolic events [115]. Methimazole is an oral antithyroid medication that when used topically depigments the skin without effecting the thyroid gland [117]. More studies are needed to determine the long-term effects of this treatment.

The Pigmentary Disorders Academy (PDA) created a treatment algorithm for melasma that has been used to guide therapy. According to the PDA, first-line treatment should be topical therapy with primarily triple or dual combination depigmenting agents that include hydroquinone. Second-line options include chemical peels, either alone or in combination with topical lightening therapy. Per PDA, lasers and light sources should be used only in select cases for melasma.

Lichen Planus Pigmentosus

Lichen planus pigmentosus (LPP) is a rare, uncommon variant of lichen planus and is more prevalent in skin of color [111, 119, 120]. Lesions often appear in a symmetrical pattern as violaceous, gray to black macules and patches which are typically present on the face [111] (Fig. 10.10). There is a variant of LPP called LPP inversus which is typically found in the flexural skin folds and intertriginous areas, primarily the axillae [120]. The frequency and etiology of this disease are unknown but may be associated with UVR, hepatitis C virus, and various topical agents [120–122]. As far as pathogenesis, LPP is similar to lichen planus (LP) in that it has an abnormal immune response, where CD8 T cells attack epidermal keratinocytes and lead to pigmentary incontinence [123]. LPP occurs mainly in females in their third to fourth decades of life. LPP presents as dark brown macules that are present in sun-exposed areas and flexural folds [119]. Pathology will show epidermal basal cell layer vacuolation, a few necrotic keratinocytes, and a lichenoid lymphocytic infiltration [111].

There is currently no gold standard option for the treatment of LPP. Management options include use of topical medications like hydroquinone, corticosteroids, calcineurin inhibitors, keratolytics, vitamin A derivatives, and chemical peels [124]. The most commonly used topical agent is tacrolimus. Systemic corticosteroids can be used for severe cases and should be tapered over time; dapsone and isotretinoin can also be used for severe cases [123]. Laser therapy has been shown to improve the appearance of LPP, and more research is needed on this area.

Erythema Dyschromicum Perstans

Erythema dyschromicum perstans (EDP) is a dermatosis of unknown etiology and is commonly seen in darker skin types, especially the Latin American population [124, 125]. The other name for EDP is ashy dermatosis [111]. EDP presents as blue-gray macules and patches and may have a pale area around the lesion which is considered a halo effect [124] (Fig. 10.11). Lesions may also have active

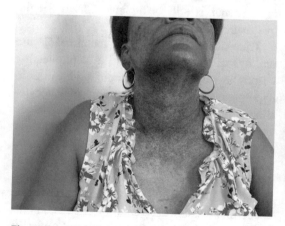

Fig. 10.10 Lichen planus pigmentosus

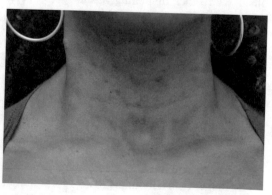

Fig. 10.11 Erythema dyschromicum perstans

erythematous borders that disappear and leave oval gray macules and patches. LPP often affects sun-protected areas, though may involve the trunk, the upper extremities, and the neck [111]. Pigmentary changes can be chronic, and there is no widely accepted treatment available. Pathology will reveal a lichenoid dermatitis with basal layer vacuolization and will also appear similar to LP.

There is no widely accepted therapy for EDP, and there has been a history of varying effectiveness of topical treatments. Promising results have been reported with laser therapy used in conjunction with topical tacrolimus which targets the exact location of the pigment in EDP [125].

Clofazimine is a hypochlorous acid that decreases inflammation and has been reported to be a good treatment option for some patients [126].

Drug-Induced Hyperpigmentation

There are some common medications that are known to cause hyperpigmentation (Table 10.1) [126–129]. These lesions classically present as hyperpigmented macules and patches, often on sun-exposed areas, though they can be found on any part of the body (Fig. 10.12). Drug-induced hyperpigmentation can either resolve after dis-

Table 10.1 Common drugs associated with skin hyperpigmentation

Drug name	Mechanism of action	Classification	Presentation
Minocycline	Tetracycline that inhibits protein synthesis and bacterial growth by binding to the 30S ribosomal subunit	Antibiotic	Type I: black blue discoloration in old scars Type II: common lower extremities Type III: generalized dark, brown pigment
Zidovudine	Nucleoside reverse transcriptase inhibitor (NRTI); inhibits thymidine kinase	Antiretroviral therapy	Diffuse melanonychia; mucocutaneous hyperpigmentation
Bleomycin	Glycopeptide antibiotic; inhibits DNA, RNA, protein synthesis in G2 and M phase	Antineoplastic	Transverse melanonychia; hyperpigmentation over joints and palmer creases
Busulfan	Alkylating agent; interferes with DNA intercalation and RNA transcription	Antineoplastic	Generalized hyperpigmentation
Chlorpromazine	Antagonizes dopamine D2 receptors in the brain	Antipsychotic	Slate-gray discoloration in sun-exposed areas
Oral contraceptives	Combination pills with estrogen and progestin or progestin-only pills	Hormonal contraceptive	Melasma; increased pigment of the nipples
Hydantoins	Stabilizes neuronal membranes and decreases seizure activity by increasing efflux of sodium ions	Anticonvulsant	Slate-gray discoloration in sun-exposed areas
Cyclophosphamide	Interferes with malignant cell growth by cross-linking tumor cell DNA	Antineoplastic	Diffuse hyperpigmentation of the skin and mucous membranes; pigment involved nails
Amiodarone	Inhibits adrenergic stimulation and affects sodium, potassium, and calcium channels	Anti-dysrhythmics	Slate-gray to violaceous discoloration in sun-exposed areas
Clofazimine	Bacteriocidal effects on *Mycobacterium*; also exerts anti-inflammatory properties	Antitubercular agent	Violet, brown to blue discoloration
Hydroxychloroquine sulfate	Unknown; may impair complement-dependent antigen-antibody reactions	Antimalarial	Gray to blue/black pigmentation usually on the lower extremities, face, and sclera
Procarbazine	Inhibits protein, DNA, and RNA synthesis	Antineoplastic	Generalized hyperpigmentation
Doxorubicin	Intercalates between DNA base pairs and impairs topoisomerase II function	Antineoplastic	Hyperpigmentation over small hand joints; involves palmer creases

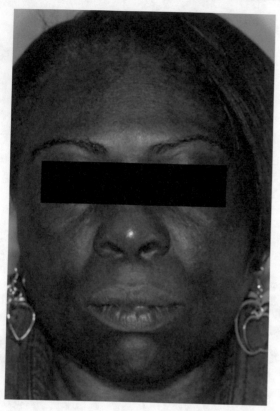

Fig. 10.12 Drug-induced hyperpigmentation

known to accumulate in the skin and mucous membranes as well as the teeth and nails. There are three types of hyperpigmentation associated with minocycline. Type 1 appears after an inflammatory process and typically presents on the sun-exposed skin of the face as a blue-black color. Type 2 appears on normal skin and is normally present on the shins and upper extremities. Type 3 is more generalized and presents as a dark brown color. There have also been many reported cases discussing neoplastic agents leading to skin hyperpigmentation. For treatment of drug-induced hyperpigmentation, the first line of action is to stop the offending agent. Skin-lightening agents have been also used to treat the lesions but are commonly ineffective because most drug-induced pigment is located in the dermis, which cannot be reached by topical lightening agents. Laser therapy using the Q-switched Nd:YAG laser and Q-switched ruby laser have shown some promising results [126].

Table 10.2 briefly describes other common metabolic and miscellaneous causes of hyperpigmentation [130–150] (Fig. 10.13).

continuation of the medication or can persist for months to years. Minocycline is a common culprit for inducing hyperpigmentation and is

Metabolic and Other Miscellaneous Causes of Hyperpigmentation (Table 10.2)

Table 10.2 Miscellaneous causes of hyperpigmentation

Diagnosis	Etiology	Epidemiology	Presentation	Histology	Management
Hyperpigmentation due to Addison's disease [24–28]	Increased production of adrenocorticotropic hormone (ACTH) which is a type of melanocortin 1 receptor agonist that is highly expressed on melanocytes	Seen in majority of adult patients and 67% of pediatric patients	Generalized bronze hyperpigmentation more prevalent in the axilla, areolas, perineum, and palmer creases. Can also involve mucosal surfaces	Increase amount of melanin in basal epidermal keratinocytes and moderate melanophages	Treat the underlying disease with replacement of deficient glucocorticoids and mineralocorticoids
Hyperpigmentation due to hyperthyroidism [28, 29]	Not well understood but likely due to melanocyte stimulation from thyroid hormones	Present in 2% of patients with hyperthyroidism; common in Graves' disease	Localized or generalized hyperpigmentation common in the creases of palms, soles, and mucosal surfaces. Fine hair; mild alopecia	Increased melanosis of the basal layer and greater deposition of hemosiderin in the dermis	Treat the underlying disease
Hyperpigmentation due to chronic renal disease [24, 30–32]	May be due to increased production of urochrome pigments, carotenoids, and melanocyte-stimulating hormone	Common in patients receiving hemodialysis	Generalized hyperpigmentation of gray to yellow to brown skin color	Basement membrane thickening, endothelial cell activation, and chronic inflammatory infiltrate	Treat the underlying disease, adequate photoprotection
Hemochromatosis [33]	Increased melanogenesis and iron deposit accumulation in the skin	Occurs in 70% of affected patients	Generalized bronze hyperpigmentation mainly affecting the face and hands	Increased melanin in the epidermis and melanophages in the dermis. Iron deposits in deeper part of the dermis	Treat the underlying cause with phlebotomy or chelation
Diabetic dermopathy [34, 35]	Likely due to microangiopathic complications of diabetes, but the exact mechanism is unknown	Affects 70% of adults with diabetes mellitus. Most common cutaneous manifestation in diabetics	Small, oval, red-brown atrophic macules and patches more commonly seen on the lower extremity. Atrophy or scarring can be present after resolution	Atrophy of rete ridges, pigmentation of basal cells, and moderate hyperkeratosis and dermal perivascular plasma cells	Appropriate wound care to prevent infection and aid in healing. The lesions are asymptomatic and often resolve spontaneously without treatment. Patients should be worked up for diabetes

(continued)

Table 10.2 (continued)

Diagnosis	Etiology	Epidemiology	Presentation	Histology	Management
Hyperpigmentation due to B12 deficiency [36–38]	Not fully understood but may be related to reduced glutathione-stimulating hormone leading to increased tyrosinase activity; high levels of biopterin which increases phenylalanine utility; defect in the transport of melanin and incorporation into keratinocytes	Common in B12 deficiency and more prevalent in patients with darker skin tones	Generalized hyperpigmentation more pronounced on the extremities and flexural folds. Less commonly in the oral mucosa and nails	Epidermal thinning, vacuolization of keratinocytes, increased number of melanocytes and melanophages in the dermis	Repletion of vitamin B12 orally, intravenously, or intramuscularly
Acanthosis nigricans [34, 39–41]	Elevated insulin concentrations lead to activation of IGF-1 receptors of keratinocytes and fibroblasts leading to proliferation	Most commonly associated with insulin resistance and people of Hispanic, African, or Native American descent. Common in children and in patients with a family history of diabetes mellitus	Diffuse, velvety hyperpigmented plaques found in the axillae, neck, inframammary folds, and inguinal folds	Thickened stratum corneum with thickened, elongated dermal projections and hyperkeratosis	Weight loss, retinoids, adapalene, calcipotriol, and laser therapy. Important to identify any underlying condition by obtaining basic labs and evaluating the patient's risk

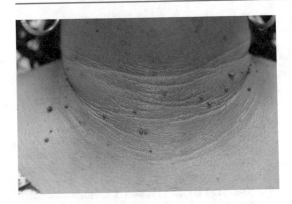

Fig. 10.13 Acanthosis nigricans

References

1. Vachiramon V, Thadanipon K. Postinflammatory hypopigmentation. Clin Exp Dermatol. 2011;36:708–14.
2. Verma S, Patterson JW, Derdeyn AS, et al. Hypopigmented macules in an Indian man. Arch Dermatol. 2006;142:1643–8.
3. Rowley MJ, Nesbitt LT Jr, Carrington PR, Espinoza CG. Hypopigmented macules in acantholytic disorders. Int J Dermatol. 1995;34:390–2.
4. Yang CC, Lee JY, Won TW. Depigmented extra-mammary Paget's disease. Br J Dermatol. 2004;151:1049–53.
5. Halder RM, Richards GM. Management of dyschromias in ethnic skin. Dermatol Ther. 2004;17:151–7.
6. High WA, Pandya AG. Pilot trial of 1% pimecrolimus cream in the treatment of seborrheic dermatitis in African American adults with associated hypopigmentation. J Am Acad Dermatol. 2006;54:1083–8.
7. Ruiz-Maldonado R, Orozco-Covarrubias ML. Postinflammatory hypopigmentation and hyperpigmentation. Semin Cutan Med Surg. 1997;16:36–43.
8. Grimes PE, Bhawan J, Ki J, et al. Laser resurfacing induced hypopigmentation: histologic alterations and repigmentation with topical photochemotherapy. Dermatol Surg. 2001;27:515–20.
9. Alexiades-Armenakas MR, Bernstein LJ, Friedman PM, Geronemus RG. The safety and efficacy of the 308-nm excimer laser for pigment correction of hypopigmented scars and striae alba. Arch Dermatol. 2004;140:955–60.
10. Suvanprakorn P, Dee-Ananlap S, Pongsomboon C, Klaus SN. Melanocyte autologous grafting for treatment of leukoderma. J Am Acad Dermatol. 1985;13:968–74.
11. Bisherwal K, Singal A, Pandhi D, Sharma S. Hypopigmented mycosis fungoides: clinical, histological, and immunohistochemical remission induced by narrow-band ultraviolet B. Indian J Dermatol. 2017;62(2):203–6.
12. Fatemi N, Abtahi-Naeini B, Sadeghiyan H, Nilforoushzadeh MA, Najafian J, Pourazizi M. Mycosis fungoides in Iranian population: an epidemiological and clinicopathological study. J Skin Cancer. 2015;306543:1–6.
13. Amorim G, Nieeyer-Corbellini J, Quintella DC, Cuzzi T, Ramos-e-Silva M. Hypopigmented mycosis fungoides: a 20-case retrospective series. Int J Dermatol. 2018;54:306–12.
14. Yamashita T, Abbade LP, Marques ME, et al. Mycosis fungoides and Sezary syndrome: clinical, histopathological and immunohistochemical review and update. An Bras Dermatol. 2012;87:817–28.
15. Sanches JA Jr, Moricz CZM, Neto CF. Lymphoproliferative processes of the skin. Part 2-Cutaneous T-cell and NK-cell lymphomas. An Bras Dermatol. 2006;81:7–25.
16. Rodney IJ, Kindred C, Angra K, Qutub ON, Villanueva AR, Halder RM. Hypopigmented mycosis fungoides: a retrospective clinicohistopathologic study. J Eur Acad Dermatol Venereol: JEADV. 2017;31:808–14.
17. Tan EST, Tang MBY, Tan SH. Retrospective 5-year review of 131 patients with mycosis fungoides and sezary syndrome seen at the National Skin Centre, Singapore. Australas J Dermatol. 2006;47:248–52.
18. Furlan FC, Sanches JA. Hypopigmented mycosis fungoides: a review of its clinical features and pathophysiology. An Bras Dermatol. 2013;88:954–60.
19. Castano E, Glick S, Wolgast L, et al. Hypopigmented mycosis fungoides in childhood and adolescence: a long-term retrospective study. J Cutan Pathol. 2013;40:924–34.
20. Laws PM, Shear NH, Pope E. Childhood mycosis fungoides experience of 28 patients and response to phototherapy. Pediatr Dermatol. 2014;31:459–64.
21. Breathnach SM, McKee PH, Smith NP. Hypopigmented mycosis fungoides: report of five cases with ultrastructural observations. Br J Dermatol. 1982;106:643–9.
22. Boulos S, Vaid R, Aladily T, Ivan D, Talpur R, Duvic M. Clinical presentation, immunopathology, and treatment of juvenile-onset mycosis fungoides: a case series of 34 patients. J Am Acad Dermatol. 2014;71:1117–26.
23. Kanokungsee S, Rajatanavin N, Rutnin S, Vachiramon V. Efficacy of narrowband ultraviolet B twice weekly for hypopigmented mycosis fungoides in Asians. Clin Exp Dermatol. 2012;37:149–52.
24. Carter J, Zug KA. Phototherapy for cutaneous T cell lymphoma: online survey and literature review. J Am Acad Dermatol. 2009;60:39–50.
25. Miazek N, Michalek I, Pawlowska-Kisiel M, Olszewska M, Rudnicka L. Pityriasis alba- common disease, enigmatic entity: up-to-date review of the literature. Pediatr Dermatol. 2015;32(6):786–91.
26. Jadotte YT, Jannige CK. Pityriasis alba revisited: perspectives on an enigmatic disorder of childhood. Cutis. 2011;87:66–72.

27. Wells BT, Whyte HJ, Kierland RR. Pityriasis alba: a ten-year survey and review of the literature. Arch Dermatol. 1960;85:183–9.

28. Givler DN, Givler A. Pityriasis, alba. StatPearls [Internet]. Treasure Island: StatPearls Publishing; 2018.

29. Vargas-Ocampo F. Pityriasis alba: a histologic study. Int J Dermatol. 1993;32:870–3.

30. In SI, Yi SW, Kang HY, et al. Clinical and histopathological characteristics of pityriasis alba. Clin Exp Dermatol. 2009;34:591–7.

31. Kang HY, Choi YM. FK506 increases pigmentation and migration of human melanocytes. Br J Dermatol. 2006;155:1037–40.

32. Lin RL, Janniger CK. Pityriasis alba. Cutis. 2005;76:21–4.

33. Al-Mutairi N, Hadad AA. Efficacy of 3058-nm xenon chloride excimer laser in pityriasis alba. Dermatol Surg. 2012;38:604–9.

34. Kallini J, Riaz F, Khachemoune A. Tinea versicolor in dark-skinned individuals. Int J Dermatol. 2014;53:137–41.

35. Hald M, Arendrup M, Svejgaard E, Lindskov R, Foged E, Saunte D. Evidence- based Danish guidelines for the treatment of Malassezia-related skin diseases. Acta Derm Venerol. 2015;95:12–9.

36. Hu S, Bigby M. Pityriasis versicolor. Arch Dermatol. 2010;146(10):1132–9.

37. Gupta AK, Foley KA. Antifungal treatment for pityriasis versicolor. J Fungi. 2015;1:13.

38. Karray M, McKinney W. Tinea, versicolor. StatPearls [Internet]. Treasure Island: StatPearls Publishing; 2018.

39. Gupta AK, Lane D, Paquet M. Systematic review of systemic treatments for tinea versicolor and evidence-based dosing regimen recommendations. J Cutan Med Surg. 2014;18(2):79–90.

40. Kose O, Bulent H, Riza A, Kurumlu A. Comparison of a single 400 mg dose versus a 7-day 200mg daily dose of itraconazole in the treatment of tinea versicolor. J Dermatol Treat. 2002;13:77–9.

41. Faergemann J, Todd G, Pather S, Vawda ZFA, Gillies JD, Walford T, Barranco C, Quiring JN, Briones MA. Double-blind, randomized, placebo-controlled, dose-finding study of oral pramiconazole in the treatment of pityriasis versicolor. J Am Acad Dermatol. 2009;61:971–6.

42. Balevi A, Ustuner P, Kaksi S, Ozdemir M. Narrowband UV-B phototherapy: an effective and reliable treatment alternative for extensive and recurrent pityriasis versicolor. J Dermatol Treat. 2018;29(3):252–5.

43. Want K, Nassef Y, Sahu J, Hermes H, Schwartz L. Facial involvement in progressive macular hypomelanosis. Cutis. 2018;101(4):297–300.

44. Pertersen RL, Scholtz C, Jensen A, Bruggemann H, Lomholt H. Propionibacterium acnes phylogenetic type III is associated with progressive macular hypomelanosis. Eur J Microbiol Immunol. 2017;7:37–45.

45. Thng S, Long V, Chuah S, Ta VW. Efficacy and relapse rates of different treatment modalities for progressive macular hypomelanosis. Indian J Dermatol Venerol Leprol. 2016;82(6):673–6.

46. Kim MB, Kim GW, Park HJ, Kim HS, Kim SH, Kim BS, Ko HC. Narrowband UVB treatment of progressive macular hypomelanosis. J Am Acad Dermatol. 2012;66(4):598–605.

47. Sim JH, Lee DJ, Lee JS, Kim YC. Comparison of the clinical efficacy of NBUVB and NBUVB with benzoyl peroxide/clindamycin in progressive macular hypomelanosis. J Eur Acad Dermatol Venereol: JEADV. 2011;25:1318–23.

48. Kim J, Lee DY, Lee JY, Yoon TY. Progressive macular hypomelanosis showing excellent response to oral isotretinoin. J Dermatol. 2012;39(11): 937–8.

49. Brown F, Crane JS. Idiopathic guttate hypomelanosis. StatPearls [Internet]. Treasure Island: StatPearls Publishing; 2018. p. 1–4.

50. Mazioti M. Idiopathic guttate hypomelanosis: a mini review. J Pigmentary Disord. 2015;2(10):1–4.

51. Falabella R, Escobar C, Giraldo N, Rovetto P, Gill J. On the pathogenesis of idiopathic guttate hypomelanosis. J Am Acad Dermatol. 1987;16:35–44.

52. Kakepis M, Katoulis A, Katsambas A, et al. Idiopathic guttate hypomelanosis: an electron microscopy study. J Eur Acad Dermatol Venerol. 2015;29:1435–8.

53. Gordon J, Reed KE, Sebastian KR, Ahmed AM. Excimer light treatment for idiopathic guttate hypomelanosis: a pilot study. Dermatol Surg. 2017;43:553–7.

54. Kumarasinghe SP. 3–5 cryotherapy is effective in idiopathic guttate hypomelanosis. J Dermatol. 2004;31:437–9.

55. Asawananda P, Sutthipong T, Prejawal N. Pimecrolimus for idiopathic guttate hypomelanosis. J Drugs Dermatol. 2010;9:238–9.

56. Hexsel DM. Treatment of idiopathic guttate hypomelanosis by localized superficial dermabrasion. Dermatol Surg. 1999;25:917–8.

57. Wambier CG, Wambier SPDF, Soares MTPS, Breunig J, Cappel MA, Landau M. 5-fluorouracil tattooing for idiopathic guttate hypomelanosis. J Am Acad Dermatol. 2018;78:e81–2.

58. Bishnoi A, Parsad D. Clinical and molecular aspects of vitiligo treatments. Int J Mol Sci. 2018;19(1509):1–15.

59. Ezzedine K, Silverberg N. A practical approach to the diagnosis and treatment of vitiligo in children. Pediatrics. 2016;138(1):e20154126.

60. Agarwal S, Gupta S, Ojha A, Sinha R. Childhood vitiligo: clinicoepidemiologic profile of 268 children from the Kumaun region of Utarakhand, India. Pediatr Dermatol. 2013;30(3):348–53.

61. Rodrigues M, Ezzedine K, Hamzavi I, Pandya A, Harris J. New discoveries in the pathogenesis and classification of vitiligo. J Am Acad Dermatol. 2017;77:1–13.

62. Mason CP, Gawkrodgor DJ. Vitiligo presentation in adults. Clin Exp Dermatol. 2005;30:344–5.

63. Manolache L, Benea V. Stress in patients with alopecia areata and vitiligo. J Eur Acad Dermatol Venereol. 2007;21:921–8.

64. Tokura Y, Fujiyama T, Ikeya S, et al. Biochemical, cytological and immunological mechanisms of rhododendrol-induced leukoderma. J Dermatol Sci. 2015;77:146–9.

65. Ghosh S, Mukhopadhyay S. Chemical leukoderma: a clinic-aetiological study of 864 cases in the perspective of a developing country. Br J Dermatol. 2009;160:40–7.

66. Ezzedine K, Lim HW, Suzuki T, Katayama I, Hamzavi I, Lan CC, Goh BK, Anbar T, de Castro CS, Lee AY, et al. Revised classification/nomenclature of vitiligo and related issues: the vitiligo global issues consensus conference. Pigment Cell Melanoma Res. 2012;25(3):E1–E13.

67. Ezzedine K, Le Thuaut A, Jouary T, Ballanger F, Taieb A, Bastuji-Gari S. Latent class analysis of a series of 717 patients with vitiligo allows the identification of two clinical subtypes. Pigment Cell Melanoma Res. 2014;27(1):134–9.

68. Toosi S, Orlow SJ, Manga P. Vitiligo-inducing phenols activate the unfolded protein response in melanocytes resulting in upregulation of IL6 and IL8. J Invest Dermatol. 2012;132:2601–9.

69. Richmond JM, Frisoli ML, Harris JE. Innate immune mechanisms in vitiligo: danger from within. Curr Opin Immunol. 2013;25:676–82.

70. Schallreuter KU, Moore J, Wood JM, et al. In vivo and in vitro evidence for hydrogen peroxide(H2O2) accumulation in the epidermis of patients with vitiligo and its successful removal by a UVB-activated pseudocatalase. J Investig Dermatol Symp Proc. 1999;4:91–6.

71. Alkhateeb A, Fain PR, Thody A, Bennett DC, Spritz RA. Epidemiology of vitiligo and associated autoimmune diseases in Caucasian probands and their families. Pigment Cell Res. 2003;16:208–14.

72. Silverberg JI, Silverberg NB. Clinical features of vitiligo associated with comorbid autoimmune disease: a prospective survey. J Am Acad Dermatol. 2013;69(5):824–6.

73. Sakata VM, Da Silva FT, Hirata CE, De Carvalho JF, Yamamoto JH. Diagnosis and classification of Vogt-Koyanagi-Harada disease. Autoimmun Rev. 2014;13:550–5.

74. Alezzandrini AA. Unilateral manifestations of tapeto-retinal degeneration, vitiligo, poliosis, grey hair and hypoacousia. Ophthalmologica. 1964;147:409–19.

75. Faria AR, Tarle RG, Dellatorre G, Mira MT, Castro CC. Vitiligo- part 2- classification, histopathology and treatment. An Bras Dermatol. 2014;89(5):784–90.

76. Goh BK, Pandya AG. Presentations, signs of activity, and differential diagnosis of vitiligo. Dermatol Clin. 2017;35:135–44.

77. Rodrigues M, Ezzedine K, Hamzavi I, Pandya A, Harris J. Emerging treatments for vitiligo. J Am Acad Dermatol. 2017;77:17–29.

78. De Francesco V, Stinco G, Laspina S, Parlangeli ME, Mariuzzi L, Patrone P. Immunohistochemical study before and after narrow band (311nm) UVB treatment in vitiligo. Eur J Dermatol. 2008;18:292–6.

79. Njoo MD, Bos JD, Westerhof W. Treatment of generalized vitiligo in children with narrow-band (TL-01) UVB radiation therapy. J Am Acad Dermatol. 2000;42(2 Pt 1):245–53.

80. Mohammad TF, Al-Jamal M, Hamzavi IH, et al. The vitiligo working group recommendations for narrowband ultraviolet B light phototherapy treatment of vitiligo. J Am Acad Dermatol. 2017;76:879–88.

81. Li R, Qiao M, Wang X, Zhao X, Sun Q. Effect of narrow band ultraviolet B phototherapy as monotherapy or combination therapy for vitiligo: a meta-analysis. Photodermatol Photoimmunol Photomed. 2017;33:21–31.

82. Bhatnagar A, Kanwar AJ, Parsad D, De D. Psoralen and ultraviolet A and narrow-band ultraviolet B in inducing stability in vitiligo, assessed by vitiligo disease activity score: an open prospective comparative study. J Eur Acad Dermatol Venereol. 2007;21:1381–5.

83. Linthorst Homan MW, Spuls PI, Nieuweboer-Krobotova L, et al. A randomized comparison of excimer laser vs narrow-band ultraviolet B phototherapy after punch grafting in stable vitiligo patients. J Eur Acad Dermatol Venereol. 2012;26(6):690–5.

84. Kanwar AJ, Mahajan R, Parsad D. Low-dose oral mini-pulse dexamethasone therapy in progressive unstable vitiligo. J Cutan Med Surg. 2013;17:259–68.

85. Singh A, Kanwar AJ, Parsad D. Mahajan. Randomized controlled study to evaluate the effectiveness of dexamethasone oral minipulse therapy vs oral minocycline in patients with active vitiligo vulgaris. Indian J Dermatol Venereol Leprol. 2014;80(1):29–35.

86. Singh H, Kumaran MS, Bains A, Parsad D. A randomized comparative study of oral corticosteroid minipulse and low-dose oral methotrexate in the treatment of unstable vitiligo. Dermatology. 2015;231:286–90.

87. Gokhale BB. Cyclophosphamide and vitiligo. Int J Dermatol. 1979;18:92.

88. Iannella G, Greco A, Didona D, Didona B, Granata G, Manno A, Pasquariello B, Magliulo G. Vitiligo: pathogenesis, clinical variants and treatment approaches. Autoimmun Rev. 2016;15:335–43.

89. Radmanesh M, Saedi K. The efficacy of combined PUVA and low-dose azathioprine for early and enhanced repigmentation in vitiligo patients. J Dermatol Treat. 2006;17:151–3.

90. Cavalie M, Ezzedine K, Fontas E, Montaudie H, Castela E, Bahadoran P, Taieb A, Lacour JP, Passeran T. Maintenance therapy of adult vitiligo with 0.1% tacrolimus ointment: a randomized, double

blind placebo-controlled study. J Invest Dermatol. 2015;135(4):970–4.

91. Feetham HJ, Chan JL, Pandya AG. Characterization of clinical response in patients with vitiligo undergoing autologous epidermal punch grafting. Dermatol Surg. 2012;38:14–9.

92. Agrawal K, Agrawal A. Vitiligo: repigmentation with dermabrasion and thin split-thickness skin graft. Dermatol Surg. 1995;21:295–300.

93. Gupta S, Ajith C, Kanwar AJ, Kumar B. Surgical pearl: standardized suction syringe for epidermal grafting. J Am Acad Dermatol. 2005;52:348–50.

94. Huggins RH, Henderson MD, Mulekar SV, et al. Melanocyte-keratinocyte transplantation procedure in the treatment of vitiligo: the experience of an academic medical center in the United States. J Am Acad Dermatol. 2012;66:785–93.

95. Nordlund JJ, Forget B, Kirkwood J, Lerner AB. Dermatitis produced by applications of monobenzone in patients with active vitiligo. Arch Dermatol. 1985;121:1141–4.

96. Lim HW, Grimes PE, Agbai O, et al. Afamelanotide and narrowband UV-phototherapy for the treatment of vitiligo: a randomized multicenter trial. JAMA Dermatol. 2015;151:42–50.

97. Passeron T. Medical and maintenance treatments for vitiligo. Dermatol Clin. 2017;35:163–70.

98. Rashighi M, Harris JE. Interfering with the IFN-gamma/CXCL 10 pathway to develop new targeted treatments for vitiligo. Ann Transl Med. 2015; 3:343.

99. King BA, Craiglow BG. Tofacitinib citrate for the treatment of vitiligo: a pathogenesis-directed therapy. JAMA Dermatol. 2015;151(10):1110–2.

100. Harris JE, Rashighi M, Nguyen N, et al. Rapid skin repigmentation on oral ruxolitinib in a patient with coexisting vitiligo and alopecia areata (AA). J Am Acad Dermatol. 2016;74:370–1.

101. Ramien ML, Ondrejchak S, Gendron R, et al. Quality of life in pediatric patients before and after cosmetic camouflage of visible skin conditions. J Am Acad Dermatol. 2014;71(5):935–40.

102. Tedeschi A, Dall'Oglio F, Micali G, Schwartz RA, Janniger CK. Corrective camouflage in pediatric dermatology. Cutis. 2007;79(2):110–2.

103. Rothstein B, Joshipura D, Saraiya A, et al. Treatment of vitiligo with the topical Janus kinase inhibitor ruxolitinib. J Am Acad Dermatol. 2017;76:1054–60.

104. Grimes P, Nashawati R. The role of diet and supplements in vitiligo management. Dermatol Clin. 2017;35:235–43.

105. De Cuyper C. Permanent makeup: indications and complications. Clin Dermatol. 2008;26:30–4.

106. Shokeen D. Postinflammatory hyperpigmentation in patients with skin of color. Cutis. 2016;97(1):E9–E11.

107. Nouveau S, Agrawal D, Kohl M, Bernard F, Misra N, Nayak CS. Skin hyper pigmentation in Indian population: Insights and best practice. Indian J Dermatol. 2016;61(5):487–95.

108. Davis E, Callender V. Postinflammatory hyperpigmentation: a review of the epidemiology, clinical features, and treatment option in skin of color. J Clin Aesthet Dermatol. 2010;3(7):20–31.

109. Lynne C, Kraft J, Lynde C. Topical treatments for melasma and post inflammatory hyper pigmentation. Skin Therapy Lett. 2006;11(9):1–6.

110. Callender VD, Surin-Lord SS, Davis EC, Maclin M. Postinflammatory hyperpigmentation etiologic therapeutic considerations. Am J Clin Dermatol. 2011;12(2):87–99.

111. Silpa-archa N, Kohl I, Chaowattanapanit S, Lim H, Hamzavi I. Postinflammatory hyperpigmentation: a comprehensive review. J Am Acad Dermatol. 2017;77(4):591–605.

112. Liz N, Vafaie J, Kihiczak N, Schwartz R. Postinflammatory hyperpigmentation: a common but troubling condition. Int J Dermatol. 2004;43:362–5.

113. Cestari T, Arellano I, Hexsel D, Ortonne JP, Latin American Pigmentary Disorders Academy. Melasma in Latin America: options for therapy and treatment algorithm. Eur Acad Dermatol Venereol. 2009;23:760–72.

114. Oma A, Hamzavi I, Jagdeo J. Laser treatments for postinflammatory hyperpigmentation: a systemic review. JAMA Dermatol. 2017;153(2):199–206.

115. Ball Arefiew KL, Hantash BM. Advances in the treatment of melasma: a review of the recent literature. Dermatol Surg. 2012;38(7):971–84.

116. Passeron T. Melasma pathogenesis and influencing factors-an overview of the latest research. J Eur Acad Dermatol Venereol. 2013;27(1):5–6.

117. Ogbechie-Gode OA, Elbuluk N. Melasma: an up-to-date comprehensive review. Dermatol Ther. 2017;7:305–18.

118. Mansouri P, Farshi S, Hashemi Z, Kasraee B. Evaluation of the efficacy of cysteamine 5% cream in the treatment of epidermal melasma: a randomized double-blind placebo-controlled trial. British Journal of Dermatology. 2015;173:209–17.

119. Rodrigues M, Panda A. Melasma: clinical diagnosis and management options. Aust J Dermatol. 2015;56:151–63.

120. Bourra H, Leila B. Lichen planus pigmentosus. Pan Afr Med J. 2013;15:55.

121. Ghosh A, Coondoo A. Lichen planus pigmentosus: the controversial consensus. Indian J Dermatol. 2016;61(5):482–6.

122. Vachiramon V, Suchonwanit P, Thadanipon K. Bilateral linear lichen planus pigmentosus associated with hepatitis C virus infection. Case Rep Dermatol. 2010;2:169–72.

123. Weston G, Payette M. Update on lichen planus and its clinical variants. Int J Women's Dermatol. 2015;1(3):140–9.

124. Robles-Medez JC, Rizo-Frias P, Herz-Ruelas ME, Pandya AG, Candiani JO. Lichen planus pigmentosis and its variants: review and update. Int J Dermatol. 2017;57(5). Wiley Online Library.

125. Osswald SS, Proffer LH, Sartori CR. Erythema dyschromicum perstans: a case report and review. Cutis: Chatham. 2001;68(1):25–8.

126. Mulinari-Brenner FA, Guilherme MR, Werner B. Frontal fibrosing alopecia and lichen planus pigmentosus: diagnosis and therapeutic challenge. An Bras Dermatol. 2017;92(5):79–81.

127. Wolfshohl JA, Geddes ERC, Stout A, Friedman PM. Improvement of erythema dyschromicum perstans using a combination of the 1,550-nm erbium-doped fractionated laser and topical tacrolimus ointment. Laser Surg Med. 2016;49(1). Wiley Online Library.

128. Pandya A, Guevara IL. Disorders of hyperpigmentation. Dermatol Clin. 2000;18(1):91–8.

129. Skorin L. Minocycline-induced hyperpigmentation of the skin, sclera, and palpebral conjunctiva. Can J Opthalmol. 2017;52:e79–81.

130. Bahloul E, Jallouli M, Garbaa S, Marzouk S, Masmoudi A, Turki H, et al. Hydroxychloroquine-induced hyperpigmentation in systemic disease prevalence, clinical features and risk factures: a cross-sectional study of 41 cases. Lupus. 2017;26:1304–8.

131. Cohen PR, Eichenfield DZ. Amitriptyline-induced cutaneous hyperpigmentation: case report and review of pscychotropic drug-associated mucocutaneous hyperpigmentation. Dermatol Online J. 2016;22(2):6.

132. Lause M, Kamboj A, Faith EF. Dermatologic manifestations of endocrine disorders. Transl Pediatr. 2017;6(4):300–12.

133. Michels A, Michels N. Addison disease: early detection and treatment principles. Am Fam Physician. 2014;89(7):563–8.

134. Neiman LK, Chanco Turner ML. Addison's disease. Clin Dermatol. 2006;24:276–80.

135. Fernandez-Flores A, Cassarino DS. Histopathologic findings of cutaneous hyperpigmentation in Addison disease and immunostain of the melanocytic population. Am J Dermatopathol. 2017;39:924–7.

136. Banba K, Tanaka N, Fujioka A, Tajima S. Hyperpigmentation caused by hyperthyroidism: differences from the pigmentation of Addison's disease. Clin Dermatol. 1999;43:196–8.

137. Leonhardt JM, Heymann WR. Thyroid disease and the skin. Dermatol Clin. 2002;20(3):473–81.

138. Amatya B, Agrawal S, Dhali T, Sharma S, Pandey SS. Pattern of skin and nail changes in chronic renal failure in Nepal: a hospital-based study. J Dermatol. 2008;35:140–5.

139. Becker S, Walter S, Witzke O, et al. Edema, hyper pigmentation, induration: 3 skin signs heralding danger in patients on maintenance hemodialysis. Medicine. 2016;95(12):1–6.

140. Onelmis H, Sener S, Sasmaz S, Ozer A. Cutaneous changes in patient with chronic renal failure on hemodialysis. Cutan Ocul Toxicol. 2013;31(4):286–91.

141. Fistarol SK, Itin PH. Disorders of pigmentation. J German Soc Dermatol. 2010;8:187–202.

142. Levy L, Zeichner JA. Dermatologic manifestation of diabetes. J Diabetes. 2012;4:68–76.

143. Morgan AJ, Schwartz RA. Diabetic dermopathy: a subtle sign with grave implications. J Am Acad Dermatol. 2008;58(3):447–51.

144. Vera-Kellter C, Andino-Navarrete R, Navajas-Galimany L. Vitamin B12 deficiency and its numerous skin manifestations. Actas Dermosifiliogr. 2015;106:762–4.

145. Brescoll J, Daveluy S. A review of vitamin b12 deficiency in dermatology. Am J Clin Dermatol. 2015;16:27–33.

146. Demir N, Dogan M, Koc A, Kaba S, Bulan K, Ozkol HU, et al. Dermatological findings of vitamin B12 deficiency and resolving time of these symptoms. Cutan Ocul Toxicol. 2014;33(1):70–3.

147. Higgins SP, Freemark M, Prose NS. Acanthosis nigricans: a practical approach to evaluation and management. Dermatol Online J. 2008;14(9). Retrieved from https://escholarship.org/uc/item/7mf6g290.

148. Abraham C, Rozmus CL. Is acanthosis nigricans a reliable indicator for risk of type 2 diabetes in obese children and adolescents? A systematic review. J Sch Nurs. 2012;28(3):195–205.

149. Brickman WJ, Binns HJ, Jovanovis BD, Kolesky S, Mancini AJ, Metzger BE. Acanthosis nigricanss: A common finding in overweight youth. Pediatr Dermatol. 2007;24(6):601–6.

150. Schwartz RA. Efficacy of topical 0.1% adapalene gel for the use in the treatment of childhood acanthosis nigricans: a pilot study. Dermatol Ther. 2015;28:266.

Hair Loss in Women of Color

Oma N. Agbai and Jodie Raffi

Introduction

"People of color" refers to a large group of people with pigmented skin from several different racial and ethnic origins, including but not limited to Africans, African Americans, African Caribbeans, Chinese, Japanese, Navajo Indians, Indians, Pakistanis, and Arabs. Already comprising a sizeable section of the American population, this group is predicted to grow dramatically over the next several decades, with patients of color comprising near 50% of the US population by the year 5050. These demographic changes emphasize the importance of understanding the cultural practices and dermatologic needs of this population [1]. One important area in which dermatologist expertise will be invaluable is hair loss. Unlike Caucasians and Asians, epidemiological data in African American women reveals alopecia among the group's top ten dermatologic conditions [2].

Hair is central to identity and appearance and may play a role in thermoregulation and photoprotection. Thus, it is no surprise that hair loss can have a detrimental psychological impact. The effect of alopecia extends beyond outward appearance; a majority of women in one study reported a change in their daily activities and loss of self-confidence due to their hair loss [3]. Studies in women with androgenetic alopecia demonstrate a reduced quality of life and reduced self-esteem at both the time of hair loss and for extended periods thereafter. Regardless of ethnicity or the underlying pathophysiology of hair loss, alopecia is likely to negatively impact a patient and encourage them to seek dermatologic help.

With a higher rate of alopecia in women of color (WOC) and the negative psychosocial impact of hair loss, it is imperative that all dermatologists are up to date on how to prevent, counsel, and treat hair-related concerns effectively in this population. This chapter will explain the structural qualities of hair in WOC and how it differs from the hair of Caucasians, including the follicle and shaft shape, the density of hair, and the intra-shaft interactions of the hair, all of which bear importance on the overall quality and strength of the hair. We will also discuss hair practices in WOC and how these practices may increase risk of certain types of hair loss. Finally, we will focus on the presentation, pathophysiology, and management of the types of alopecia that present uniquely in WOC.

O. N. Agbai
University of California, Davis, Department of Dermatology, Sacramento, CA, USA

J. Raffi (✉)
UC Irvine School of Medicine, Department of Dermatology, Beverly Hills, CA, USA

© Springer Nature Switzerland AG 2021
B. S. Li, H. I. Maibach (eds.), *Ethnic Skin and Hair and Other Cultural Considerations*, Updates in Clinical Dermatology, https://doi.org/10.1007/978-3-030-64830-5_11

Structural Differences of Hair Between Patients of Color and Caucasian Patients

Hair of different ethnicities can be separated into three groups based on differences in shaft and follicular architecture: African, Caucasian, and Asian [4]. The hair shaft is composed of a cortex surrounded by several layers of cuticular cells [5]. The chemical structure of the shaft itself, specifically the keratin and the amino acid configurations, is similar across ethnicities [2, 4]. However, Black hair reserves some distinctions. It is more densely pigmented than Caucasian hair [1], and unlike Caucasian hair, it contains melanosomes in the outer root sheath and in the bulb of vellus hairs [1]. The size of the melanin granules in Black hair is also larger than in that of individuals with a fair complexion [1, 6].

There are four major types of hair patterns: helical, spiral, straight, and wavy [1]. The majority of Africans have spiral hair, a quality that makes the hair more difficult to comb [2]. Unlike in Asians or Caucasians, the African hair follicle is sharply curved, contributing to the frizzy, curly appearance of the hair. It also results in the growing hair emerging from the skin obliquely, leading to higher rates of conditions such as pseudofolliculitis barbae [4]. Under magnification, African hair is described as an oval-twisted rod with many random twists and irregular direction changes; in cross section, the shaft has a flattened, elliptical morphology [1, 2]. The diameter of the hair shaft is highly irregular [2], reducing gradually as the hair descends from the scalp. Additionally, there are fewer sebaceous glands in the scalp of individuals of African descent, compared with other ethnicities, resulting in drier, more brittle hair.

Caucasian hair, in contrast, is of a more straight or gently curved shape [5] with an oval cross section and oval follicle [5]. It has a larger diameter than that of African hair [2]. Studies have shown that Caucasian hair grows faster than African hair (0.330 vs 0.259 mm/day, respectively) [7]. However, there is marked similarity in the cuticle thickness, shape and size of scale, and cortical cells between African and Caucasian hair [1].

Structural studies of African hair compared to Caucasian hair have revealed a number of differences. For example, African hair may display microscopic signs of structural damage such as longitudinal fissures leading to splits along the shaft, which ultimately cause more frequent knotting of African hair. A majority of African hairs removed by combing were found to be fractured at the top rather than containing an attached root, indicating breakage of the shaft rather than natural shedding of intact hair during grooming. Additionally, most of the tips of the African hair studied were frayed or serrated, rather than appearing smooth or cut (as during a haircut) [8]. Examination of the in situ hair relationships in African and Caucasian women demonstrated greater intertwining of hairs in African hair, developing into a mat-like structure of hair, whereas Caucasian hair formed fewer single-strand knots and had fewer interlocking knots and weaves between adjacent hairs. These differences may explain why less sebum is able to coat African hair, resulting in drier, less shiny hair with lesser tensile strength [9]. They also explain why there is increased breakage with combing of African hair, making long hair difficult to achieve [7, 10].

Hair density and the total number of hair follicles are notably lower in African than Caucasian hair [1]. Some authors have also observed fewer elastic fibers attaching the hair follicles to the dermis in the Black subjects compared with White subjects [1, 11]. This differential may provide an explanation for certain types of alopecia, such as traction alopecia and central centrifugal cicatricial alopecia [1], which occur more commonly in African than Caucasian women [2, 9]. In addition, African hair has been shown to contain a fewer lipids than Caucasian hair, rendering it more vulnerable to damage by UV radiation [12]. Integral lipids in the hair cuticle offer a degree of protection from UV damage by imparting hydrophobicity, moisturization, and stiffness to hair that reinforces the structural integrity of the strands. These findings, along with reduced tensile strength and less moisture compared to Caucasian hair, explain why African hair is more easily susceptible to breakage [2, 12]. Overall, however, the composition of lipids in the hair is similar across racial type [2].

Hair Care Practices in Women of African Descent

Hair care practices are influenced by current trends as well as ease of style and maintenance [3]. There are several culture-specific hair practices common in women of African descent that induce hair damage either by introducing excess tension at the root of the hair follicles or by direct insult to the hair shaft, potentially contributing to alopecia in women of African descent.

Certain hairstyles subject the hair root to excess tension, including cornrows, weaves, dreadlocks, sisterlocks, braids, and twists. The prolonged periods of traction increase the risk of traction folliculitis and traction alopecia [9, 13]. Cornrows is a hairstyle that involves splitting hair into sections and then braiding it to produce rows of braids (Fig. 11.1). Cornrows and braids are low-maintenance hairstyles that enable less frequent use of chemical or thermal hair treatment and allow the hair a period to "rest" and "grow out" after being chemically relaxed (Fig. 11.2) [13]. A hair weave is a style that sews or glues additional human or synthetic hair to the base of the cornrowed hair, with the added hair worn loose (Fig. 11.3) [9]. Hair wefting is another type of hair extension in which a group of hairs brought together in a band of threads is thereby clipped, glued, or sewn to the hairline for extended periods of time [14]. Dreadlocks, or "locs," is a hairstyle that involves the hair knotting into individual twist-like structures (Fig. 11.4, left) [9]. This is a permanent style that remains until the hair is cut [13]. The dreadlocks are styled by twisting or "palm-rolling" the root with a balm or wax to lock the hair together [9, 13]. Sisterlocks are created in a similar fashion but with much thinner and smaller locs (Fig. 11.4, right) [13]. While the loc style avoids the use of chemical or heat processing, it induces tension at the roots, especially if the sections are small, the locs over-twisted at the root, or if grown very long [9].

Straight hair, a sought-after style in this group due to its increased manageability, is achieved either by thermal or chemical means [2, 9]. Thermal techniques, such as hot combing or pressing, introduce heat to the shaft leading to short-term rearrangement of hydrogen bonds within hair strands. Hot combing is a technique introduced in the early twentieth century that has become less popular since the advent of chemical straighteners [3]. After washing and drying, an oil or pomade is first applied throughout the hair, and then a hot metal comb heated to 300 to 500 °F is pulled through the length of the hair. The thermal straightening effect is temporary, lasting until the hair is washed [3]. This method is associated with damage to the hair shaft as well as scalp burns, potentially causing acquired trichorrhexis nodosa [3]. The use of hot combing plus braiding is a common hairstyle initiated as early as childhood or adolescence [1].

Hair straightening is also achieved with the use of a flat iron, which consists of two flat ceramic plates heated to 180–450 °F pressed along the length of the hair [2]. Despite temperatures nearly as high as hot combing, flat irons may result in less damage due to even heating and better temperature control [9]. Furthermore, as opposed to oils and pomades used with hot combs, silicone heat-protectant lubricators are often used with flat irons to protect the hair from damage [9]. In addition to these two methods,

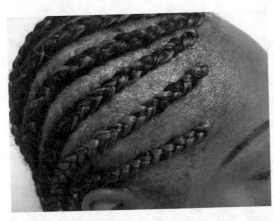

Fig. 11.1 Cornrow hairstyle. (Reproduced with permission from Ref. [15])

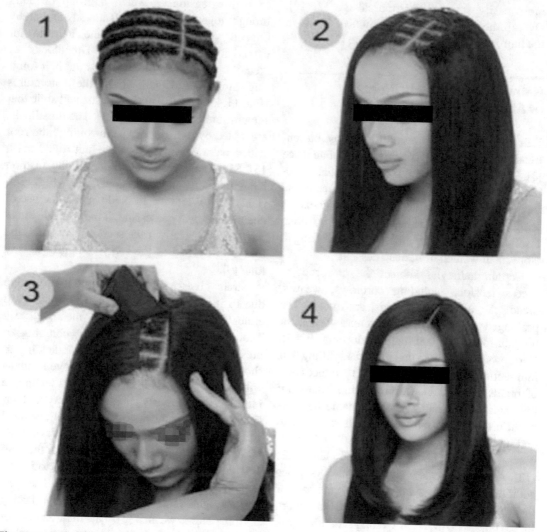

Fig. 11.2 (Was 4) Tight braids inducing folliculitis and early traction alopecia. (Reproduced with permission from Ref. [15])

women also use curling irons, hair rollers, and hair dyes, all of which may contribute to hair damage [1].

Chemical straightening, a method used by 90% of African American women at some point, is much more commonly used than hot combing. Unlike the temporary effect of thermal straightening, chemical straightening rearranges disulfide bonds within the shaft to produce permanently straight hair. Chemical relaxers are highly alkaline substances containing sodium hydroxide or guanidine hydroxide, the latter used in no-lye formulas [9, 16]. This method, often performed up to 6–12 times per year, is seen as an easier way to reduce the curliness of the hair [3]. However, it is not without risks, as it frequently leads to frail, damage-susceptible hair, irritant contact dermatitis, and acquired trichorrhexis nodosa, especially with improper use [1]. The resultant hair fragility may be due to a lower cysteine content in relaxed hair, a component of the disulfide bond that is essential for hair strength [9]. Use with concurrent permanent hair dye can induce breakage [17]. The Brazilian keratin treatment, another method of chemical straightening lasting about 2–2.5 months, involves covering the

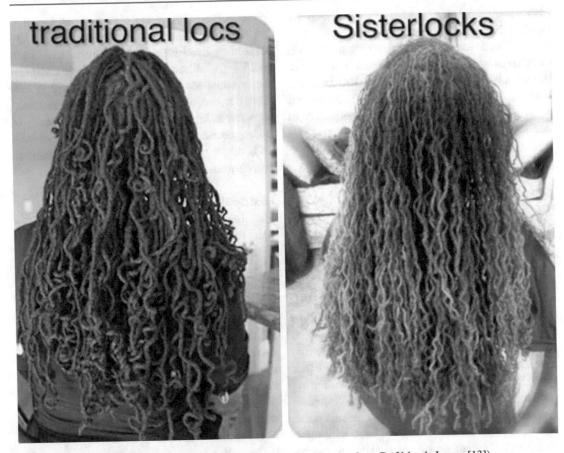

Fig. 11.3 (Was 2) Sew-in weave hairstyle. (Reproduced with permission from Dr. Yolanda Lenzy [13])

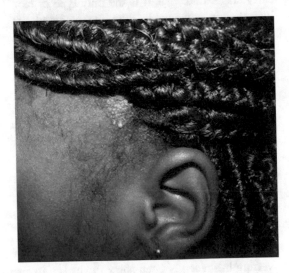

Fig. 11.4 (Was 3) Left: Traditional locs. Right: sister-locks. (Reproduced with permission from Dr. Yolanda Lenzy [13])

hair with a liquid keratin and formaldehyde preparation and sealing the solution to the hair with a flat iron. Formaldehyde exposure during the use of Brazilian keratin is the main health risk to both the client and the hair stylist, and the heat from the flat iron is also damaging the hair [2, 4].

African American women typically shampoo once every 1–2 weeks, compared with the every-other-day or once-weekly washes in Caucasian women [7]. In addition to naturally low hair sebum levels, necessitating less frequent washing, shampooing often may contribute to dry hair and risk for breakage. Less frequent shampooing also allows longer preservation of the time-consuming and expensive hairstyles [2]. This is of importance to dermatologists, as treatments involving shampooing or wetting the hair may not be adopted easily in this group [4].

Furthermore, infrequent shampooing allows for product buildup, which contributes to hair shaft dryness and reduced tensile strength. Product buildup may also lead to or worsen scalp conditions such as seborrheic dermatitis or cause irritant contact dermatitis [4, 7]. The use of emollients may provide a false impression of healthy hair and also result in less frequent shampooing [3].

Alopecia

Alopecia is a condition that has a wide range of etiologic subtypes, certain forms of which are far more common in women of color. Alopecia can be categorized into two major groups, non-scarring or scarring (also referred to as "cicatricial"). Non-scarring alopecias of special focus to the WOC population include traction alopecia, trichorrhexis nodosa, and seborrheic dermatitis, the latter of which can be associated with hair loss. It is important to be familiar with non-scarring forms of alopecia as prompt diagnosis can have a profound impact on the clinical course and total eventual hair loss associated with these diseases. Examples of cicatricial alopecias include central centrifugal cicatricial alopecia, discoid lupus erythematosus, lichen planopilaris, and frontal fibrosing alopecia. Generally, management of these diseases focuses on symptom relief and halting the progression of hair loss. Unfortunately, the underlying cause and strategies for management of many alopecias remains to be studied and delineated with greater confidence [18].

Traction Alopecia

Traction alopecia (TA) is a pattern of traumatic hair loss highly associated with hair care practices and increased hair follicle vulnerability [14]. It occurs most commonly in females of African ethnicity [2, 6, 19]. The primary insult occurs when tension is applied to the hair for prolonged periods or in a repetitive manner [2]. Regularly styling the hair in a manner that involves tight pulling is the central risk factor to TA. The combination of traction and chemically relaxed or dyed hair significantly increases the risk of TA, although the frequency of chemical use has not been found to affect the risk [2, 6, 19]. Genetics, too, may play a role; TA has been found to occur at higher rates with a family history of androgenetic alopecia [15]. The use of shampoo and other hair products does not appear to increase risk of TA [15].

Histopathology

Histology early on shows a normal density of hair follicles, retained hair sebaceous glands, higher numbers of telogen and catagen hairs, and trichomalacia. Over time, the number of terminal follicles will be fewer, although vellus hairs appear unaffected. Loss of hair follicles is accompanied by concentric fibrosis [14]. Overall, there is little inflammation in TA. Biopsy of transverse sections of scalp showing a low-power pattern of miniaturization and follicular dropout with retained sebaceous glands should point toward a diagnosis of TA [15]. This method is preferable over vertical sections in differentiating TA from scarring alopecias such as cicatricial alopecia. TA is the only type of alopecia that has a reversible early stage. Likewise, it is the only type of hair loss that is preventable with the potential for eradication [15]. A proposed staging system delineates TA into a reversible "prealopecia stage," a reversible stage with alopecia, and a stage with permanent, irreversible alopecia [14].

Etiology

The patient history may point to the use of tight hairstyles that put tension on the hair root or hair treatments that increase the vulnerability to traction-related damage. The physician should evaluate for a history of tight ponytails, buns, chignons, braids, twists, weaves, cornrows, dreadlocks, sisterlocks, and hair wefts in addition to the usage of religious hair coverings [2, 14]. Wefting has recently been shown to cause TA in some cases [14]. Some patients with TA report symptoms with hairdressing, which may include scalp tenderness, stinging, crusting, and follicular papules [15]. Finally, a history of treatment

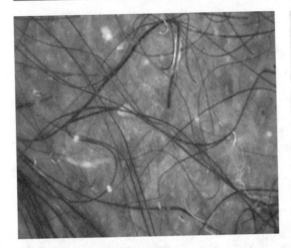

Fig. 11.5 Peripilar casts. (Reproduced with permission from Ref. [21])

with hair dyes or chemical relaxers may be readily apparent or elicited upon questioning the patient.

Clinical Features

Physical exam findings are dependent on the clinical stage of TA. At the earliest stage, scalp traction results in perifollicular erythema, which may evolve into follicular papules or pustules. These findings are most prominent in the area with the greatest traction. However, the patient may not be aware of these lesions as they can be missed without close inspection [15]. As the traction continues, affected hair shafts become enveloped by a yellow-white material called a peripilar cast (Fig. 11.5) [2, 20, 21]. Peripilar casts on the hair shaft indicate that TA is ongoing or persistent [15]. Beyond this point, clinically evident hair loss develops. In the late stages of TA, dermal scarring and permanent alopecia develop. The scalp at this stage demonstrates a reduction of follicular ostia in affected areas [2, 20].

The most common locations subject to traction and the development of TA are the marginal hairline (along the frontal and temporal scalp) and anterior and superior to the ears [2, 14]. The "fringe sign," which can aid in the diagnosis of TA, refers to hair loss at the marginal hairline with some preserved hairs along the frontal and/ or temporal hairline (Fig. 11.6) [2, 20]. Less common variants of TA have been found to affect

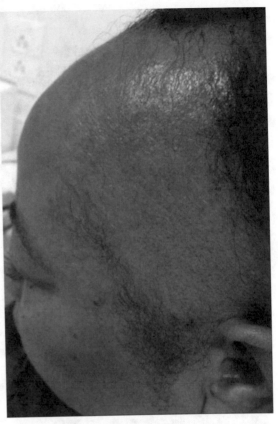

Fig. 11.6 Fringe sign. (Reproduced with permission from Ref. [15])

other areas of the scalp (Fig. 11.7). When due to wefted hair extensions, TA may present with a "horseshoe" pattern (Fig. 11.8) [14]. Reports of TA in Hispanic women with a history of tight ponytail use and ballerinas and Japanese women commonly styling their hair into a tight bun have demonstrated hair loss localized to the temporal or occipital scalp [22, 23]. TA may also appear in linear, curved, or geometric shapes [15].

Differential Diagnosis

Not all TA patients present with a clear-cut history of high tension hairstyles. In the case of unclear history of hair tension or unclear clinical presentation, other diagnoses to consider include androgenetic alopecia, telogen effluvium, trichotillomania, and central centrifugal cicatricial alopecia. Long-term or repetitive hair wefting may induce TA that appears similar to scarring alopecia [14]. Consider frontal fibrosing alopecia

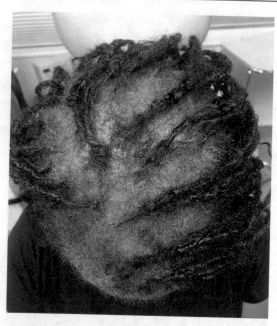

Fig. 11.7 Sisterlocks on a scalp affected by traction alopecia. (Image courtesy of Oma Agbai, MD)

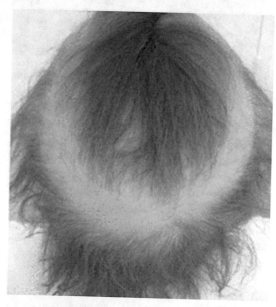

Fig. 11.8 Horseshoe traction alopecia. Alopecia of occipital and temporoparietal scalp corresponds to area where patient used glued-in hair wefts. (Reproduced with permission from Ref. [14])

(FFA) and alopecia areata (AA) ophiasis pattern in cases confined to the marginal hairline [24]. Unlike TA, AA and FAA may also involve the eyebrows, body hair, skin, and nails. Follicular

markings, which are decreased in TA, remain present in AA and are absent in FFA. Accurate diagnosis requires biopsy [15]. See Table 11.1 for a comparison of the clinical features of TA, AA, and FAA.

Management

Management of TA is also dependent on the stage of the disease. A proposed prevention strategy involves notifying at-risk patients to limit tension hairstyles to a short time duration (maximum 2 weeks) infrequent use, created in a painless manner and on natural hair [15]. In early stages, TA is reversible; thus, the clinician plays an important role in counseling the patient of the risk of progressive, permanent hair loss [25]. Once TA is noted, the patient should avoid chemical relaxers, dyes, and heat and lessen or avoid tension in their hairstyles. Early intervention includes suppression of follicular inflammation with topical and/or intralesional corticosteroids [26]. This may be combined with topical minoxidil [2, 19]. Oral or topical antibiotics can be beneficial at this stage given their anti-inflammatory properties [26]. Once there is scarring of the dermis or permanent alopecia, treatment necessitates surgical interventions such as hair transplantation [26, 27].

Acquired Trichorrhexis Nodosa

Trichorrhexis nodosa (TN) is a form of alopecia resulting from the loss of cuticle cells on the hair shaft. The congenital form of TN is rare, while acquired TN is much more common and caused by trauma to the hair during grooming practices [2, 28]. Without the protective cuticle, the cortical fibers of the hair shaft become fragile and fray longitudinally [2].

Etiology

Causes of acquired TN include a variety of hair care practices that induce trauma to the hair. Repeated chemical treatment, such as the use of relaxers, dyes, bleaches, perms, or shampoos have been implicated in TN. Relaxers have been found to directly weaken the hair cuticle and

Table 11.1 A comparison of clinical features of traction alopecia, alopecia areata, and frontal fibrosing alopecia

	Traction alopecia	Alopecia areata	Frontal fibrosing alopecia
Follicular markings (ostia)	Decreased (especially in late stage)	Retained	Absent/decreased
Perifollicular erythema	May be present in early stages	None	Typically present
Perifollicular scale	Scale or casts may be present in early or ongoing traction	None	Can be present
Hair findings	Fringe sign	Exclamation point hairs	Lonely hair sign
Dermoscopy	Vellus hairs, mobile hair casts, pinpoint white dots	Pinpoint white dots, yellow dots rarer in pigmented skin, exclamation mark hairs, and black dots	Absence of vellus hairs, black dots, and peripilar casts at new hairline
Appearance of scalp skin	Unchanged	May be slightly erythematous	Atrophic, sclerotic with accentuation of veins
Eyebrows	Unaffected	May be affected	Often affected
Body hair	Unaffected	May be affected	May be affected
Nail findings	None	Pits	None, pterygium (rare)
Skin findings	None	None	Lichen planus/lichen planus pigmentosus, facial papules, prominent facial veins
Mucosal findings	None	None	Oral lichen planus/Wickham striae may be present

Reproduced with permission from Ref. [15]

compromise the hair shaft itself by reducing the cysteine levels [2, 19]. Thermal hair tools including flat irons and hot combs damage the cuticle leading to increased fragility and breakage. Aggressive hair brushing or combing also introduces damage to the cuticle and contribute to TN. Medical conditions such as iron deficiency anemia and hypothyroidism may also lead to TN [2, 28].

Clinical Features

Hair affected by TN is characterized by a dry, lusterless, brittle quality with whitish spots along the shaft [2, 28]. TN is most often localized to the distal shaft, with focal narrowing observed along the length of the shaft. A normal hair cuticle contains cells organized in a neat fashion similar to roof tiles. Under magnification, cuticle cells affected by TN appear disrupted, and the underlying cortical fibers split into many small fibers [2, 28].

Management

Minimization or cessation of traumatizing processes is the priority in managing TN. The use of hot combs and flat irons should be limited to once weekly or less, temperatures under 175 °C, and use on dry hair [2, 29]. Frequency of chemical relaxers and dye use should be minimized, and these products should be applied by a licensed hair stylist. The combination of dyeing and chemically relaxing hair should be avoided if possible as it leads to a notably increased risk of hair breakage. In routine hair care, efforts should be made to reduce friction by the use of conditioners, hair oils, and combs with straight elongated bristles [2].

Central Centrifugal Cicatricial Alopecia

Central centrifugal cicatricial alopecia (CCCA) is a form of scarring alopecia affecting the crown and vertex of the head. It is most often seen in women of African ethnicity, with many fewer cases observed in men of African descent. Known historically by names such as "hot comb alopecia" and "follicular degeneration syndrome," CCCA is the most common cause of permanent hair loss in this ethnic group [9, 30]. The disease most often presents in middle age [30]. It is characterized by hair loss originating at the vertex of the scalp that proceeds centrifugally, often in a symmetric manner [30].

Etiology

The cause of CCCA is not known. Although it was initially believed to be caused by trauma from hot comb use, subsequent studies have failed to demonstrate a causal effect between hot comb use and CCCA [9]. Studies have also failed to find correlation between chemical relaxer use and CCCA but have yielded mixed results with regard to traction-inducing hairstyles [9, 19, 30–32]. One theory suggests that CCCA originates as female pattern hair loss (FPHL), given the pattern I and pattern II distribution of hair loss, which is subsequently negatively influenced by hair grooming practices. Although CCCA and FPHL may appear similar, in late stages CCCA distinguishes itself by scarring and follicular dropout [30]. Other investigatory findings point toward a potential hereditary component, either due to a genetic predisposition or shared exposures, although more evidence is warranted in this area. Interestingly, studies show that scalp sebum maintains a pro-inflammatory state even in unaffected hair, with a greater amount of IL-1 alpha than IL-1 antagonist. It is theorized that after an initial event of premature desquamation of the inner root sheath (PDIRS), the inner follicle is more susceptible to invasion by cosmetics and microorganisms, with eventual inflammation and scarring [9].

Histopathology

CCCA is characterized by chronic perifollicular lymphocytic inflammation leading to eventual scarring of the scalp. Early in the course of the disease, hair follicles are surrounded by a lymphocytic infiltrate and perifollicular fibroplasia. PDIRS is a central histologic finding in CCCA, although it can also be found in other types of primary scarring alopecia. There is also a reduction in the number of terminal hair follicles with a concurrent increase in fibrous tracts [9]. Early biopsies may be interpreted as "lichen planopilaris" or "pseudopelade," given the scarring and

follicular destruction [30]. An active phase in which the affected area increases in size may last years but ultimately ceases naturally [30]. Late in the disease, pathological findings include obliteration of pilosebaceous units, dermal scarring, and dermal lymphocytic and plasma cell infiltrate. Biopsy of end-stage CCCA will demonstrate fibrosis with little remaining inflammation [30]. Although these findings are useful in the diagnosis of CCCA, they are not unique to this disease and cannot distinguish it from other primary scarring alopecias such as lichen planopilaris, discoid lupus erythematosus, and folliculitis decalvans [9, 30]. Therefore, every effort should be made to evaluate the patient early in the disease course and to correlate the histopathologic findings with the patient's history and clinical presentation [30].

Clinical Features

Patients with CCCA present with hair loss originating on the crown or vertex of the head, spreading outward in a centrifugal pattern (Fig. 11.9) [9, 30]. The patient may describe burning, itching, or tenderness in the affected area. However, not all patients experience symptoms and thus often present late after slow, insidious hair loss is noticed by others [31]. Early stages may demonstrate erythema or follicular pustules; late disease lacks observable inflammation. As the disease progresses, the number of visible follicles decreases, and the scalp appears smooth and shiny. Some individual strands may remain [9]. For a comparison of dermoscopic features of CCCA, lichen planopilaris, and frontal fibrosing alopecia, see Table 11.2.

Differential Diagnosis

Lichen planopilaris (LPP) can occur anywhere on the scalp but may look similar to CCCA especially in cases that begin on the vertex with centrifugal spread. Unlike CCCA, affected areas of LPP originate as hyperkeratotic follicular papules with perifollicular erythema. The lesions progress radially, ultimately resulting in dappled areas of scarred hair loss surrounded by unaffected hair. Frontal fibrosing alopecia (FFA) tar-

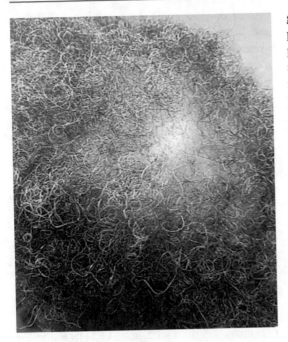

Fig. 11.9 Central centrifugal cicatricial alopecia. (Image courtesy of Oma Agbai, MD)

Table 11.2 Dermoscopic features of cicatricial alopecias

LPP	Peripilar white or silver scales
	Peripilar erythema
	Keratotic plugs
	Elongated, concentric blood vessels
	Violaceous-blue interfollicular areas
	Big irregular white dots
FFA	Peripilar white scales
	Peripilar erythema
	Predominance of follicular ostia
	Background of ivory white
	Lack of follicular ostia
	Eyebrows show regularly distributed gray dots
DLE	Peripilar white scales
	Peripilar erythema
	Keratotic plug
	Large yellow dots (keratotic material)
	Thick arborizing vessels
	Scattered dark brown discoloration
	Follicular red dots
CCCA	One or two hairs emerging together
	Peripilar white gray halo
	Lack of follicular ostia

Open access from Bolduc C, Sperling L, Shapiro J. Primary cicatricial alopecia: Lymphocytic primary cicatricial alopecias, including chronic cutaneous lupus erythematosus, lichen planopilaris, frontal fibrosing alopecia, and Graham-Little syndrome. Reproduced with permission from Ref. [61]

gets the eyebrows and frontotemporal hairline. It presents later than CCCA, most often in postmenopausal women in their 60s or 70s. It is slowly progressive and may also spread down the inferior temporoparietal hairline ("ophiasis-like pattern"). In some patients it may occur with nearby LPP or discoid lupus erythematosus [30, 33]. Folliculitis decalvans is characterized by patches of scarring alopecia surrounded by pustules. The hair loss begins in distinct round or oval areas but may merge into a large central area, mimicking CCCA. Lastly, discoid lupus erythematosus typically affects young to middle-aged females. While it characterized affects the sun-exposed face, ears, trunk, and limbs, the scalp may be involved. Some patients present with only scalp lesions, which can range from papules to sclerotic plaques. Affected areas are well circumscribed, erythematous, scaling, and pruritic. They may also display atrophy, telangiectasia, dyspigmentation, and follicular plugging. Key in distinguishing this process from CCCA is its tendency to recur within the confines of a previous patch [30].

Management

There is no established definitive treatment of CCCA. Therapy should be aimed at symptom relief and halting the progression of the disease [26]. Hair regrowth, if achieved, should be viewed as an extra benefit, though not assured. Patients should be advised to decrease or avoid trauma to the scalp during hair grooming. This includes decreasing the use of thermal hair appliances and loosening tight braids and weaves. Intervals between reapplication of relaxers should be increased as much as possible (at least every 8–12 weeks). Some sources recommend temporary cessation of heat or chemical processing and the avoidance of occlusive scalp greases to allow the scalp to heal [26, 30].

Medical management involves daily topical corticosteroids until symptom remission, with subsequent maintenance at 3 days per week. Intralesional steroids aimed at the periphery of the hair loss (including unaffected areas for prevention) can be administered at a dose range of 2.5–10 mg/mL every 4–8 weeks, for 6 months or longer [26, 31, 34]. Topical minoxidil should be tried for the potential of avoiding future scarring and nurturing recovering follicles; once inflammation has cleared, topical 2% or 5% solution or 5% foam can be used [30]. The use of oral tetracyclines and antimalarial medications for their anti-inflammatory properties has been reported with variable success [9]. Prior to initiating antibiotics, any pustules should be cultured to evaluate for a fungal infection or resistant *Staphylococcus*. In late-stage disease, surgical intervention may be considered. Hair transplantation should only be initiated once inflammatory infiltrate has cleared and hair loss has not progressed for at least 12 months [30]. While keloids are not as common a complication as previously thought, the scarring of the scalp due to CCCA renders transplantation more complicated and decreases the survival of the hair grafts [26].

Lichen Planopilaris

Lichen planopilaris (LPP) is an uncommon primary scarring alopecia of unknown etiology. It is considered a follicular variant of lichen planus [35]. Chronic lymphocytic inflammation in LPP targets the upper third of the hair follicle, with eventual destruction of the follicular stem cells and permanent hair loss [36]. Of new patients presenting with hair loss, LPP is estimated to account for 1.15–7.59% of cases [37]. It occurs more often in women and commonly presents during 30 and 60 years of age [35, 37]. Frontal fibrosing alopecia (FFA) and Graham-Little-Piccardi-Lassueur syndrome (GLPLS) are clinical variants of LPP. FFA, a scarring of alopecia presenting as a receding band the frontotemporal hairline, will be discussed in the following section. GLPLS is recognized by the combination of scarring patches of scalp alopecia, spinous follicular papules on the limbs and trunk, and a non-scarring alopecia in the axillary and pubic areas [35].

Histopathology

Biopsy demonstrates perivascular infiltrate with a lichenoid dermatitis enveloping the follicular infundibulum and isthmus [30]. Early lesions feature destruction of the sebaceous epithelium and arrector pili muscles; as the disease progresses, follicles may fuse, and the inner sheath may degenerate. In late disease, inflammation is less prominent, and perifollicular hyalinization and lamellar fibrosis are notable in the upper and lower dermis and follicle [35, 38]. With the aid of dermoscopy, perifollicular scaling can be visible on the proximal hair shaft of active lesions [35]. Lesions later in the course may be characterized by fibrotic white dots, absence of follicular ostia, pili torti, and honeycomb hyperpigmentation [35].

Clinical Presentation

Lichen planopilaris may manifest as multifocal patches or diffuse areas of hair loss throughout the scalp. The lesional margins spread outward creating smooth, pale, atrophic polygonal alopecic areas (Figs. 11.10 and 11.11). Follicular markings are absent. The hairs at the margins display perifollicular erythema and scaling [30, 36, 38]. Lichen planus on the body may occur prior to, during, or after LPP affects the scalp. The trunk and limbs may also display follicular hyperkeratosis. Symptoms are variable and can include moderate to severe discomfort, pruritus, pain, or burning. Active disease can be deter-

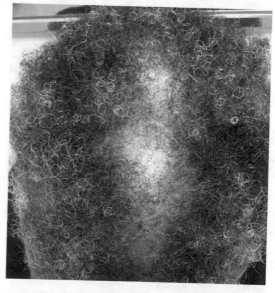

Fig. 11.10 Lichen planopilaris in a mature African American woman. (Image courtesy of Oma Agbai, MD)

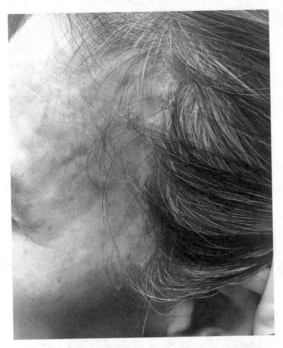

Fig. 11.11 Overlapping lichen planopilaris and frontal fibrosing alopecia in a mature Asian woman. (Image courtesy of Oma Agbai, MD)

mined with a positive pull test for anagen hairs. LPP tends to progress slowly, often leaving enough hair for styling to conceal the alopecic areas [38].

Differential Diagnosis

LPP can resemble alopecia areata, particularly in the early stages of disease. The differential diagnosis for LPP also includes discoid lupus, CCCA, and folliculitis decalvans, necessitating a close look at clinical, dermoscopic, and histologic findings [35]. Histologically, subepidermal lymphocytic infiltrate in LPP surrounds the isthmus and infundibulum (the upper portion) of the hair follicle but does not penetrate the deeper follicle as seen in alopecia areata [35]. Common dermoscopic features of alopecia areata include dystrophic hairs, yellow dots, cadaverized hairs (appearing as black dots), and exclamation mark hairs [39]. LPP is more commonly characterized by perifollicular scales [35].

Management

Current treatment modalities are aimed at slowing the disease progression and symptom relief [38]. Treatment includes high-potency topical steroids such as clobetasol propionate. However, topical therapy with corticosteroids or immunomodulators such as pimecrolimus and tacrolimus are often ineffective as monotherapy [36]. Oral immunosuppression is often required, with hydroxychloroquine as a common choice [30, 36]. Areas of active disease can be treated with intralesional corticosteroids such as triamcinolone acetonide suspension 10 mg/ml. Oral corticosteroids, azathioprine, antimalarial medications, dapsone, isotretinoin, and cyclosporine may also be used [30, 38]. Recent literature suggests that mycophenolate mofetil is safe and effective in the treatment of recalcitrant LPP [36].

Frontal Fibrosing Alopecia

Frontal fibrosing alopecia (FFA), a clinical variant of LPP, is a primary scarring alopecia associated with progressive regression of the frontotemporal hairline [2]. Despite the differing overarching hair loss patterns of alopecia, FFA and LPP are similar in histology and certain clinical features. FFA most often affects women of postmenopausal age and occurs more commonly in Caucasian and Asian women, although it has been reported in women of African descent [2, 40]. It can also occur in men and premenopausal women [2].

Etiology

Although FFA appears to be increasingly common, little is known about the etiology or pathology of this condition [41]. Given the predilection for postmenopausal women and recent studies demonstrating benefit from antiandrogenic therapy, it is theorized that FFA may be due to a hormonal cause [41]. Other findings point toward a potential autoimmune etiology, as FFA has been associated with other autoimmune disorders such as vitiligo and thyroid dysfunction. A high prevalence of hypothyroidism in some studies has prompted the suggestion to include thyroid studies in the workup of FFA [42, 43]. The paucity of data and low apparent prevalence of FFA in African Americans may be due to misdiagnosis as traction alopecia, a common cause of hair loss in this group [2, 40]. Given significant overlapping clinical histories and pathologic features between FFA and TA, making the correct diagnosis can be challenging [40].

Histopathology

Scalp biopsy in FFA appears histologically identical to that of lichen planopilaris, necessitating clinicopathologic correlation [41]. A lymphocytic infiltrate surrounds the infundibulum and isthmus of the hair follicle. Long-term inflammation ultimately leads to follicular destruction and fibrosis [23].

Clinical Presentation

FFA is characterized by a band-like receding frontotemporal hairline and that may also involve hair loss of the eyebrows, eyelashes, axillary region, pubic region, limb, scalp, and vellus hairs (Figs. 11.11 and 11.12). Eyebrow loss, which can be the presenting sign, is another central feature and occurs in up to 75% of patients [2, 41, 44, 45]. The patient may initially develop pruritus, noninflammatory perifollicular papules, and red follicular spots on the forehead [2, 41, 43, 45].

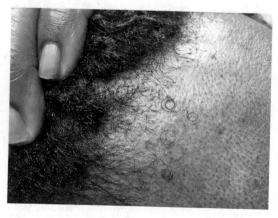

Fig. 11.12 Frontal fibrosing alopecia. (Image courtesy of Oma Agbai, MD)

Perifollicular erythema, follicular keratotic plugs, and follicular dropout visible on dermoscopy are indicative of active disease [2, 46]. Follicular inflammation is associated with and eventually replaced by scarring with a loss of follicular markings [23, 47]. The presence of one or a few terminal hairs on the forehead despite the regression of the marginal hairline, the "lonely hair sign," is another clue pointing to a diagnosis of FFA [48]. Clinical course is variable but commonly progresses slowly until self-stabilization [43, 45, 47].

Differential Diagnosis

The most important confounding diagnosis in FFA is traction alopecia [40], which is a common cause of alopecia in this group. Please refer to Table 11.1 for a comparison of clinical features of FFA and TA. Lichen planopilaris is similar to FFA, although the pattern of hair loss is distinct. Eyebrow loss, axillary hair loss, and follicular keratotic papules are features common in both conditions. Histologic appearance of the two conditions is equivalent, precluding this technique as a method of differentiating the two conditions [47]. FFA may also be difficult to distinguish from the ophiasis pattern of alopecia areata, with both conditions involving band-like hair loss in the fronto-parieto-temporal regions. Both may affect the eyebrows, although this occurs most consistently in FFA. Close clinical examination of FFA will demonstrate scarring with follicular loss, perifollicular erythema, and follicular keratotic plugs. In cases where biopsy is required, the ophiasis pattern of alopecia areata exhibits peribulbar lymphocytic infiltration, follicular miniaturization, and telogen arrest; the ophiasis pattern specifically may show fewer hair follicles and replacement by fibrosis. Histology of FFA more reliably exhibits fibrosis and scaring with a lichenoid interface infiltrate around the upper follicle in active lesions [49].

Lastly, cutaneous sarcoidosis not only may mimic alopecia but has been known to stimulate scarring alopecia. Sarcoidosis-induced alopecia has been reported most commonly in African American women between 23 and 78 years of age and most often presents simultaneously with facial, pulmonary, and lymph node involvement [50]. When occurring on the scalp, cutaneous sarcoidosis usually presents as localized with indurated papules, plaques, and erythema with scale [50]. These lesions may resemble not only FFA but also CCCA, discoid lupus, and lichen planopilaris, making biopsy essential for diagnosis. On biopsy, FFA will demonstrate granulomas surrounding the hair follicle, while sarcoidosis demonstrates noncaseating granulomas present in the dermis with or without follicles [51]. Evaluation for systemic sarcoidosis is indicated in patients with cutaneous sarcoidosis-induced alopecia [50].

Management

Efforts to establish effective therapy for FFA have been elusive, and there is currently no gold standard treatment [2, 41]. The current goal of management is to prevent further hair loss. Without any intervention, the marginal hairline recedes at a rate of 0.95–1.08 cm/year [2, 40, 46] and tends to self-stabilize [43, 45, 47]. Varying success has been reported with the use of topical and intralesional corticosteroids, topical calcineurin inhibitors, hydroxychloroquine, mycophenolate mofetil, and oral 5-alpha-reductase inhibitors [2, 44, 45, 47]. Some authors suggest a trial of triamcinolone acetonide 20 mg/ml in patients with evidence of inflammatory activity [47]. Recent evidence suggests that oral finasteride and dutasteride may be a beneficial maintenance therapy after the use of intralesional corticosteroids has cleared any perifollicular erythema or follicular hyperkeratosis [2, 41, 43]. Furthermore, PPAR-gamma agonists may be a promising treatment option for frontal fibrosing alopecia and lichen planopilaris.

Discoid Lupus Erythematosus

Discoid lupus erythematosus (DLE) is a clinical variant of cutaneous lupus erythematosus (CLE) and is one of the most prevalent causes of scarring alopecia [52]. In those presenting solely with discoid lesions, an estimated 17–30% will ultimately show signs of systemic lupus erythematosus (SLE). 8–28% of patients with diagnosed SLE exhibit discoid lesions. Discoid lesions limited to the head indicate a lower likelihood of future SLE (5%) compared with discoid lesions below the neck (20%) [53]. DLE generally affects the face, ears, neck, and scalp, with over half of patients presenting with scalp lesions [52]. DLE occurs more commonly in both people of color and females [54, 55]. Importantly, quality of life studies in CLE have demonstrated poorer outcomes in females, patients of color, and those of low socioeconomic status [55].

Histopathology

Histopathology shows vacuolization of the basal epidermis and increased dermal mucin. Direct immunofluorescence shows granular deposition of IgG and C3 along the follicular epithelium and dermoepidermal junction [56]. Lesions also demonstrate basement membrane thickening [57].

Clinical Features

Lesions typically appear as erythematous plaques with follicular plugging, scale, central hypopigmentation, and epidermal atrophy [52, 56]. One author has observed two African American patients with DLE presenting hyperpigmented scaly plaques of the scalp (Agbai, unpublished clinical observation). A classic sign on trichoscopy is follicular red dots, but branching vessels, large yellow dots, and speckled brown discoloration may also be seen [56]. Patients may be asymptomatic or experience tenderness or pruritus in affected areas [56]. Late-stage lesions eventually develop into atrophic, fibrotic areas with absent follicular markings and central hypopigmentation in the late stages (Fig. 11.13) [52]. Without treatment this condition leads to irreversible alopecia.

Differential Diagnosis

Differentiating alopecia caused by DLE from that of LPP can be challenging, as the two share several clinical and histological characteristics. The presence of follicular plugging and central hypopigmentation in alopecic areas is suggestive of DLE, whereas perifollicular erythema and scale favor a diagnosis of LPP. Interface dermati-

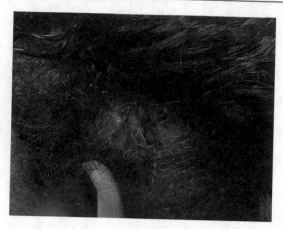

Fig. 11.13 Hyperpigmented papules within an alopecic patch in a middle-aged African American woman with discoid lupus erythematosus. (Image courtesy of Oma Agbai, MD)

tis on histology is more telling of LPP as opposed to DLE. Perivascular inflammation is more suggestive of LPP than DLE unless it is deep and dense. Excess mucin in LPP is located perifollicularly, while in DLE it is in the dermis. Thickening of the basement membrane in LPP is minimal but prominent in DLE [57].

Management

Early treatment is essential as scarring of the hair follicles leads to permanent alopecia [56]. Smoking cessation and the use of sunscreen may exert a protective and preventive effect against the formation of new lesions [56]. Management of early DLE includes the use of potent topical, intralesional, and oral corticosteroids. Oral antimalarials and topical calcineurin inhibitors are also effective [52, 56]; calcineurin inhibitors are particularly useful on affected areas showing thinning or atrophy [56]. Mycophenolate mofetil, methotrexate, retinoids, dapsone, and thalidomide have also been used but lack sufficient data [56].

Seborrheic Dermatitis

Seborrheic dermatitis (SD) is a chronic inflammatory condition of the scalp, face, and upper chest that leads to erythema, flaking, scaling, and pruritus [58]. While not classically associated with hair loss, some evidence shows a connection between the long-term subclinical inflammation in chronic SD and increased telogen shedding. Cicatricial hair loss has also been reported in some patients with SD [59]. Awareness of the relationship between seborrheic dermatitis and hair loss is significant in the care of WOC as seborrheic dermatitis numbers are among the top five dermatologic diagnoses in African American patients. Caucasian and Asian patients, by contrast, experience seborrheic dermatitis much less frequently, with SD being the ninth most common dermatologic diagnosis in Asians and not among the top ten in Caucasians [2, 60]. The general incidence of SD is 1–3% in the postpubertal population, with a higher proportion of cases in men [58].

Histopathology

In patients with SD, the fungus *Malassezia* is thought to play a pathogenic role in disruption of seborrheic skin [58]. It is also theorized that an inflammatory reaction is stimulated in the SD scalp when local deposits of immunoglobulins attract and activate leukocytes. Chronic, subclinical inflammation near the follicle is believed to interrupt the hair cycle in the short term but cause scarring in the long term [59]. Common features of scalp biopsy in a case report of patients with SD and hair loss included a mild spongiotic dermatitis, focal parakeratosis of hair follicles, parakeratosis in the deep follicular infundibulum, and scattered perivascular and perifollicular lymphocytes. Mild chronic perifolliculitis with fibrosis was also observed. Unlike other cicatricial alopecias, the patients described in this report demonstrated a mild, diffuse scarring with follicular dropout. No lichenoid inflammation, trichomalacia, or any features of androgenetic alopecia were noted [59].

Clinical Features

Seborrheic dermatitis can affect the scalp, face, retroauricular area, and upper chest. In adults with scalp involvement, it appears as areas of mild des-

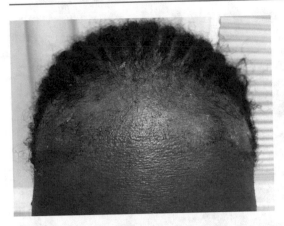

Fig. 11.14 Seborrheic dermatitis associated with alope-cia. (Image courtesy of Oma Agbai, MD)

Table 11.3 Pigmentary findings and management considerations in patients of color compared with Caucasian patients with seborrheic dermatitis

	Skin of color	Caucasian
Pigmentary alterations	Hypopigmentation more common; resolves with therapy	Erythema more common
Lifestyle modifications	Increase frequency of hair washing to 1–2 times weekly	Not necessary as washing daily or every other day more common
Therapeutic considerations	Prescription shampoos such as ketoconazole may be excessively drying for women, leading to hair fragility	More flexibility with prescription shampoo
	Topical ointments such as tacrolimus 0.1% ointment or topical corticosteroids can be used	Topical ointments not as useful due to greasiness
	Topical fluocinolone oil can be used overnight prior to shampoo as well as between washes as spot treatment	

quamation or greasy, honey-colored crusts with associated hair loss (Fig. 11.14). A scaly, erythematous margin of SD from the scalp can appear at the frontotemporal hairline, called "corona seborrheica." Pruritus often also accompanies SD of the scalp [58]. Table 11.3 demonstrates differing pigmentary alterations seen in patients of color and Caucasian patients, as well as differing management modalities in these two populations.

Differential Diagnosis

Patients with tinea capitis, especially children, may present similarly, with scaly patches of hair loss. However, the patches will contain black dots that are short, broken hairs. Diagnosis of tinea can be made with potassium hydroxide microscopic preparation of the hair shaft or scalp scale or fungal culture [58]. Seborrheic dermatitis must also be distinguished from scalp psoriasis, which presents as sharply demarcated erythematous or hyperpigmented plaques with thick micaceous scale.

Management

SD is a chronic condition that requires ongoing management. Goals of treatment include alleviating pruritus, reducing or eliminating visible signs of SD, and long-term maintenance. Topical antifungal and anti-inflammatory therapies are used

to target *Malassezia* excess and scalp inflammation. Common agents also used are coal tar, lithium gluconate or succinate, and phototherapy. If the affected area is large or the lesions are recalcitrant to topical therapy, systemic agents may be used. See Table 11.4 for specific treatment recommendations [58].

Conclusion

Certain forms of alopecia have unique clinical presentations in WOC. Furthermore, the relative incidence of different forms of alopecia in WOC is distinct from those affecting Caucasian patients. A better understanding of the diagnostic and management nuances in this patient population may optimize diagnostic accuracy, treatment adherence, and management outcomes.

Table 11.4 Treatment of seborrheic dermatitis [58]

Medication			Dose/formulation	Regimen	Mechanisms	Side effects
Topical	Antifungals	Ketoconazole	2% shampoo, cream, gel, or foam	Scalp or skin: twice/week × 4 weeks and then once/week for maintenance	Inhibition of fungal cell wall synthesis	ICD (irritant contact dermatitis) in <1% of patients. Itching, burning sensation, and dryness in 3% of patients
		Bifonazole	1% shampoo, cream or ointment	Scalp: every other day or once daily. Skin: once daily		ICD in 10% of patients
		Miconazole	Cream	Skin: 1–2 times daily		ICD, itching, burning sensation
		Ciclopirox olamine	1.5% shampoo, cream, gel, or lotion	Scalp: 2–3 times/week × 4 weeks and then once/week for maintenance. Skin: twice daily	Inhibition of metal-dependent enzymes	ICD in <1% of patients. Itching, burning sensation in 2% of patients
		Selenium sulfide	2.5% shampoo	Scalp: twice/week × 2 week and then once/week × 2 weeks. Repeat after 4–6 weeks	Cytostatic and keratolytic	ICD in ~3% of patients. Orange-brown scalp discoloration
		Zinc pyrithione	1% shampoo	Scalp: 2–3 times/week	Increased cellular copper interferes with iron-sulfur proteins	ICD in ~3% of patients
	Corticosteroids	Hydrocortisone	1% cream	Skin: 1–2 times daily	Anti-inflammatory, anti-irritant	Risk of skin atrophy, telangiectasias, folliculitis, hypertrichosis, and hypopigmentation with prolonged use
		Betamethasone dipropionate	0.05% lotion	Scalp and skin: 1–2 times daily		
		Desonide	0.05% lotion, gel	Scalp and skin: 1–2 times daily.		
		Fluocinolone	0.01% shampoo, lotion, or cream	Scalp or skin: once or twice daily		
	Immunomodulators	Pimecrolimus	1% cream	Skin: 1–2 times daily	Inhibition of cytokine production by T-lymphocyte	Risk of skin malignancy and lymphoma with prolonged use
		Tacrolimus	0.1% ointment	Skin: 1–2 times daily × 4 weeks and then twice/week for maintenance		
	Miscellaneous	Coal tar	4% shampoo	Scalp: 1–2 times/week	Antifungal, anti-inflammatory, keratolytic, reduces sebum production	Local folliculitis, ICD on fingers, psoriasis aggravation, skin atrophy, telangiectasias, hyperpigmentation. Risk of squamous cell carcinoma with prolonged use
		Lithium gluconate/succinate	8% ointment or gel	Skin: twice daily × 8 weeks	Anti-inflammatory via increased IL-10 and decreased TLR2 and TLR4 in keratinocytes	ICD in <10% of patients
		Metronidazole	0.75% gel	Skin: twice daily × 4 weeks	Anti-inflammatory via inhibition of free radical species	Rare contact sensitization with prolonged use
		Phototherapy	UVB: cumulative dose of 9.8 J/cm2	Three times/week × 8 weeks or until clearing	Immunomodulation and inhibition of cell proliferation	Burning, itching sensation during/after therapy. Risk of genital tumor with prolonged use
Systemic		Itraconazole	Oral: 200 mg	Once daily × 7 days and then once daily × 2 days/month for maintenance	Inhibition of fungal cell wall synthesis. Anti-inflammatory via inhibition of 5-lipoxygenase metabolites	Rare liver toxicity
		Terbinafine	Oral: 250 mg	Once daily × 4–6 weeks or 12 days monthly × 3 months	Inhibition of cell membrane and cell wall synthesis	Rare tachycardia and insomnia

Note: Shampoos, foams, and lotions are better suited for treating seborrheic dermatitis and dandruff on the scalp; gels, creams, and ointments are used to treat seborrheic dermatitis on body locations other than the scalp.

References

1. Taylor SC. Skin of color: biology, structure, function, and implications for dermatologic disease. J Am Acad Dermatol [Internet]. Elsevier. 2002 [cited 2018Aug15]; 46(2 Suppl Understanding):S41–62.

2. Lawson CN, Hollinger J, Sethi S, Rodney I, Sarkar R, Dlova N, Callender VD. Updates in the understanding and treatments of skin & hair disorders in women of color. Int J Womens Dermatol [Internet]. 2017 [cited 2018Aug15];3(1 Suppl):S21–37.

3. McMichael AJ. Ethnic hair update: past and present. J Am Acad Dermatol [Internet]. Elsevier. 2003 [cited 2018Aug18];48(6):S127–33.

4. Lindsey SF, Tosti A. Alopecias – practical evaluation and management. Curr Probl Dermatol [Internet]. 2015 [cited2018Aug15]. Karger;47:139–49.

5. Khumalo NP, Ngwanya RM. Traction alopecia: 2% topical minoxidil shows promise. Report of two cases. J Eur Acad Dermatol Venereol [Internet]. 2007 [cited 2018Aug16];21:433–4.

6. Khumalo NP, Jessop S, Gumedze F, Ehrlich R. Hairdressing and the prevalence of scalp disease in African adults. Br J Dermatol [Internet]. 2007 [cited 2018Aug16];157:981–88.

7. Lewallen R, Francis S, Fisher B, Richards J, Li J, Dawson T, et al. Hair care practices and structural evaluation of scalp and hair shaft parameters in African American and Caucasian women. J Cosmet Dermatol [Internet]. Wiley Online Library. 2015 [cited 2018Aug16];14(3):216–23.

8. Khumalo NP, Doe PT, Dawber RPR, Ferguson DJP. What is normal black African hair? a light and scanning electron-microscopic study. J Am Acad Dermatol [Internet]. 2000 [cited 2018Sept15]. Science Direct;43(5):814–20.

9. Ogunleye TA, McMichael A, Olsen EA. Central centrifugal cicatricial alopecia: what has been achieved, current clues for future research. Dermatol Clin [Internet]. Elsevier. 2014 [cited 2018Aug18];32(2):173–81.

10. Khumalo NP, Jessop S, Gumedze F, Ehrlich R. Determinants of marginal traction alopecia in African girls and women [Internet]. Elsevier. 2008 [cited 2018Aug16];59:432–8.

11. Montagna W, Carlisle K. The architecture of black and white facial skin. J Am Acad Dermatol [Internet]. 1991 [cited 2018Aug20];24:929–37.

12. Ji JH, Park TS, Lee HJ, Kim YD, Pi LQ, Jin XH, Lee WS. The ethnic differences of the damage of hair and integral hair lipid after ultra violet radiation. Ann Dermatol [Internet]. 2013 [cited 2018Aug16];25:54–60.

13. Griffin M, Lenzy Y. Contemporary African-American hair care practices. Pract Dermatol [Internet]. 2015 [cited 2018Aug21].

14. Ahdout J, Mirmirani P. Weft hair extensions causing a distinctive horseshoe pattern of traction alopecia. J Am Acad Dermatol [Internet]. Elsevier. 2012 [cited 2018Aug20];67:e294–5.

15. Mirmirani P, Khumalo NP. Traction alopecia: how to translate study data for public education—closing the KAP gap? Dermatol Clin [Internet]. Elsevier. 2014 [cited 2018Aug20];32(2):153–61.

16. Swee W, Klontz KC, Lambert LA. A nationwide outbreak of alopecia associated with the use of a hair-relaxing formulation. Arch Dermatol. [Internet] 2000 [cited 2018Aug19];136(9):1104–8.

17. Grimes PE. Skin and hair cosmetic issues in women of color [Internet]. Elsevier. 2005 [cited 2018Aug19];18(4):659–65.

18. McMichael AJ. Scalp and hair disorders in African-American patients: a primer of disorders and treatments. J Cosmet Dermatol [Internet]. 2003 [cited 2018Aug19]. 16:37–41.

19. Khumalo NP, Jessop S, Gumedze F, Ehrlich R. Hairdressing is associated with scalp disease in African schoolchildren [Internet]. Wiley Online Library; 2007 [cited 2018Aug16];157(1):106–10.

20. Samrao A, Price VH, Zedek D, Mirmirani P. The "Fringe Sign" – a useful clinical finding in traction alopecia of the marginal hair line. Dermatol Online J [Internet]. 2011 [cited 2018Aug21];17(11):1.

21. Tosti A, Miteva M, Torres F, Vincenzi C, Romanelli P. Hair casts are a dermoscopic clue for the diagnosis of traction. Br J Dermatol [Internet]. Wiley Online Library. 2010 [cited 2018Aug21];163(6).

22. Trueb RM. "Chignon alopecia": a distinctive type of nonmarginal traction alopecia. Cutis [Internet]. 1995 [cited 2018Aug21];55:178–9.

23. Samrao A, Chen C, Zedek D, Price VH. Traction alopecia in a ballerina: clinicopathologic features. Arch Dermatol [Internet]. 2010 [cited 2018Aug22];146:930–1.

24. Heath CR, Taylor SC. Alopecia in an ophiasis pattern: traction alopecia versus alopecia areata. Cutis [Internet]. 2012 [cited 2018Aug22];89:213–6.

25. James J, Saladi RN, Fox JL. Traction alopecia in Sikh male patients. J Am Board Fam Med [Internet]. 2007 [cited 2108Aug22];20:497–8.

26. Callendar 2004 Callender VD, McMichael AJ, Cohen GF. Medical and surgical therapies for alopecias in black women. Dermatol Ther [Internet]. 2004 [cited 2018Aug20];17:164–76.

27. Ozcelik D. Extensive traction alopecia attributable to ponytail hairstyle and its treatment with hair transplantation. Aesthet Plast Surg [Internet]. Springer; 2005 [cited 2018Aug22];29:325–7.

28. Miyamoto M, Tsuboi R, Tsunao OH-I. Case of acquired trichorrhexis nodosa: scanning electron microscopic observation. J Dermatol [Internet]. 2009 [cited 2018Aug22];36(2).

29. Mirmirani P. Ceramic flat irons: improper use leading to acquired trichorrhexis nodosa. J Am Acad Dermatol [Internet]. 2010 [cited 2018Aug23];62:145–7.

30. Whiting DA, Olsen EA. Central centrifugal cicatricial alopecia. Dermatol The [Internet]. 2008 [cited 2018Aug23]. Wiley Online Library;21(4):268–78.

31. Gathers RC, Jankowski M, Eide M, Lim HW. Hair grooming practices and central centrifugal cicatricial

alopecia. J Am Acad Dermatol [Internet]. 2009 [cited 2018Aug23]. Elsevier;60(4):574–8.

32. Kyei A, Bergfeld WF, Piliang M, Summers P. Medical and environmental risk factors for the development of central centrifugal cicatricial alopecia: a population study. Arch Dermatol [Internet]. 2011 [cited 2018Aug23];147(8):909–14.

33. Whiting DA. Cicatricial alopecia: clinicopathological findings and treatment. Clin Dermatol [Internet]. 2001[cited 2018Aug23]. Elsevier;9(2):211–25.

34. Gathers RC, Lim HW. Central centrifugal cicatricial alopecia: past, present, and future. J Am Acad Dermatol [Internet]. 2009 [cited 2018Aug23];60(4):660–8.

35. Errichetti E, Figini M, Croatto M, Stinco G. Therapeutic management of classic lichen planopilaris: a systematic review. Clin Cosmet Investig Dermatol [Internet]. 2018 [cited 2018Aug24]. Dove Press;2018(11):91–102.

36. Cho BK, Sah D, Chwalek J, Rosenborough I, Ochoa B, Chiang C, Price VH. Efficacy and safety of mycophenolate mofetil for lichen planopilaris. J Am Acad Dermatol [Internet]. 2010 [cited 2018Aug24]. Elsevier;62(3):393–7.

37. Chiang C, Sah D, Cho BK, Ochoa B, Price VH. Hydroxychloroquine and lichen planopilaris: efficacy and introduction of Lichen Planopilaris Activity Index scoring system. J Am Acad Dermatol [Internet]. 2010 [cited 2018Aug24]. Elsevier;62(3):387–92.

38. Mirmirani and price Wiley A, Price VH. Short course of oral cyclosporine in lichen planopilaris. J Am Acad Dermatol [Internet]. 2003 [cited 2018Aug24]. Elsevier;49(4):667–71.

39. Rubegni P, Mandato F, Fimiani F. Frontal fibrosing alopecia: role of dermoscopy in differential diagnosis. Case Rep Dermatol. [Internet]. 2010 [cited 2018Sept14];2(1):40–45.

40. Miteva M, Whiting D, Harries M, Bernardes A, Tosti A. Frontal fibrosing alopecia in black patients [Internet]. 2012 [cited 2018Aug24]. Wiley Online Library;167(1):208–10.

41. Ladizinski B, Bazakas A, Selim A, Olsen EA. Frontal fibrosing alopecia: a retrospective review of 19 patients seen at Duke University. J Am Acad Dermatol [Internet]. 2013 [cited 2018Aug24];68:749–55.

42. MacDonald A, Clark C, Holmes S. Frontal fibrosing alopecia: a review of 60 cases. J Am Acad Dermatol [Internet]. 2012 [cited 2018Aug25]. Elsevier;67(5):955–61.

43. Vañó-Galván S, Molina-Ruiz AM, Serrano-Falcón C, Arias-Santiago S, Rodrigues-Barata AR, Garnacho-Saucedo G, Martorell-Calatayud A, Fernández-Crehuet P, Grimalt R, Aranegui B, Grillo E, Diaz-Ley B, Salido R, Pérez-Gala S, Serrano S, Moreno JC, Jaén P, Camacho FM. Frontal fibrosing alopecia: a multicenter review of 355 patients. J Am Acad Dermatol [Internet]. 2014 [cited 2018Aug24];70:670–8.

44. Samrao A, Chew AL, Price V. Frontal fibrosing alopecia: a clinical review of 36 patients. Br J Dermatol [Internet]. 2010 [cited 2018Aug26];163:1296–300.

45. Tan KT, Messenger AG. Frontal fibrosing alopecia: clinical presentations and prognosis [Internet]. 2008 [cited 2018Aug25]. Wiley Online Library;160(1):75–9.

46. Toledo-Pastrana T, Hernández MJ, Camacho Martínez FM. Perifollicular erythema as a trichoscopy sign of progression in frontal fibrosing alopecia. Int J Trichol [Internet]. 2013 [cited 2018Aug25];5:151–3.

47. Moreno-Ramirez D, Camacho Martinez F. Frontal fibrosing alopecia: a survey in 16 patients. J Eur Acad Dermatol Venereol [Internet]. 2005 [cited 2018Aug25];19:700–5.

48. Tosti A, Miteva M, Torres F. Lonely hair: a clue to the diagnosis of frontal fibrosing alopecia. Arch Dermatol [Internet]. 2011 [cited 2018Aug25];147:1240.

49. Kossard S, Kwong RA. Alopecia areata masquerading as frontal fibrosing alopecia. Aust J Dermatol [Internet]. 2006 [cited 2018Aug15];47(1):63–6.

50. House NS, Welsh JP, English JC. Sarcoidosis-induced alopecia. Dermatol Online J [Internet]. 2012 [cited2018Sept25];18(8)4.

51. Ranasinghe G, Hogan S, Ibrahim I, et al. Sarcoidosis presenting as frontal fibrosing alopecia: a master mimicker or a coincidental finding? Am J Dermatopathol [Internet]. 2018 [cited2018Sept25];40(1):73–5.

52. Milam EC, Ramachandran S, Franks AG Jr. Treatment of scarring alopecia in discoid variant of chronic cutaneous lupus erythematosus with tacrolimus lotion, 0.3%. JAMA Dermatol [Internet]. 2015 [cited 2018Aug26];151(10):1113–6.

53. Skare TL, Stadler B, Weingraber E, De Paula DF. Prognosis of patients with systemic lupus erythematosus and discoid lesions. An Bras Dermatol [Internet]. 2013 [cited 2018Sept15];88(5):755–8.

54. Drenkard C, Parker S, Aspey LD, Gordon C, Helmick CG, Bao G, Lim SS. Racial disparities in the incidence of primary chronic cutaneous lupus erythematosus in the Southeastern United States: the Georgia Lupus Registry. Arthritis Care Res [Internet]. 2019 [cited 2018 Sept 16];71(1):95–103.

55. O'Brien JC, Chong BF. Not just skin deep: systemic disease involvement in patients with cutaneous lupus. J Investig Dermatol Symp Proc [Internet]. 2017 [cited 2018Sept15];18(2): S69–S74.

56. Udompanich S, Chanprapaph K, Suchonwanit P. Hair and scalp changes in cutaneous and systemic lupus erythematosus. Am J Clin Dermatol [Internet]. 2018 [cited 2018Aug26]. Springer;19(5):679–94.

57. Nambudiri VE, Vleugels RA, Laga AC, Goldberg LJ. Clinicopathologic lessons in distinguishing cicatricial alopecia: 7 cases of lichen planopilaris misdiagnosed as discoid lupus. J Am Acad Dermatol [Internet]. 2014 [cited 2018Aug27]. Elsevier;71(4):e135–8.

58. Borda LJ, Wikramanayake TC. Seborrheic dermatitis and dandruff: a comprehensive review. J Clin Invest Dermatol [Internet]. 2015 [cited 2018Aug28]. Avens Online;3(2):10.

59. Pitney L, Weedon D, Pitney M. Is seborrhoeic dermatitis associated with a diffuse, low-grade folliculitis and progressive cicatricial alopecia? Aust J Dermatol

[Internet]. 2015 [cited 2018Aug27]. Wiley Online Library;57(3):e105–7.

60. Davis SA, Narahari S, Feldman SR, Huang W, Pichardo-Geisinger RO, McMichael AJ. Top dermatologic conditions in patients of color: an analysis of nationally representative data. J Drugs Dermatol. [Internet]. 2012 [cited 2018Aug28];11(4):466–73.

61. Bolduc C, Sperling L, Shapiro J. Primary cicatricial alopecia: lymphocytic primary cicatricial alopecias, including chronic cutaneous lupus erythematosus, lichen planopilaris, frontal fibrosing alopecia, and Graham-Little syndrome. J Am Acad Dermatol [Internet]. 2016 [cited 2018Sept30];75(6):1081–99.

Ethnic Skin Disorders

12

Aya J. Alame, Titilola Sode, Cynthia O. Robinson, Donald A. Glass II, and Katherine Omueti Ayoade

Acne Keloidalis Nuchae

Acne keloidalis nuchae (AKN) is characterized by a scarring folliculitis that typically presents at the nape of the neck in postpubertal African American males that forms keloid-like scars and cicatricial alopecia (see Fig. 12.1). Though the etiology is unclear, potential triggers include chronic irritation or blockage of hair follicles related to hair care practices. The predilection for AKN to localize to the nuchal and occipital areas is uncertain, but some have attributed this pattern to increased mast cells and dermal papillary dilatation, in addition to friction from scalp skin folds and neck gear [1]. Histopathology demonstrates neutrophils and lymphocytes around the isthmus of the hair follicle, with eventual destruction of sebaceous glands, chronic granulomatous inflammation, collagen deposition, and fibrosis.

Epidemiologic studies of AKN demonstrate a strong male predominance. A retrospective study at the University Hospital of the West Indies showed that in a population of 1031 patients, the male-to-female ratio was 7:1 [2], while others have reported a ratio up to 20:1 [1]. This skew toward affecting postpubertal age men has led to the hypothesis that androgens may play a role in the pathogenesis of AKN via a stimulatory effect on sebaceous glands or the sensitivity of hair follicles to the hormones themselves [3]. AKN also primarily affects individuals of African descent. In Nigeria, reports have shown a prevalence ranging from 0.7% to 9.4% [1], suggesting a genetic influence in the pathogenesis of AKN; however, no significant association has been demonstrated in the literature [1]. Studies have shown a significant association between components of metabolic syndrome like diabetes mellitus, hypertension, hypercholesterolemia, and obesity with the extension of lesions beyond the nape and occipital scalp [2]. A case series of four Indian patients demonstrated an association between AKN and acanthosis nigricans [4]. Furthermore, a study of 36 individuals in Latin America showed that 61% of patients with AKN had metabolic syndrome in accordance with the parameters set by the International Diabetes Federation [5, 6].

Management of this condition is primarily preventative and involves avoiding frequent haircuts, close shaving, tight neck gear, and greasy

A. J. Alame · D. A. Glass II · K. O. Ayoade (✉)
University of Texas Southwestern Medical Center, Department of Dermatology, Dallas, TX, USA
e-mail: katherine.ayoade@utsouthwestern.edu

T. Sode
U.S. Dermatology Partners Dallas Hillcrest, Dallas, TX, USA

U.S. Dermatology Partner Dallas Presbyterian, Dallas, TX, USA

C. O. Robinson
Dermatology Associates of Uptown, Cedar Hill, TX, USA

© Springer Nature Switzerland AG 2021
B. S. Li, H. I. Maibach (eds.), *Ethnic Skin and Hair and Other Cultural Considerations*, Updates in Clinical Dermatology, https://doi.org/10.1007/978-3-030-64830-5_12

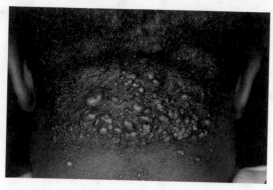

Fig. 12.1 Keloid papules on the occipital scalp. (Image is courtesy of the Betty E. Janes Clinical Image Library, Department of Dermatology, UT Southwestern Medical Center. Submitted by courtesy of Dr. Donald Glass II)

hair products. For the treatment of hard papules, triamcinolone injections may be used, while for maintenance, topical antimicrobial agents, steroids, and retinoids are utilized [7]. Therapy with the erbium-doped yttrium aluminum garnet (Er:YAG) laser and long-pulsed 1064 nm neodymium-doped yttrium aluminum garnet (Nd:YAG) laser has demonstrated utility in treating AKN [7–10]. In a small ($n = 13$) single-blinded, randomized controlled study evaluating the 1064 nm Nd:YAG laser and topical steroids compared to topical steroids alone, the laser-treated side of the scalp demonstrated an improvement in the appearance of papules, while larger plaques and nodules were more difficult to treat [10]. Moreover, another study examined the efficacy of the Nd:YAG laser compared to the Er:YAG laser; while both treatment groups showed a statistically significant decrease in the number of papules and in the size of plaques, the Er:YAG group also demonstrated a significant decrease in the number of plaques [8]. In addition, in a prospective randomized split-scalp study, Okoye et al. demonstrated the use of targeted UVB as a treatment modality. In their study, the clinical appearance of AKN significantly improved [11]. Lastly, case reports have described radiation therapy as an effective treatment for refractory AKN [12].

Overall, the current understanding of AKN consists of an inflammatory reaction to chronic irritation resulting in scarring and alopecia that predominantly affects men of African descent. Its etiology is complex and is likely a combination of several factors (including traumatic, hormonal, metabolic, and genetic) that need further elucidation. Treatments are targeted at reducing exposure to triggers and/or controlling inflammation.

Keloids

Keloids are benign growths characterized by an abnormal response to wound healing by dermal fibroblasts, with excessive deposition of collagen [13] and increased expression of growth factors like TGF-ß [14]. They develop in response to inflammation from traumatic events to the skin such as acne, piercings, and surgery [14] (see Figs. 12.2, 12.3, and 12.4). Unlike hypertrophic scars, keloids are not confined to the boundaries of the skin wound, do not typically spontaneously regress, and are often characterized as pruritic and/or painful. Keloids tend to develop in areas of high skin tension such as the presternal region, though they can also occur on earlobes. On histopathology, keloids show increased glycosaminoglycan content with pathognomonic thick, hyalinized whorls of collagen [14].

Keloids predominantly affect individuals of African descent, occurring about 20 times more often in this population than Caucasians. Other individuals with skin of color, Hispanics and Asians, are also disproportionately affected [15]. In an analysis of medical visits for keloids in the National Ambulatory Medical Care Survey from 1990 to 2009, there were about 8.5 million visits for keloids. Among these patients, African Americans made the highest number of visits for keloids, about three times as many as non-Hispanic whites [15]. There is believed to be no gender predisposition, though women may be more likely to present at office visits for keloids [15]. In a recent study using admixture mapping and exome analysis, researchers at Vanderbilt identified a region on chr15q21.2–22.3 associated with an increased risk for keloids in African Americans [16]. The strongest association within this region was with gene MYO1E, which encodes for myosin. Outside this region, there

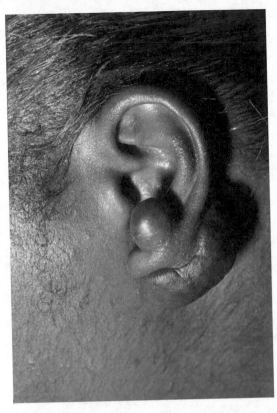

Fig. 12.2 Keloid nodules involving the earlobe. (Image is courtesy of the Betty E. Janes Clinical Image Library, Department of Dermatology, UT Southwestern Medical Center. Submitted by courtesy of Dr. Donald Glass II)

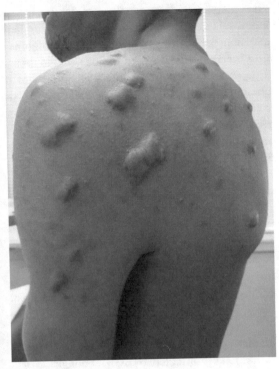

Fig. 12.3 Keloid plaques on the trunk. (Image is courtesy of Dr. Donald Glass II, Department of Dermatology, UT Southwestern Medical Center)

was also an association with MYO7A, another myosin-encoding gene. The identification of these genes suggests a role for cytoskeleton behavior in the abnormal migration of fibroblasts in keloid formation [16].

Despite their benign nature, studies have demonstrated that keloids carry significant morbidity. A cross-sectional study of adults with keloids using online surveys consisting of the Patient and Observer Scar Assessment Scale (POSAS) and health-related quality of life assessments showed that almost half of patients reported severe emotional symptoms related to having keloids [17]. This accentuates the effect that keloids can have on quality of life. In light of the disproportionate number of African Americans who are affected, healthcare providers have the opportunity to make a positive impact on the psychosocial consequences related to this condition.

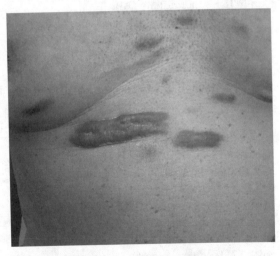

Fig. 12.4 Keloids on the chest and abdomen. (Image is courtesy of Dr. Donald Glass II, Department of Dermatology, UT Southwestern Medical Center)

While preventing unnecessary trauma is the most effective way to manage or prevent keloid formation in predisposed individuals, intralesional injection of corticosteroid remains a first-line therapeutic option for the treatment of keloids [18]. Other treatments include surgical excision, which must be followed by combination therapy including the use of silicone dressings, intralesional corticosteroids, intralesional chemotherapy (5-fluorouracil, bleomycin), or topical imiquimod to prevent reoccurrence. Other treatment modalities include pressure therapy, radiation therapy, cryotherapy, and lasers including Nd:YAG and pulse dye lasers [18].

Idiopathic Guttate Hypomelanosis

Idiopathic guttate hypomelanosis (IGH) is an acquired leukoderma that manifests as hypopigmented macules on sun-exposed areas such as extensor surface of the forearms and pretibial areas. This condition commonly affects individuals greater than age 40, and the prevalence increases with age [19]. Women and men appear to be equally affected by IGH. Though IGH is more prevalent among individuals with lighter skin color, it is more prominent on dark skin and may therefore present a significant cosmetic burden in these individuals [20].

The etiology is unclear; however, it is hypothesized that factors such as ultraviolet exposure, aging, and genetics play a role. Histology of IGH shows a decrease in the number of melanocytes, with the remaining melanocytes demonstrating fragmented or absent dendrites and fewer melanosomes [21].

Several different therapies are used such as corticosteroids, topical retinoids, and laser therapy, though the effectiveness of these therapies is debated [19]. A randomized control study ($n = 26$) evaluated the utility of 0.1% tacrolimus ointment compared to placebo in treating IGH, using a colorimeter to measure changes in skin color [21]. After 6 months, differences in colorimeter measurement from baseline reached statistical significance in the group treated with tacrolimus, suggesting it may be an effective treatment to promote repigmentation in IGH lesions [21]. Alternatively, newer studies have shown that the use of 5-fluorouracil tattooing of IGH lesions may induce melanocyte migration

and repigmentation [22, 23]. IGH does not require treatment. Patients who seek the attention of dermatologists may choose to explore any of the previously mentioned therapy options for aesthetics or cosmetic reasons after being reassured of the benign nature of the condition [24].

Vitiligo

Vitiligo is an autoimmune disorder that results from the destruction of skin melanocytes, resulting in depigmented macules and patches, often occurring in visible areas such as the face and extremities, causing emotional and psychological distress [25, 26] (see Fig. 12.5). In the genetically susceptible individual, the onset of vitiligo may be preceded by several factors including severe sunburn, cutaneous trauma, pregnancy, and significant psychological distress [25].

Epidemiologic studies of vitiligo have demonstrated a prevalence of about 0.5–2%, affecting men and women equally, without a preference for any race [25]. A retrospective study of 246 patients with vitiligo at the Department of Dermatology in Cotonou, Benin, showed a prevalence of 0.9%, the mean age of the study population was 25.9 years old, and men and women were affected in a 1:1 ratio. The sites of lesions were most often present on the head, with the lips being the most commonly affected site. The most common form of vitiligo represented was vitiligo

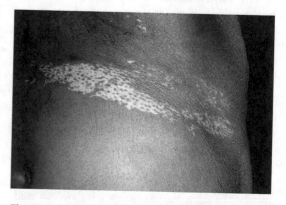

Fig. 12.5 Vitiligo lesion with repigmentation. (Image is courtesy of the Betty E. Janes Clinical Image Library, Department of Dermatology, UT Southwestern Medical Center. Submitted by courtesy of Dr. Donald Glass II)

vulgaris at 52.4%, with 36.2% of the population affected by localized vitiligo, 9.8% with segmental vitiligo, and 1.6% with vitiligo universalis [27].

A study of the genetics underlying vitiligo used genome-wide association studies and identified about 50 genetic loci associated with risk of vitiligo [26]. The proteins encoded by these regions of the genome were regulators of the immune system, cellular apoptosis, and melanocyte function, underscoring the role of autoimmunity leading to destruction of melanocytes in the condition [28]. Indeed, in a cross-sectional study of 1098 patients at Henry Ford Hospital system in Detroit, Michigan, demonstrated a higher prevalence of autoimmune diseases among individuals with vitiligo. These conditions included thyroid disease, alopecia areata, inflammatory bowel disease, systemic lupus erythematous, linear morphea, and Sjogren syndrome [29].

The diagnosis of vitiligo can be made clinically. Determination of disease activity is important to access prognosis and select the right treatment. Koebner phenomenon, trichrome lesions, inflammatory vitiligo, as well as confetti-like lesions are important to identify during a clinical exam as they are markers of very active disease [30]. When tissue is obtained, histopathology will demonstrate an absence of melanocytes, and in early lesions there may be a subtle interface dermatitis consisting of CD8+ cytotoxic T-cell lymphocyte infiltrates in close approximation to melanocytes [25, 31].

Like many of the pigmented dermatoses, in skin of color patients, vitiligo may be more aesthetically burdensome, especially as the depigmentation induced by vitiligo threatens racial identity [32]. In fact, a meta-analysis of 25 studies including 2708 patients showed that individuals with vitiligo are at a higher risk of suffering from depression [33]. Although vitiligo affects individual of all races with comparable representation among men and women, the psychological burden in patients with skin of color underscores the importance of addressing this condition effectively in this population.

Current treatments for vitiligo include topical and systemic immunosuppressants, phototherapy, and surgical techniques which together may slow or halt disease progression and improve repigmentation of affected areas [26]. Of these listed, phototherapy is the mainstay of treatment with NB-UVB being the most successful form due to its immunosuppressive effects and its ability to induce melanocyte differentiation and melanin production [34]. In patients with signs of active disease, a short course of an oral corticosteroid, such as dexamethasone, may be warranted [34]. Adjunct supportive therapy includes the use of vitamin C, E, and alpha-lipoic acid. Their antioxidant properties may be useful in reducing triggering factors that lead to depigmentation when used in combination with topical and systemic treatments, as well as phototherapy [34]. Emerging therapies for vitiligo include the topical and oral JAK inhibitors, ruxolitinib and tofacitinib, in addition to therapeutic targets to interferon gamma, CXCL9/10, and CXCR3 [34]. Mini-punch grafting, blister grafting, and non-cultured epidermal suspension (NCES) are viable options for patients with stable disease [34]. Lastly, but certainly not least, patients with widespread vitiligo (>50% body surface area) that is resistant/refractory to therapy can be counseled about using monobenzylether of hydroquinone to depigment the remaining pigmented areas [34]. Patients who tend to respond well to therapy include younger patients, patients with darker skin types, and patients with depigmentation that primarily involves the face, ears, neck, axilla, and hair-bearing areas [34]. This bodes well for African American patients and should be part of the counseling of these patients (Fig. 12.6).

Post-inflammatory Hyperpigmentation

Post-inflammatory hyperpigmentation (PIH) is a reactive hypermelanosis that occurs in the setting of inflammatory skin conditions such as eczema, acne, and psoriasis, or skin trauma such as picking or burns, or cosmetic procedures [35] (see Fig. 12.7). Among African Americans, PIH is one of the most common dermatological diagnoses, with up to 20% of diagnoses being related to PIH

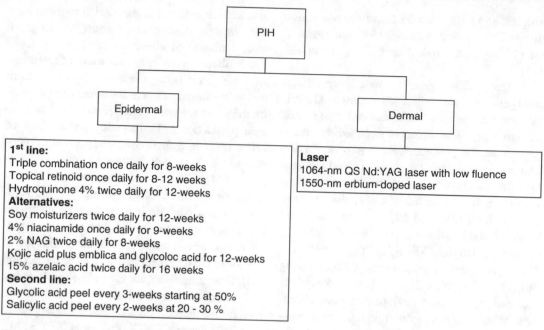

Fig. 12.6 Outlines first-line and alternative treatment regimens for post-inflammatory hyperpigmentation, classified by epidermal or dermal histopathologic pattern. NAG N-acetyl glucosamine, QS Nd:YAG Q-switched neodymium-doped yttrium aluminum garnet. (Adapted from Chaowattapanit et al. [38], with permission)

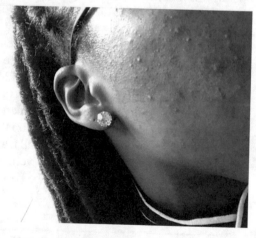

Fig. 12.7 Post-inflammatory hyperpigmentation in a female with acne. (Image is courtesy of Dr. Titilola Sode)

[36]. While this condition is prevalent in ethnicities with darker skin types, it affects fair-skinned individuals as well [36].

The basis underlying this hyperpigmentation is likely related to the activity of growth factors such as keratinocyte growth factor and interleukin-1 alpha inducing excessive melanogenesis

[37]. Histopathology shows increased melanin in the epidermal and dermal layers, and in the presence of inflammation, hypertrophy and hyperplasia of melanocytes may be visible [38].

PIH typically lacks associated symptoms and systemic findings aside from cosmetic or psychosocial concern [39]. Indeed, in a study evaluating the psychosocial impact of PIH after acne, a survey of 200 Nigerian undergraduates showed a significant impact on quality of life in patients with acne and hyperpigmentation compared to those without hyperpigmentation [40]. In addition, hyperpigmentation was associated with anxiety in 26.5% and emotional distress in 35.4% of individuals with hyperpigmentation compared to 10.3% in those without hyperpigmentation [40]. While asymptomatic, these studies suggest that healthcare providers should consider treating the condition as it does impact on the quality of life of patients.

There are two clinical forms of PIH: epidermal and dermal. Epidermal hyperpigmentation tends to be light to dark brown, whereas dermal hyperpigmentation tends to have a blue-gray coloration [38]. The depth of dermal melanophages is the most important factor in the response to treatment [38].

Treatments for PIH are focused on preventative measures and therapies to lighten the affected areas after they develop [38, 39]. Some preventative therapies include using lightening agents, anti-inflammatory agents, and topical retinoids prior to procedures and using photoprotection regularly [35]. Hydroquinone is the standard skin-lightening agent, and combination products containing hydroquinone, retinoic acid, and corticosteroids are the most effective medical treatment for PIH [38]. Common short-term side effects of hydroquinone include irritation, contact dermatitis, and post-inflammatory hypopigmentation. Ochronosis is the most common long-term complication, usually occurring in African patients who have been exposed to high concentrations (>4%) of hydroquinone along with exposure to high doses of sunlight, although it has also been reported to occur with a low concentration (2%) [38]. Figure 12.6 provides additional treatment regimens for PIH [38].

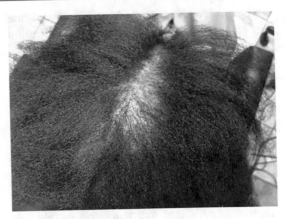

Fig. 12.8 Female with CCCA. (Image is courtesy of Dr. Katherine Ayoade, Department of Dermatology, UT Southwestern Medical Center)

Central Centrifugal Cicatricial Alopecia

Central centrifugal cicatricial alopecia (CCCA) refers to a progressive scarring alopecia in which the hair follicle is destroyed and replaced with fibrous tracts that typically starts at the crown of the scalp and expands outwards (see Fig. 12.8). Hair breakage may be an early sign of disease [41] (see Fig. 12.9). CCCA primarily affects middle-aged women of African ancestry with a prevalence ranging between 2.7% and 5.7% [42, 43]. The etiology of this condition is unknown. Originally named "hot comb" alopecia [44], studies have classically demonstrated a strong association between the use of traumatic hairstyling such as tight braids and hair extensions [45]. A recent microarray analysis of gene expression in five individuals with biopsy-proven CCCA showed an upregulation of genes associated with fibroproliferative disorders. These include genes encoding platelet-derived

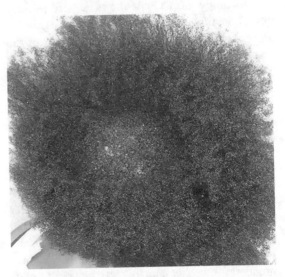

Fig. 12.9 Hair breakage in early CCCA. (Image is courtesy of Dr. Katherine Ayoade, Department of Dermatology, UT Southwestern Medical Center)

growth factor, collagen, and matrix metallopeptidases [46]. To better understand the role of genetics in CCCA, a study identified 14 families with 31 immediate family members with histologic features consistent with CCCA, suggesting the possibility of an autosomal dominant inheritance pattern with partial penetrance [47]. The hypothesis of a genetic predisposition to this scarring disorder was further supported by a recent study where exome sequencing in a group of 16 women with CCCA identified missense mutation in the gene *PADI3*, which encodes peptidyl-arginine deaminase, type III, an enzyme that plays a role in posttranslational modification of proteins integral to the developing hair shaft. This gene was mutated in an additional 9 out of 42 patients who underwent sequencing of *PADI3*. An analysis of these groups compared to a comparable group of women of African ancestry demonstrated a significantly higher prevalence of mutated *PADI3* among the patients with CCCA [48]. Mutations in *PADI3* lead to another hair disorder known as uncombable hair syndrome – a non-scarring hair disorder. Thus, the authors hypothesize that mutations in this hair shaft gene coupled with environmental trauma, such as traumatic grooming styles, may increase the probability of developing CCCA.

Histology of CCCA shows a perifollicular lymphocytic infiltrate, concentric lamellar fibroplasia, and premature desquamation of the inner root sheath [42]. Using a dermatoscope, the presence of a peripilar white or gray halo was highly specific and sensitive for CCCA and corresponded to the lamellar fibrosis of the outer root sheath visible on histopathology [49]. These findings suggest a suitable site for biopsy.

Therapeutic options for CCCA are limited. The goal of therapy is to quench the inflammatory process, preventing progression, and administer treatment options targeted as follicular rescue of follicles that are not scarred. Combination therapy works best. Topicals including antiseborrheic shampoos, recommended for weekly use, followed by use of a conditioner as well as a topical class I–II high-potency steroids, administered once or twice daily, are used to mitigate the inflammatory progress. In addition, intralesional injections of corticosteroids 2.5 mg–7.5 mg/cc by the author (KOA) are administered every 8 weeks until clinical signs and symptoms of inflammation have ceased; this usually occurs within 4–6 months. Alternatively, systemic anti-inflammatory agents such as doxycycline 100 mg twice daily, typically for 3 months, can be prescribed. For follicular rescue, laboratory tests to screen for thyroid function, vitamin D deficiency, zinc deficiency, and iron deficiency, including complete blood count, iron studies, ferritin, and erythrocyte sedimentation rate, are performed, and therapy is initiated if evidence of a deficiency is discovered. In addition to supplements for nutritional deficiencies, topical minoxidil and more recently in the author's experience (KOA), oral minoxidil, dose 0.625–2.5 mg, have shown improvement. There are anecdotal reports in the literature of using systemic hydroxychloroquine, mycophenolate mofetil, cyclosporine, and antiandrogens for 6–9 months when topicals are unsuccessful [42]. More recently platelet-rich plasma (PRP) has been shown to help some patients [50]. In patients in whom scalp inflammation is absent or well controlled for at least 9–12 months, hair transplantation can be considered [51]. The treatment of patients with CCCA is not complete without counseling about grooming practices unique to persons of African descent. In patient counseling, it is advised that these patients limit or stop traumatic grooming practices including traction-inducing hairstyles such as tight braids, tight cornrows, and weaves, as well as frequent use of chemical relaxers and frequent application of heat for hair straightening. It is also advised to limit the use of non-medicated oils, pomades, and grease on the scalp as these may exacerbate seborrheic dermatitis and or folliculitis, further contributing to the inflammatory process. Instead, patients are encouraged to use their favorite oils on the distal hair shaft which is prone to dryness.

Future research aimed at better understanding the genetics of CCCA may allow for the development of more effective therapies for this condition.

Traction Alopecia

Traction alopecia (TA) is a form of hair loss associated with the use of traction-inducing hair practices. These hairstyle practices include grooming hair into tight buns, ponytails, braids, dreadlocks, sister locks, wearing weaves and other hair extensions, as well as the use of tight overnight rollers [52, 53]. In the patient of African descent, hair that has been chemically relaxed and subjected to these traction grooming styles is most prone to

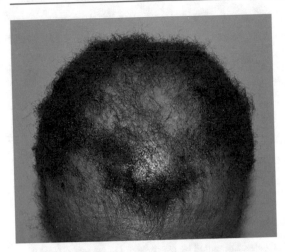

Fig. 12.10 Female with CCCA and traction alopecia. (Image is courtesy of Dr. Katherine Ayoade, Department of Dermatology, UT Southwestern Medical Center and Dr. Cynthia Robinson)

developing this form of alopecia [52, 53]. Though TA has been noted in most races, there appears to be a high prevalence among individuals of African descent, with a prevalence ranging between 1.0% of black adults in an outpatient dermatology clinic in London and 37% of black women at a primary care center in Cape Town, South Africa [53]. The wide variability in prevalence between populations with similar level of genetic risk may be due to the different hairstyle practices [53]. Women are most frequently affected, and the incidence increases with age [54]. Clinically, due to the nature of these hairstyles, the frontotemporal region is most frequently affected, though there are also instances of the posterior hairline being affected [55] (see Fig. 12.10). There may be mild perifollicular erythema, scaling, and pustules in early TA. Symptoms of pruritus or tenderness may be mild or absent. As the follicles atrophy, only short thin vellus hairs remain. Permanent follicular hair loss can occur if chronic tension persists [56]. On examination with a dermatoscope, there are broken hairs, miniaturized hairs, pinpoint white dots, reduced hair density and hair casts. Hair casts are 2–7 mm long, freely moveable, gray-white cylinders wrapped around the proximal hair shaft of hairs surrounding areas under tension [55].

The histopathology of early TA shows trichomalacia, increased numbers of telogen and catagen hairs, a normal number of terminal follicles, and preserved sebaceous glands. At some point there may be "follicular dropout" of the terminal hairs where the follicles seem to have disappeared but the vellus-sized hairs are intact. With long-standing TA, sebaceous glands are present but may be decreased, and vellus-sized hairs may be seen. There is a decrease in the number of terminal follicles, which are replaced with fibrotic fibrous tracts. Inflammation is little to absent in long-standing TA but may be mild in some cases of early TA [57].

Treatment for traction alopecia mainly consists of cessation of traumatic and traction-inducing hairstyling and encouraging loose hairstyles. In addition, reports have demonstrated hair regrowth with using topical minoxidil and intralesional and topical steroids in persons demonstrating inflammation in early TA. Hair transplants are an option for refractory cases [55, 56].

Dermatosis Papulosa Nigra

Dermatosis papulosa nigra (DPN) refers to benign epidermal growths that appear as pigmented filiform papules and often present on the face and neck [58, 59] (see Fig. 12.11). This condition primarily affects individuals with darker skin color, such as individuals of African and Asian descent, affecting up to one-third of African Americans in the United States, with a female predominance. DPN typically affects individuals starting in adolescence, with the number and size of the lesions increasing with age and peaking during the sixth decade [58].

The etiology is unknown; however, it is believed to be a variant of seborrheic keratoses, with genetic analyses of DPN showing mutations in FGFR3, which have been previously reported in seborrheic keratoses [60]. Other studies have reported an association between DPN and a positive family history [61]. There is also a hypothesized link to UV exposure due to the distribution of DPN on sun-exposed areas and the observation that individuals who use topical lightening

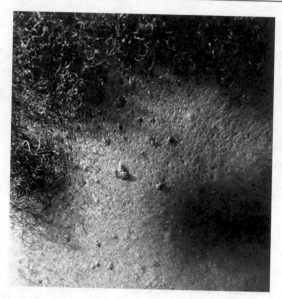

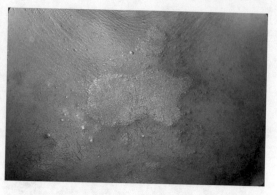

Fig. 12.12 Seborrheic dermatitis on the chest. (Image is courtesy of the Betty E. Janes Clinical Image Library, Department of Dermatology, UT Southwestern Medical Center. Submitted by courtesy of Dr. Donald Glass II)

Fig. 12.11 Dermatosis papulosa nigra on the temple. (Image is courtesy of Dr. Katherine Ayoade, Department of Dermatology, UT Southwestern Medical Center)

agents had more severe DPNs [58]. On histology, DPNs are characterized by hyperkeratosis, irregular acanthosis, horn cysts, and marked hyperpigmentation of the basal layer [61].

Treatment of DPNs classically consists snip excision, light curettage, and light electrodesiccation. Studies have shown the use of carbon dioxide lasers in the ablation of DPN to be as effective as electrodesiccation with high patient satisfaction and a low rate of post-procedural complications such as change in pigmentation and scarring [62].

Seborrheic Dermatitis

Seborrheic dermatitis (SD) is an inflammatory skin disorder characterized as a yellow greasy scaly dermatitis with underlying erythema affecting the sebaceous regions of the body, including the face, scalp, chest, and back [63] (see Fig. 12.12). Several factors appear to play a role in the etiology of SD including the skin microbiota, immune system, and genetics. Several studies have evaluated the relationship between *Malassezia* spp., a yeast that naturally exists on skin as typical skin flora, and SD. In the setting of

SD, it appears that *Malassezia* yeast causes inflammation that contributes to hyperproliferation of the stratum corneum leading to scaling [63, 64]. A systematic review of the literature addressing the role of genetics in SD identified 11 gene mutations or protein deficiencies that were involved in SD or a SD-like phenotype in humans or animal models [65]. In humans, four of these genes are associated with immune system function and differentiation, and a fifth gene was involved in epidermal differentiation [65].

The prevalence of SD ranges between 1% and 3% in immunocompetent individuals and up to 10% in the immunocompromised. Men are more often affected than women, and it occurs in infants as well as the third and fourth decades of age [63, 66]. Some studies suggest there may be an increased incidence among African Americans, up to 6.5%, and West Africans, up to 6%, and seborrheic dermatitis is one of the five most common diagnoses among black patients [67]. Surveys assessing the quality of life of individuals with SD have demonstrated a significantly negative impact for patients with SD and dandruff compared to those without dandruff, emphasizing the importance of treating this condition effectively [68].

Management of SD mostly consists of emollients to loosen the scales and remove them with a cloth or comb. Other treatments include coal tar shampoo, topical antifungals, topical corticosteroids, and calcineurin inhibitors [64]. Among patients with skin of color, the management of seborrheic dermatitis should be adjusted to account for differences in hair texture and hair washing frequency [67].

References

1. Ogunbiyi A. Acne keloidalis nuchae: prevalence, impact, and management challenges. Clin Cosmet Investig Dermatol. 2016;9:483–9.
2. East-Innis A, et al. Acne keloidalis nuchae: risk factors and associated disorders – a retrospective study. Int J Dermatol. 2017;56(8):828–32.
3. George A, et al. Clinical, biochemical and morphologic features of acne keloidalis in a black population. Int J Dermatol. 1993;32(10):714–6.
4. Verma S, Wollina U. Acne keloidalis nuchae: another cutaneous symptom of metabolic syndrome, truncal obesity, and impending/overt diabetes mellitus? Am J Clin Dermatol. 2010;11(6):433–6.
5. Loayza E, et al. Acne keloidalis nuchae in Latin American women. Int J Dermatol. 2015;54(5):183–5.
6. Loayza E, et al. Acne keloidalis nuchae in Latin America: is there a different phenotype? Int J Dermatol. 2017;56(12):1469.
7. Al Aboud D, Badri T. Acne keloidalis nuchae. Teasure Island: StatPearls Publishing; 2018.
8. Gamil H, et al. Successful treatment of acne keloidalis nuchae with erbium:YAG laser: a comparative study. J Cosmet Laser Ther. 2018;20:419.
9. Tawfik A, Osman M, Rashwan I. A novel treatment of acne keloidalis nuchae by long-pulsed alexandrite laser. Dermatol Surg. 2018;44(3):413–20.
10. Woo D, et al. Prospective controlled trial for the treatment of acne keloidalis nuchae with a long-pulsed neodymium-doped yttrium-aluminum-garnet laser. J Cutan Med Surg. 2018;22(2):236–8.
11. Okoye G, et al. Improving acne keloidalis nuchae with targeted ultraviolet B treatment: a prospective, randomized, split-scalp comparison study. Br J Dermatol. 2014;171(7):1156–63.
12. Millan-Cayetano J, et al. Refractory acne keloidalis nuchae treated with radiotherapy. Australas J Dermatol. 2017;58(1):11–3.
13. He Y, et al. From genetics to epigenetics: new insights into keloid scarring. Cell Prolif. 2017;50(2):e12326.
14. Chike-Obi C, Cole P, Brissett A. Keloids: pathogenesis, clinical features, and management. Semin Plast Surg. 2009;23(3):178–84.
15. Davis S, Feldman S, McMichael A. Management of keloids in the United States, 1990–2009: an analysis of the National Ambulatory Medical Care Survey. Dermatol Surg. 2013;39(7):988–94.
16. Velez Edwards D, et al. Admixture mapping identifies a locus at 15q21.2-22.3 associated with keloid formation in African Americans. Hum Genet. 2014;133(12):1513–23.
17. Kouwenberg C, et al. Emotional quality of life is severely affected by keloid disease: pain and itch are the main determinants of burden. Plast Reconstr Surg. 2015;136(4S):150–1.
18. Mayo T, Glass D. Keloids. In: Pandya A, Jackson-Richards D, editors. Dermatology atlas for skin of color. Berlin, Heidelberg: Springer; 2014. p. 249–53.
19. Juntongjin P, Laosakul K. Idiopathic guttate hypomelanosis: a review of its etiology, pathogenesis, findings, and treatments. Am J Clin Dermatol. 2016;17(4):403–11.
20. Brown F, Crane J. Idiopathic guttate hypomelanosis. Treasure Island: StatPearls Publishing; 2018.
21. Rerknimitr P, Disphanurat W, Achariyakul M. Topical tacrolimus significantly promotes repigmentation in idiopathic guttate hypomelanosis: a double-blind, randomized, placebo-controlled study. J Eur Acad Dermatol Venereol. 2013;27(4):460–4.
22. Wambier C, et al. 5-Fluorouracil tattooing for idiopathic guttate hypomelanosis. J Am Acad Dermatol. 2018;78(4):81–2.
23. Arbache S, et al. Activation of melanocytes in idiopathic guttate hypomelanosis after 5-fluorouracil infusion using a tattoo machine: preliminary analysis of a randomized, split-body, single blinded, placebo controlled clinical trial. J Am Acad Dermatol. 2018;78(1):212–5.
24. Omueti-Ayoade K, Pandya A. Idiopathic guttate hypomelanosis. In: Pandya A, Jackson-Richards D, editors. Dermatology atlas for skin of color. Berlin, Heidelberg: Springer; 2014. p. 17–20.
25. Rodrigues M, et al. New discoveries in the pathogenesis and classification of vitiligo. J Am Acad Dermatol. 2017;77(1):1–13.
26. Rodrigues M, et al. Current and emerging treatments for vitiligo. J Am Acad Dermatol. 2017;77(1):17–29.
27. Degboe B, et al. Vitiligo on black skin: epidemiological and clinical aspects in dermatology, Cotonou (Benin). Int J Dermatol. 2017;56(1):92–6.
28. Spritz R, Andersen G. Genetics of vitiligo. Dermatol Clin. 2017;35(2):245–55.
29. Gill L, et al. Comorbid autoimmune diseases in patients with vitiligo: a cross-sectional study. J Am Acad Dermatol. 2016;74(2):295.
30. Goh B, Pandya A. Presentations, signs of activity, and differential diagnosis of vitiligo. Dermatol Clin. 2017;35(2):135–44.
31. Ezzedine K, et al. Vitiligo. Lancet. 2015;386(9988):74.
32. Porter J, Beuf A. Racial variation in reaction to physical stigma: a study of degree of disturbance by vitiligo among black and white patients. J Health Soc Behav. 1991;32(2):192–204.
33. Lai Y, et al. Vitiligo and depression: a systematic review and meta-analysis of observational studies. Br J Dermatol. 2017;177(3):708–18.
34. Dina Y, McKesey J, Pandya A. Disorders of hypopigmentation. J Drugs Dermatol. 2019;18(3):115–6.
35. Sofen B, Prado G, Emer J. Melasma and post inflammatory hyperpigmentation: management update and expert opinion. Skin Therapy Lett. 2016;21(1):1–7.

36. Passeron T, et al. Development and validation of a reproducible model for studying post-inflammatory hyperpigmentation. Pigment Cell Melanome Res. 2018;31(5):649–52.

37. Cardinali G, Kovacs D, Picardo M. Mechanisms underlying post-inflammatory hyperpigmentation: lessons from solar lentigo. Ann Dermatol Venereol. 2012;139:148–52.

38. Chaowattanapanit S, et al. Postinflammatory hyperpigmentation: a comprehensive overview: epidemiology, pathogenesis, clinical presentation, and noninvasive assessment technique. J Am Acad Dermatol. 2017;77(4):591–605.

39. Savory S, Pandya A. Post-inflammatory hyperpigmentation. In: Pandya A, Jackson-Richards D, editors. Dermatology atlas for skin of color. Berlin, Heidelberg: Springer; 2014. p. 21–5.

40. Akinboro A, et al. The impact of acne and facial post-inflammatory hyperpigmentation on quality of life and self-esteem of newly admitted Nigerian undergraduates. Clin Cosmet Investig Dermatol. 2018;11:245–52.

41. Callender VD, et al. Hair breakage as a presenting sign of early or occult central centrifugal cicatricial alopecia: clinicopathologic findings in 9 patients. Arch Dermatol. 2012;148(9):1047–52.

42. Dlova N, et al. Central centrifugal cicatricial alopecia: new insights and a call for action. J Investig Dermatol Symp Proc. 2017;18(2):54–6.

43. Ogunleye T, McMichael A, Olsen E. Central centrifugal cicatricial alopecia: what has been achieved, current clues for future research. Dermatol Clin. 2014;32(2):173–81.

44. LoPresti P, Papa C, Kligman A. Hot comb alopecia. Arch Dermatol. 1968;98(3):234–8.

45. Gathers R, et al. Hair grooming practices and central centrifugal cicatricial alopecia. J Am Acad Dermatol. 2009;60(4):574–8.

46. Aguh C, et al. Fibroproliferative genes are preferentially expressed in central centrifugal cicatricial alopecia. J Am Acad Dermatol. 2018;79(5):904–12.

47. Dlova N, et al. Autosomal dominant inheritance of central centrifugal cicatricial alopecia in black South Africans. J Am Acad Dermatol. 2014;70(4):679–82.

48. Malki L, et al. Variant PADI3 in central centrifugal cicatricial alopecia. N Engl J Med. 2019;380(9):833–41.

49. Miteva M, Tosti A. Dermatoscopic features of central centrifugal cicatricial alopecia. J Am Acad Dermatol. 2014;71(3):443–9.

50. Dina Y, Aguh C. Use of platelet-rich plasma in cicatricial alopecia. Dermatol Surg. 2018;45:979.

51. Callender V, Lawson C, Onwudiwe O. Hair transplantation in the surgical treatment of central centrifugal cicatricial alopecia. Dermatol Surg. 2014;40(10):1125–31.

52. Tosti A, et al. Hair casts are dermoscopic clue to diagnosis of traction alopecia. Br J Dermatol. 2010;163(6):1353–5.

53. Billero V, Miteva M. Traction alopecia: the root of the problem. Clin Cosmet Investig Dermatol. 2018;11:149–59.

54. Khumalo N. The "fringe sign" for public education on traction alopecia. Dermatol Online J. 2012;18(9):16.

55. Akingbola C, Vyas J. Traction alopecia: a neglected entity in 2017. Indian J Dermatol Venereol Leprol. 2017;83(6):644–9.

56. Jackson-Richards D. Traction alopecia. In: Pandya A, Jackson-Richards D, editors. Dermatology atlas for skin of color. Berlin, Heidelberg: Springer; 2014. p. 95–8.

57. Samrao A, et al. The "Fringe Sign" – a useful clinical finding in traction alopecia of the marginal hair line. Dermatol Online J. 2011;17(11):1.

58. Xiao A, Ettefagh L. Dermatosis papulosa nigra. Treasure Island: StatPearls Publishing; 2019.

59. Metin S, et al. Dermatosis papulosa nigra: a clinically and histopathologically distinct entity. Clin Dermatol. 2017;35(5):491–6.

60. Hafner C, et al. FGFR3 and PIK3CA mutations in stucco keratosis and dermatosis papulosa nigra. Br J Dermatol. 2010;162(3):508–12.

61. Bhat R, et al. A clinical, dermoscopic, and histopathological study of Dermatosis Papulosa Nigra (DPN) – an Indian perspective. Int J Dermatol. 2017;56(9):957–60.

62. Ali F, et al. Carbon dioxide laser ablation of dermatosis papulosa nigra: high satisfaction and few complications in patients with pigmented skin. Lasers Med Sci. 2016;31(3):593–5.

63. Ijaz N, Fitzgerald D. Seborrhoeic dermatitis. Br J Hosp Med. 2017;78(6):C88.

64. Clark G, Pope S, Jaboori K. Diagnosis and treatment of seborrheic dermatitis. Am Fam Physician. 2015;91(3):185–90.

65. Karakadze M, Hirt P, Wikramanayake T. The genetic basis of seborrhoeic dermatitis: a review. J Eur Acad Dermatol Venereol. 2017;32(4):529–36.

66. Dessinioti C, Katsambas A. Seborrheic dermatitis: etiology, risk factors, and treatments: facts and controversies. Clin Dermatol. 2013;31(4):343–51.

67. Elgash M, et al. Seborrheic dermatitis in skin of color: clinical considerations. J Drugs Dermatol. 2019;18(1):24–7.

68. Szepietowski J, et al. Quality of life in patients suffering from seborrheic dermatitis: influence of age, gender and education level. Mycoses. 2009;52(4):357–63.

Part III

Other Considerations

Multicultural Competence and Other Considerations

Edward W. Seger, Amy J. McMichael,
Steven R. Feldman, and William W. Huang

Introduction

Previous discussion on the pathophysiology of ethnic skin and hair provides a foundation for the clinician to successfully identify and treat dermatologic disorders in a diverse patient population. In addition to the basic science of skin disease, the diversity that exists between patients of different cultures, ethnicities, and regions of the world must color the approach to patient care. Individuals view life (and health and medicine) through the lens of the camera that they are provided, and a practitioner must be fluent in navigating this cultural terrain without unnecessary bias.

The lack of diversity within the field of dermatology is striking: only 3% of practicing dermatologists are black, and 4% Hispanic, despite combining to account for almost 30% of the total population of the United States [1]. These limitations matter, as patients visiting a physician who shares a common racial, cultural, or language background perceive better care [2]. While efforts are underway to recruit diverse and talented individuals to pursue the specialty, determining how these patient perceptions may act as a predictor of good care can improve how to improve perceptions of providers of all ethnicities. The purpose of this chapter is to provide a background in the multicultural competence in healthcare and its impact within dermatology.

Defining Cultural Competence

Culture is the fabric of meaning in terms of which human beings interpret their experience and guide their action. – Clifford Geertz

There are many ways to describe what the term culture means. Broadly speaking, culture is the set of beliefs and traits that are shared by individuals of a common social, religious, or ethnic background. This term is distinct from race as patients from many racial and ethnic backgrounds often share a similar culture. Personal identity is often derived at least in part from physical and cosmetic features, making cultural competence particularly important within the field of dermatology. The way we style our hair, the clothes that we wear, and the way that we otherwise present ourselves to the world are inherently linked to the social cues to which we are exposed. Our culture is everything that surrounds us, and it impacts how we perceive disease and how we view the medical system.

E. W. Seger · A. J. McMichael · S. R. Feldman (✉)
W. W. Huang
Wake Forest School of Medicine,
Department of Dermatology,
Winston-Salem, NC, USA
e-mail: sfeldman@wakehealth.edu

© Springer Nature Switzerland AG 2021
B. S. Li, H. I. Maibach (eds.), *Ethnic Skin and Hair and Other Cultural Considerations*, Updates in Clinical Dermatology, https://doi.org/10.1007/978-3-030-64830-5_13

Understanding Bias

Bias is a representation of the opinions that one carries, either positive or negative, toward an individual or a group of people. Gender, religion, race, and cultural background are all subject to bias. In general terms, bias is categorized as either conscious (explicit) or unconscious (implicit) [3]. The formation of personal bias is through a combination of stereotyping and prejudice. Stereotyping is the association of a particular group (such as ethnic, social, or cultural) with a predetermined set of traits. Usually these opinions result from the environment in which a person resides and are a reflection of opinions of others around them. Stereotyping primarily is discussed with negative connotations, but group generalization with a "positive" sentiment similarly fits the criteria. In comparison, prejudice is always negative and is a view commonly formed through social conditioning that unfairly affects a particular group or individual.

It is important to understand the impact of these biases in everyday life. Patients with skin tones and hairstyles that do not conform to regional norms are often discriminated against, even if unintentionally, based on external appearance. Similarly, the homeless and the disabled are often subjected to unnecessary bias. Medicine is not immune, and healthcare may be modified based on a provider's preconceived views. This can lead to patients who are undertreated or subjected to additional suffering [4]. Moreover, these preconceived views may lead to missed diagnoses if the provider falsely believes the patient has a primary desire for secondary gain.

Ethnic and Cultural barriers in Healthcare

Alongside these professional biases, there are inherent cultural differences in healthcare delivery and views about disease. These factors often prevent patients from even seeking care. Providers should be aware of these limitations that will impact how patients present and how much success is achieved with treatment. (Table 13.1)

Definition of Illness

Western clinicians are trained with a scientific and data-driven understanding of what disease is, but this approach is relatively new. For instance, ancient Chinese medicine often views illness from a holistic and energy-based approach [5]. Similarly, religious patients may view their illness within the confines of their beliefs [6]. There are several important implications to these situations. Patients may prefer to use local remedies despite the availability of scientifically proven options. They may also be resistant to treatment if it conflicts with their beliefs, as is the case with Jehovah's Witnesses' frequent refusal of blood transfusions. It is often necessary to find a delicate balance between these beliefs and care plans. Framing a disease within the context of their beliefs may improve success. In patients with more rigid views, acceptable supportive care may be pursued.

Table 13.1 Cultural barriers in healthcare

Definition of illness	Cultures define disease differently. Religious, social, and regional norms can all affect when a patient presents for care and what treatments they are willing to undergo
Access to care	Geographic and financial considerations impact the pursuit of care. Minority groups are less likely to be insured and with the means to pay for care. Similarly, many regions of the world do not have access to adequate healthcare within a reasonable distance
Comprehension	The health system is often only practiced within the confines of the regional language. Beyond the patient interview, navigating the initiation of care as well as discharge and treatment plans is more difficult for patients who are not native speakers
Adherence	Alongside comprehension, complex and expensive treatment plans are more difficult to follow. Moreover, patients who do not reside in the local area may have more difficulty with follow-up
Patient/provider	The ethnicity and cultural background of a patient matter. Providers who share cultural similarities with a patient are viewed by patients more favorably which may impact treatment outcomes

Access to Care

Even when patients attempt to seek out care, many barriers exist. Global healthcare infrastructure has tremendous variability. Patients from impoverished regions such as Africa, South America, and India often do not have adequate healthcare facilities. The result is a persistence of preventable disease and increased mortality resulting from a lack of access to appropriate treatment. While this global discrepancy is unfortunately well established, there remains similar issues within the Western world. Patients of a lower socioeconomic status are less likely to have a primary care physician than counterparts with more resources [7]. These disparities cause a division along ethnic lines. White patients are more likely to seek out preventative care than similar patients who are black or Hispanic [8]. If we know that certain groups are not utilizing health services, then the question must be asked why?

Distance may be partially to blame, and urban environments with an abundance of primary care providers produce a smaller discrepancy in care among ethnic groups [9]. Cost is another reason for not seeking care [10, 11]. Underrepresented minorities are more likely to be uninsured and with lower income as compared to their white counterparts [12]. Universal healthcare coverage in the United Kingdom improved these inequalities, but these systems are still not perfect [13]. Irrespective of insurance, undocumented costs exist as well such as loss of pay for missing work and lack of accessible childcare. All of these factors play a role in patients delaying care until it is absolutely necessary. This is an issue within dermatology as well. For example, a substantially higher proportion of melanomas are diagnosed at later stages in Hispanic patients when compared to white counterparts [14]. Even in benign instances, patients are often subjected to more time living with easily treated skin and hair conditions simply because they cannot afford to access care.

Barriers to Comprehension

When patients surpass these financial limitations, communication barriers persist. The most obvious of these is language. Accessing healthcare is daunting even without trying to navigate the system primarily speaking a foreign language. Quality of care is perceived as higher if the provider speaks the patient's native language, probably a result of improved ability to develop a rapport and understanding [15]. Professional interpreters help but do not completely remove the language barriers [16, 17]. Having access to multilingual paperwork is important, in particular when they are receiving educational materials or treatment plans. These modifications work as less adverse events resulting from medication misuse were reported when native language discharge instructions were provided [18].

Barriers to Adherence

Effective treatment requires patient understanding after the clinician leaves the room. Considerations for compliance include the cost of treatment, complexity of medication regimen, and patient availability for follow-up. Providers often do not pay attention to the costs of the therapies that they are prescribing, despite the fact that this is one of the most common reasons patients are non-adherent [11]. This results in patients not filling prescriptions or not utilizing medication at the appropriate frequency and amount. Complexity of medication regimen is also implicated in lack of adherence and errors in usage [19]. Patients may benefit from simplifying these regimens and utilizing easily accessible and affordable therapies. In dermatology, beyond internal toxicities, cosmetic side effects may be important to consider. For example, isotretinoin is effective at improving acne but may also lead to hair loss. These side effects may impact a patient's willingness to start or maintain a treatment irrespective of its efficacy. Finally, returning to clinic may be difficult. Patients who visit the region for the sole purpose of medical care may not be easily able to follow-up. If intermediate providers in proximity to the patient's locale are not established, adherence may suffer. Even for patients nearby, extended wait times for appointments can reduce attendance [20]. Minimization of these barriers of adherence will likely improve dermatologic outcomes across all cultural groups.

Patient-Provider Interactions

There is an association between effective patient-provider communication and health outcomes and patient satisfaction. Vising a provider with a shared culture (beliefs, values, and language) was associated with higher levels of trust, satisfaction, and intention to adhere to therapies [21]. Social and cultural differences can limit effective communication in the medical interview. For example, in female patients treated for acne, Caucasian women were most concerned with lesional clearance from treatment, compared to clearance of hypo- or hyperpigmentation which was the greatest concern in non-white/Caucasian respondents [22]. Regardless of the competence of the physician, patients from different cultures may have different outcome goals and desires, and their opinion of the quality of care will be impacted by these views. Similarly, accommodating patients with a strong gender preference when possible may ease anxiety and enable them to discuss sensitive topics more easily.

Despite the importance of limiting barriers of interaction, some cultural components remain important. The prevalence of disease varies around the world, and the differential diagnosis will change on regional, social, and ethnic history. For example, a suspected infectious etiology in a person who returned from South America will vary between someone who has not recently traveled. Similarly, genetic diseases are seen in clusters of similar populations. Finally, cultural differences in healthcare result in patients who may not have been vaccinated for common disease or have had even basic preventative care.

Interventions Aimed at Improving Ethnic and Cultural Care

There are many ways to improve cultural competency and healthcare disparities. Broadly these approaches can be classified as provider centered, patient centered, and community centered. Research performed within these areas has tremendous relatability and can be utilized as best needed for each practice. (Table 13.2).

Provider-Centered Approaches

Cultural competence for a healthcare provider involves realization and minimization of personal biases along with a social understanding of the patients they treat. Educational resources and online modules are easily implemented and may provide a basic framework for understanding. These forms of learning are not perfect and often neglect the true fluidity of culture. Focusing on the historical context of a society, as well as tangible attributes such as lifestyles, occupations, nutrition, and health risks, may provide more benefit to the practitioner. Similarly, health out-

Table 13.2 Interventions aimed at improving cultural care

Provider	Improving a provider's competence and familiarity with other cultures through education, group activities, and increased exposure can improve patient care and patient satisfaction
Patient	Interventions aimed at patient comprehension can improve care. Translating care plans to a native language and working within the confines of an individual's health infrastructure may improve outcomes
Community	Outreach programs such as free health screenings and educational seminars both increase awareness and provide a platform to establish care for patients
Educational	Medical education focusing more time into teaching students about the impact of culture in medicine improves awareness. Exposure to a diverse patient population during school and residency provides a background for treating patients from different cultures

comes are important, recognizing that incidence and prevalence of disease changes among different groups are essential. Within dermatology, we know that specific conditions affect patients with different hair types differently so it is beneficial to have a basic cultural competency as it relates to hair type, which may impact patients of different ethnicities differently. Finally, faith is a major component of many patients' lives, and a working understanding of local religions may aid understanding. It is difficult to understand the cultural intricacies of every patient you interact with. Focusing on commonly encountered cultures as well as identifying personal weaknesses may provide the most benefit. Activities that require personal engagement such as small group discussions and simulations may be even better for comprehension. These discussions are opportunities to recognize personal biases and how it impacts care. They may also help serve to better prepare the provider for dealing with culturally sensitive questions and situations.

Another form of improving cultural competence is by actively seeking out opportunities to engage with different cultures. This can be accomplished through work or volunteering in areas with diverse patient populations. Moreover, these endeavors may improve clinical diagnostic skills through increased exposure and comfort. Use of role models within healthcare can also be beneficial. Particularly in larger institutions, there are often colleagues from different social and cultural upbringings and those with interests in the culture of medicine. Finally, and perhaps easiest, is simply inquiring with patients. Showing an interest and a desire to learn more will likely be well received and is an opportunity to develop a deeper rapport with the patient going forward.

Patient-Centered Approaches

Approaches targeting the patient revolve around recognizing what roadblocks or barriers to care exist. Accessible translators and paperwork in multiple languages can improve medical comprehension. Particularly in dermatology, where prescription of several medications simultaneously

is common, a concerted effort to write out easy-to-follow care plans and using techniques such as "ask-tell-ask" have the potential to improve medical outcomes. In areas with high rates of missed appointments, phone call reminders are an easy way to encourage patients to attend. Post-visit communication such as follow-up calls and online messaging similarly improve medication adherence, possibly by increasing patient engagement in the treatment plan, creating accountability, and increasing the perception that the provider cares about the patient [23].

Individuals from resource-poor countries often come to the United States specifically for healthcare. Management of these patients is difficult as a result of the potential lack of follow-up. A care plan for disease management when they are away could be established. This includes understanding of the regional health infrastructure and access to suitable intermediate care providers. Similarly, it is important to select medications carefully to ensure that they can be acquired when the patient heads back home.

Health literacy and personal views about disease also vary among different cultures. This does not mean that patients do not want to learn as half of minority patients surveyed from a free healthcare clinic had never performed a self-skin examination, yet almost all wanted to learn more about how to prevent skin cancer [24]. Targeted educational programs including pamphlets, online resources, and information sessions can help interested patients learn more about their disease and provide a framework to prepare questions that may arise. Moreover, this increased patient engagement may also improve adherence and health outcomes.

Community Outreach Approaches

The easiest way to promote health and well-being on a larger social scale is with outreach programs. For example, providing free skin checks in low-resource areas is an inexpensive and effective way to screen for high-risk lesions in patients who were otherwise not imminently seeking out dermatologic care. Moreover, simultaneous monitoring for common health concerns such as high blood pressure and diabetes is easily done on the same day. As this may be the first time that patients are seeking care, we can use this as an opportunity to establish dermatologic and primary care services for follow-up and preventative monitoring. Utilizing in neighborhood resources such as churches, local schools, and community centers has the potential to be well attended due to their easily accessible locations and familiarity to the patient.

These outreach programs are also educational. The free nature of these screening sessions is well advertised but also can provide awareness for additional free or low-cost health services that may be available. By attempting to increase healthcare utilization, patients may be less apt to wait until absolutely necessary before seeking out care. Community sessions can also be implemented with series of patient-targeted lectures and group discussions on common health problems. These are informative and also provide more opportunities for patient engagement and potential improvements in adherence.

On a global scale, free clinics provide essential services to underserved areas. The focus on many of these initiatives is not only to assist in the treatment of patients but also to help train local providers in dermatological management. Emphasis is often on providing care in resource-poor areas, with a reliance on low cost and easily accessible treatments and diagnostic modalities. For hair and skin specifically at both the community and global level, education is often the most important factor. It may not be perfect as the use of low-tension hairstyles and natural skin and hair products is easy to recommend but will likely have some resistance based on cultural norms in the region.

Health Education Approaches

Professional health programs are continuously seeking to improve competence of the future generation of doctors, nurses, and healthcare providers. Cultural education is common, both to acquaint students to each other and to the patients

that they will be providing care for. Similar to provider education, small group discussion and patient interaction can aid in improving knowledge and competence. A focus on education at the start of these health programs will hopefully have far-reaching future implications which make care more accessible for all individuals.

In medical and residency training, often efforts are made to provide a diverse educational experience to their trainees. This may include rotations through different health systems and in areas with different ethnic populations. Aside from improved competence in diagnosing diseases across a spectrum of skin tones, this serves to emphasize the differences in prescribing and obtaining medications that exist in different areas.

Additional Considerations for Vulnerable Populations

Throughout history many groups have been subjected to marginalization by society resulting from a difference in personal ideology, lifestyle, or simply due to indifference within the communities that they reside. Accordingly, these patients have a more difficult time accessing healthcare and often face discriminatory practices when they do seek care. Health workers should recognize that these barriers still remain and that they can play a role in providing a safe and welcoming environment. The remainder of the chapter will briefly touch on several additional vulnerable populations as well as successful interventions that have been utilized to improve care.

Gender Identity

It has been estimated that approximately 5–10% of the population identifies as lesbian, gay, bisexual, transgender, or queer (LGBTQ). This is not a comprehensive list, and individuals identify in many ways beyond this. Social stigmatization has been persistent for individuals of these groups throughout history, which has unfortunately also involved the healthcare community. Although social and legal progress is being made, disparities in care remain. Higher rates of certain malignancies and sexually transmitted infections such as HIV and syphilis are seen in men who have sex with men (MSM) [25]. This may be from discomfort seeking care or failure to disclose sexual identity to clinicians, resulting in missed opportunities for prevention, screening, and education [26]. Youth who identify at LGBTQ are particularly hesitant on disclosing this information and are also more likely to engage in high-risk sexual behaviors and illicit drug use [27].

Rates of mental health issues such as depression, anxiety, and suicidal ideology are increased in individuals identifying as LGBTQ [28]. Resources such as counseling and mental health support may be available but are often underutilized. Advertising mental health, preventative care, and screening services to LGBTQ individuals may help lower the stigma of seeking care. Providers being competent and comfortable discussing personal and medical concerns with patients is also important. Addressing this through educational interventions aimed at improving provider knowledge helps [29]. Being cognizant that these patients face unique health challenges and risks is important. Appropriate patient education and disease prevention strategies can be discussed, in addition to informing what other medical or legal resources may be available.

A dermatologist understanding of LGBTQ-related health concerns is important, as skin and hair problems often create additional distress. For instance, transgender patients undergoing hormonal therapy will often experience changes in patterns of hair distribution [30]. Similar anxiety-provoking changes are seen in the skin of these individuals. Useful provider knowledge would include which hormonal therapies are used, what physical changes are expected, and what new skin and hair conditions may arise. Cosmetic therapies such as hair removal may be sought out in some instances, and in these cases realistic expectations and treatment options can be addressed.

Physical and Intellectual Limitations and Disabilities

The description of a disability extends far beyond those which are intellectual in origin. Physical limitations such as decreased visual acuity, deafness, and difficulty ambulating all impart barriers to care. Healthcare is difficult to navigate for an able-bodied individual, and patients with these impairments are at heightened risk for underutilization of health services [31]. Within dermatology, poor vision makes daily tasks such as personal hygiene more difficult, and these patients may be at higher risk for infection and injury. Those with low vision are also less likely to be aware of potential new skin lesions that may arise. Moreover, understanding care instructions is more difficult. Similar comprehension dilemmas face patients who have difficulty hearing. Having the patient attend healthcare visits with a family member or friend may improve adherence and minimize risks of medication misuse. Reasonable accommodations should also be made by the provider: larger font sizes and simplified instructions may improve some visual limitations, and written instructions will likely aid the hearing impaired.

For patients who have difficulty ambulating or are completely bedbound, care often must be modified. Often patients must actively seek in-house healthcare delivery, which may reduce the incidence of preventative screenings and nonurgent medical consultations. For patients who are not completely immobile but still have some difficulty, similar physical barriers to accessing healthcare persist. Facilities equipped for patients with disabilities are mandatory in most areas; however, reasonable accommodations can be made in these instances irrespective of legal requirement.

Intellectually disabled patients often have additional health concerns which require attention. In many cases, rates of malignancy and other systemic and cutaneous manifestations occur at higher rates [32]. While there is a wide range of intellectual disability, patients are at a disadvantage resulting from a lack of comprehension and often decision-making capacity. Consenting for invasive procedures and treatment plans may be left to guardians and patient advocates, which results in additional barriers to care. Provider competence for the intellectually disabled could include knowledge about common conditions causing disability, as well as methods to effectively communicate. Screening and preventative care will change when known associations exist, therapies with known systemic side effects may have to be modified. Moreover, the risks of abuse are increased in these patients and should be reported if suspected.

The Aging and Elderly

Eleven percent of the world's population is greater than 60 years old – a number projected to increase to over 20% by 2050 [33]. As individuals age, there is an increased need for medical services. There is also a gradual (or sometimes abrupt) decline in functional capacity in the aged, and assistance is often required to complete activities of daily living (ADLs) as well as more complex tasks. Moreover, this decline renders patients more susceptible to abuse from family members and caretakers. Including physical abuse, elder abuse can also include financial and emotional abuse as well as neglect. Over 15 million Americans require some form of long-term care [34]. Often these patients suffer from forms of neurodegenerative disorders which increases their susceptibility further.

Competence in providing care for the elderly requires a multifactorial approach. Physiologic differences in elderly patients render some forms of medication or therapy too toxic or nonfeasible, necessitating modification in care. If suspected, concerns for elder abuse and neglect can be referred to the appropriate agencies. Financial constraints are also common in elderly patients who often have fixed sources of income. The healthcare industry is rapidly becoming unaffordable and even with insurance coverage patients are often unable to fill prescriptions and undergo testing as a result of high copays. Discussing these costs with the patient will enable the creation of a joint care plan. Finally,

access to care changes when patients age as it becomes more difficult to visit healthcare providers. Insurance companies may offer at-home services for some individuals, but this often does not include specialty care and more invasive diagnostic testing. Furthermore, uninsured patients do not have access to these forms of healthcare yet suffer from similar (if not more) health ailments.

Incarcerated Patients

By law, individuals who are incarcerated irrespective of reason are still provided access to medical services. Despite this requirement, disparities in facilities and health outcomes are prominent [35]. Furthermore, health risks are actually increased with release from prison, as lack of discharge planning and healthcare often leaves these individuals unable to afford or access health services [36]. This population is already vulnerable, irrespective of the fact that a disproportionate number of incarcerated individuals identify as an ethnic minority group [36]. Medical competence for common medical and environmental risk factors for patients who are incarcerated may help improve care. Moreover, these patients are often accompanied by security personnel, and it may be difficult to develop rapport or discuss sensitive information. Efforts can be made to ensure the patient of the confidential nature of the encounter. Bias and cultural sensitivity training may also be encouraged in providers interacting with incarcerated patients, to ensure consistent and unbiased medical care.

Homeless, Immigrant, and Refugee Patients

Homeless patients often suffer from a wide range of untreated medical conditions. Importantly, increased rates of psychological disorders and toxic habits exist within this group of individuals which may further hinder ability to access and maintain care [37, 38]. Seeking care is often delayed due to lack of insurance and inability to pay, causing patients to present later with more advanced disease [39]. Resultantly, these patients have higher mortality rates than the general population [40]. Access to care does exist; however, it is extremely limited and often locational dependent. Urban areas see higher rates of homelessness but also generally have a larger network of hospitals that can provide access to free care. Providers can be cognizant of the disparities that homeless patients experience and provide information about available resources including and beyond access to care. With the recognition that follow-up is often more difficult in homeless patients, simplified treatment plans that do not require extensive monitoring may produce better results. Similarly, free or low-cost medications may remove the financial barrier to treatment.

Refugee and immigrant patients face a unique set of obstacles as well, particularly when they are residing in a region without documentation. The "health paradox" described with these individuals is that they often arrive in the United States with better overall health than the native population but quickly revert to similar health levels after arriving [41]. These patients are up to four times more likely to live in crowded housing than native counterparts and often have many untreated medical comorbidities [42]. Moreover, distrust of public health services by undocumented individuals may reduce healthcare usage out of fear of deportation [43]. Competence within these groups of individuals can stress the confidential nature of the healthcare visit and consider other health concerns that may arise when cultural differences exist. In addition, communication barriers are often present and should be addressed when possible.

Conclusion

A general understanding of cultural values and practices of our patients is a key element in dermatology and healthcare in general. There are fundamental differences in healthcare access and delivery between different regions of the world. Similar differences occur within the diverse American population, and discrepancies in healthcare lead to preventable adverse outcomes. An attempt to improve one's own cultural competence may have long-standing positive implications for ourselves and our patients.

Citations

1. Pandya AG, Alexis AF, Berger TG, Wintroub BU. Increasing racial and ethnic diversity in dermatology: a call to action. J Am Acad Dermatol. 2016;74(3):584–7.
2. Napoles-Springer AM, Santoyo J, Houston K, Perez-Stable EJ, Stewart AL. Patients' perceptions of cultural factors affecting the quality of their medical encounters. Health Expect. 2005;8(1):4–17.
3. McKesey J, Berger TG, Lim HW, McMichael AJ, Torres A, Pandya AG. Cultural competence for the 21st century dermatologist practicing in the United States. J Am Acad Dermatol. 2017;77(6):1159–69.
4. Green AR, Carney DR, Pallin DJ, Ngo LH, Raymond KL, Iezzoni LI, et al. Implicit bias among physicians and its prediction of thrombolysis decisions for black and white patients. J Gen Intern Med. 2007;22(9):1231–8.
5. Fung FY, Linn YC. Developing traditional chinese medicine in the era of evidence-based medicine: current evidences and challenges. Evid Based Complement Alternat Med. 2015;2015:425037.
6. Koenig HG. Religion, spirituality, and health: the research and clinical implications. ISRN Psychiatry. 2012;2012:278730.
7. Starfield B, Shi L, Macinko J. Contribution of primary care to health systems and health. Milbank Q. 2005;83(3):457–502.
8. Egede LE. Race, ethnicity, culture, and disparities in health care. J Gen Intern Med. 2006;21(6):667–9.
9. Shi L, Macinko J, Starfield B, Politzer R, Wulu J, Xu J. Primary care, social inequalities and all-cause, heart disease and cancer mortality in US counties: a comparison between urban and non-urban areas. Public Health. 2005;119(8):699–710.
10. Taber JM, Leyva B, Persoskie A. Why do people avoid medical care? A qualitative study using national data. J Gen Intern Med. 2015;30(3):290–7.
11. Steen AJ, Mann JA, Carlberg VM, Kimball AB, Musty MJ, Simpson EL. Understanding the cost of dermatologic care: a survey study of dermatology providers, residents, and patients. J Am Acad Dermatol. 2017;76(4):609–17.
12. Kirby JB, Kaneda T. Unhealthy and uninsured: exploring racial differences in health and health insurance coverage using a life table approach. Demography. 2010;47(4):1035–51.
13. van Doorslaer E, Koolman X, Jones AM. Explaining income-related inequalities in doctor utilisation in Europe. Health Econ. 2004;13(7):629–47.
14. Hu S, Parmet Y, Allen G, Parker DF, Ma F, Rouhani P, et al. Disparity in melanoma: a trend analysis of melanoma incidence and stage at diagnosis among whites, Hispanics, and blacks in Florida. Arch Dermatol. 2009;145(12):1369–74.

15. Gonzalez HM, Vega WA, Tarraf W. Health care quality perceptions among foreign-born Latinos and the importance of speaking the same language. J Am Board Fam Med. 2010;23(6):745–52.

16. Karliner LS, Jacobs EA, Chen AH, Mutha S. Do professional interpreters improve clinical care for patients with limited English proficiency? A systematic review of the literature. Health Serv Res. 2007;42(2):727–54.

17. Locatis C, Williamson D, Gould-Kabler C, Zone-Smith L, Detzler I, Roberson J, et al. Comparing in-person, video, and telephonic medical interpretation. J Gen Intern Med. 2010;25(4):345–50.

18. Wilson E, Chen AH, Grumbach K, Wang F, Fernandez A. Effects of limited English proficiency and physician language on health care comprehension. J Gen Intern Med. 2005;20(9):800–6.

19. Ingersoll KS, Cohen J. The impact of medication regimen factors on adherence to chronic treatment: a review of literature. J Behav Med. 2008;31(3):213–24.

20. Lacy NL, Paulman A, Reuter MD, Lovejoy B. Why we don't come: patient perceptions on no-shows. Ann Fam Med. 2004;2(6):541–5.

21. Street RL Jr, O'Malley KJ, Cooper LA, Haidet P. Understanding concordance in patient-physician relationships: personal and ethnic dimensions of shared identity. Ann Fam Med. 2008;6(3):198–205.

22. Callender VD, Alexis AF, Daniels SR, Kawata AK, Burk CT, Wilcox TK, et al. Racial differences in clinical characteristics, perceptions and behaviors, and psychosocial impact of adult female acne. J Clin Aesthet Dermatol. 2014;7(7):19–31.

23. Bass AM, Anderson KL, Feldman SR. Interventions to increase treatment adherence in pediatric atopic dermatitis: a systematic review. J Clin Med. 2015;4(2):231–42.

24. Jacobsen AA, Galvan A, Lachapelle CC, Wohl CB, Kirsner RS, Strasswimmer J. Defining the need for skin cancer prevention education in uninsured, minority, and immigrant communities. JAMA Dermatol. 2016;152(12):1342–7.

25. Hafeez H, Zeshan M, Tahir MA, Jahan N, Naveed S. Health care disparities among lesbian, gay, bisexual, and transgender youth: a literature review. Cureus. 2017;9(4):e1184.

26. East JA, El Rayess F. Pediatricians' approach to the health care of lesbian, gay, and bisexual youth. J Adolesc Health. 1998;23(4):191–3.

27. Mayer KH, Garofalo R, Makadon HJ. Promoting the successful development of sexual and gender minority youths. Am J Public Health. 2014;104(6):976–81.

28. Safren SA, Heimberg RG. Depression, hopelessness, suicidality, and related factors in sexual minority and heterosexual adolescents. J Consult Clin Psychol. 1999;67(6):859–66.

29. Felsenstein DR. Enhancing lesbian, gay, bisexual, and transgender cultural competence in a Midwestern primary care clinic setting. J Nurses Prof Dev. 2018;34(3):142–50.

30. Gao Y, Maurer T, Mirmirani P. Understanding and addressing hair disorders in transgender individuals. Am J Clin Dermatol. 2018;19(4):517–27.

31. Sakellariou D, Rotarou ES. Access to healthcare for men and women with disabilities in the UK: secondary analysis of cross-sectional data. BMJ Open. 2017;7(8):e016614.

32. Cooper SA, McLean G, Guthrie B, McConnachie A, Mercer S, Sullivan F, et al. Multiple physical and mental health comorbidity in adults with intellectual disabilities: population-based cross-sectional analysis. BMC Fam Pract. 2015;16:110.

33. Kanasi E, Ayilavarapu S, Jones J. The aging population: demographics and the biology of aging. Periodontol 2000. 2016;72(1):13–8.

34. Holt JD. Navigating long-term care. Gerontol Geriatr Med. 2017;3:2333721417700368.

35. Wilper AP, Woolhandler S, Boyd JW, Lasser KE, McCormick D, Bor DH, et al. The health and health care of US prisoners: results of a nationwide survey. Am J Public Health. 2009;99(4):666–72.

36. Kulkarni SP, Baldwin S, Lightstone AS, Gelberg L, Diamant AL. Is incarceration a contributor to health disparities? Access to care of formerly incarcerated adults. J Community Health. 2010;35(3):268–74.

37. North CS, Eyrich KM, Pollio DE, Spitznagel EL. Are rates of psychiatric disorders in the homeless population changing? Am J Public Health. 2004;94(1):103–8.

38. McCarty D, Argeriou M, Huebner RB, Lubran B. Alcoholism, drug abuse, and the homeless. Am Psychol. 1991;46(11):1139–48.

39. Baggett TP, O'Connell JJ, Singer DE, Rigotti NA. The unmet health care needs of homeless adults: a national study. Am J Public Health. 2010;100(7):1326–33.

40. Nusselder WJ, Slockers MT, Krol L, Slockers CT, Looman CW, van Beeck EF. Mortality and life expectancy in homeless men and women in Rotterdam: 2001–2010. PLoS One. 2013;8(10):e73979.

41. Goldman N, Pebley AR, Creighton MJ, Teruel GM, Rubalcava LN, Chung C. The consequences of migration to the United States for short-term changes in the health of Mexican immigrants. Demography. 2014;51(4):1159–73.

42. Landale NS, Thomas KJ, Van Hook J. The living arrangements of children of immigrants. Futur Child. 2011;21(1):43–70.

43. Hacker K, Anies M, Folb BL, Zallman L. Barriers to health care for undocumented immigrants: a literature review. Risk Manag Healthc Policy. 2015;8:175–83.

The Impact of Skin and Hair Disease in Ethnic Skin

Aldo Morrone

The Term "Ethnic"

Deciding to use the term "ethnic" in this chapter automatically meant removing the taboo surrounding its use, stepping up to and accepting the challenge, as well as highlighting the complexities and the problems that this term brings with it and beyond its use, conscious that this term represents a cognitive category constructed and manipulated and, therefore, ultimately an "invention" [1–3] but equally determined to put aside the idea of renouncing its use due to the "defective" and "subordinate" connotations it has assumed in the past Western intellectual tradition. This also implied avoiding inventing a new category, feeding the confusion and ambiguity that often hovers around the term itself [4, 5].

We do not want to therefore refer to the impact that skin and hair diseases have on "other" ethnicities using terms such as ethnomedicine, ethnopsychiatry and ethnodermatology but rather emphasize the interpretations of skin diseases from an individual's perspective, which is in fact rather impossible to do outside the environmental, anthropological and cultural contexts where they originate from. On the other hand, in scientific literature, the term ethnicity has been the subject of profound critical consideration, which has rightly stressed the casual and irresponsible use of terms such as ethnicity and ethnic by researchers and media outlets to explain everything relating to social and cultural dynamic of populations of the so-called developing countries or in any case "other" populations different from us. Time and time again, and way too often, it has been used to indicate the culture and traditions of "less-developed" people, in a sort of implicit distinction to the term "civilization": we will and would be a nation, a society, a culture, instead the "others" belong to an ethnic group, where the levels of society and culture are less differentiated and evolved. Moreover, an ethnic group is believed to be, in a certain sense, by nature non-compliant to history, thus designating a level closer to a sort of naturalization of the cultural constitution rather than to its historicized configuration, thus indicating a constitutive core of relative resistance to identity change.

This ethnic aspect does not only concern Western populations but all of us. This highlights how inevitable symbolic aspects of culture are largely and unconsciously ingrained in us and how it influences our behaviour in resisting somewhat changes and being noncompliant to them and, more generally, moulds us into feeling we belong to something, rather than something that belongs to us, something that recalls our sense of belonging to something not as an individual in question, but rather constantly to something we are embodied in one flesh. It is something

A. Morrone (✉)
San Gallicano Dermatological Institute IRCCS, Rome, Italy
e-mail: aldo.morrone@ifo.gov.it

© Springer Nature Switzerland AG 2021
B. S. Li, H. I. Maibach (eds.), *Ethnic Skin and Hair and Other Cultural Considerations*, Updates in Clinical Dermatology, https://doi.org/10.1007/978-3-030-64830-5_14

we are drawn, belong to, or participate in, almost independently from one individual's will [6–9].

Therefore, the title "The Impact of Skin and Hair Diseases in Ethnic Skin" aims to focus on cutaneous diseases of men and women belonging to all ethnic groups, that is, all "distinct human groups based on their geographical, linguistic and cultural characteristics", groupings and characteristics that obviously have one fluid, non-crystallized and dynamic nature, indicating people and realities engaged in continuous negotiation and reinterpretation [10, 11]. Alternatively, circumstances may sometimes force them to daily fragmentation and recomposition of their identity. fragments of cultures that tell each other stories every day, like a collage whose design is continually modified and reinterpreted. In regard to the first and second points, we must first refer to the use of the term *ethnos* employed by the ancient Greeks. This term was used as a political category that designated the following:

1. The Greek populations from the indistinct institutions, that is, "a form of a political social organization preceding and inferior to the *polis* [5]
2. The "barbarians", i.e. those who did not speak the Greek language [4]

In turn, by observing the use of the term, we see that from the second half of the nineteenth century, the term was created by some European scholars and theorists [12].

The century of enlightenment replaced the term "barbarian" with the word "savage", that is, an inhabitant of the forest, in order to distinguish it from the "citizen", an inhabitant of the city.

The term "ethnicity" was used ambiguously. On the one hand, it was employed as a synonym of race, nation and civilization and, on the other, as a result of a racial mixture [13–15]; the "ethnic group" was employed to express a homogeneous human grouping from a racial point of view which, following the lasting and close cohabitative relations with different races, was inclined to assimilate its language and culture [4, 5, 16]. When the idea of "nation" arose as "a closed group, defined by specific characteristics and

identified with a territory", a semantic distance resulted between the two terms and was associated with an alleged lack of political institutions, "civilized" figures and consciousness of self and of one's own destiny, particular to the concept of people's nation of the first term [4, 5].

Finally, immense approval acknowledged, in response to the administrative needs of the twentieth-century colonial policy, the ethnic model adopted by ethnology [17, 18], which defined "ethnicity" as an acephalous and segmented political-social body characterized by "complex balances of power among various institutions or social hierarchies" [5], endowed with a specific system of ideas, values and beliefs, from a fixed and immutable nature.

In regard to the third point, we must look at the affirmation of the ethnic revival aimed at rediscovering "authentic roots", preservation of a threatened culinary identity and together with the explosion of studies, cultural events (markets, food, musical and theatrical performances, photographic and pictorial exhibitions) and commercial services (supermarkets, clothing stores, restaurants, book stores) dedicated to the regional-local-suburban "diversity" and to the political movements narrating exasperated localisms, as well as to the political model of "multicultural" integration.

If these events, on the one hand, bear witness to an interest in celebrating the particularism of cultural differences, at times subdued acts of censure/condemnation of subcultural and subaltern status that are often attributed to them, on the other hand, they use these particularisms to reconfirm the superiority of Western and hegemonic systems of thought and social models, which nourish their presumed "originality" and "authenticity" to reproduce themselves and confirm an impenetrable cultural distance.

Charles Darwin

Charles Darwin, in 1871, in *The Descent of Man and Selection in Relation to Sex*, stated that the human species is only one, since "races all graduated into each other" [19]. Closer to our times, in

1950, just after the Nazi horror, UNESCO made a solemn declaration stating that races did not exist. Nonetheless, prejudices are hard to get rid of. Anyone seriously thinking about it would come to the inevitable conclusion that races obviously do not exist and that the different colours of human skin and the different physical characteristics are the result of adaptation occurring in the course of thousands, millions of years of the ecological and climatic geographical conditions our ancestors lived in.

The Classification of Man into Races

In the past, the scientific desire to bring order to human knowledge led a number of researchers to attempt a classification for human beings, as well as for the flora and fauna. One of the first to take the challenge was Carl von Linné, also known as Linnaeus (1707–1778). In 1758, Linnaeus scientifically classified populations of the various continents, underlining their characteristics and differences [20]. Since the order of primates Linnaeus had invented listed a number of varieties, including the *Homo* variety we belong to, and since the *Homo* category, Linnaeus reckoned, would include two sub-varieties, the *Homo sapiens* (us) and the *Homo nocturnus* (chimpanzees), how many sub-varieties should the *Homo sapiens* species needed to include?

The naturalist decided that there should be five: *Homo sapiens monstrosus*, which collected more or less abnormal people, and four "geographical" types:

- *Homo sapiens americanus*
- *Homo sapiens europaeus*
- *Homo sapiens asiaticus*
- *Homo sapiens afer*

Being an objective scientist, Linnaeus claimed to classify human groups by applying the same rules used for any other species. We must admit that the characteristics defined by Linnaeus to distinguish geographical subspecies were ridiculous generalizations, if not mere slander, and generally completely unrelated to whatever bio-

logical trait. In that way, the *Homo sapiens americanus* is tenacious, happy, free, red, impassive and has a bad temper; the *Homo europaeus* is sporty, lively and full of inventiveness; the *Homo asiaticus* is austere, proud and mean; and the *Homo afer* is smart, slow and negligent. Linnaeus also describes clothing and the system of government: Americans paint themselves, Europeans wear tight-fitting clothes, Asians wear large garments, and Africans smear their bodies with fat. Linnaeus was obviously influenced by the time he lived in, especially in considering the Europeans greater than any other people. However, it is precisely at that time that the idea of a division in four basic human types becomes a "scientific" theory. The generation of scientists that came immediately after Linnaeus abandoned clothing as a taxonomic criterion.

It was not until the mid-twentieth century that certain scientists started to question the empirical basis of the continental-scale generalization of the human species. Today we know that the eighteenth-century subspecies are neither clear fundamental divisions of our species nor biological subdivisions. This is the main illusion introduced by Linnaeus: the scientific legitimacy of a division of men into a small number of distinct groups, apparently homogeneous.

However, though his correlation between physical and mental aspects was arbitrary, and with a clear racist connotation already, Linnaeus never used the term "race", to which he preferred the word "variety".

The first scientist to propose a classification of mankind based on the colour of skin and other visible external characters was Johann Friedrich Blumenbach (1752–1840), who today is considered the founder of anthropology. He distinguished five "varieties":

1. Caucasian (fair skin, brown hair, with non-protruding molars bones, narrow, curved and very high nose, a full-shaped, round chin), which settled in Europe – except in Lapland and in the Finnish region – in western Asia, as far as the Ganges river and in Northern Africa
2. Mongolian (yellow-brown skin, dark hair, flattened nose, narrow eyelid opening which

curves in the inner eye corner), which settled in Asian territories not occupied by Europeans and which also included the Finns, the Lapps and the Inuit people

3. Ethiopian (dark skin, woolly hair, with the lower face being narrow and protruding), which included all the peoples of Africa except those in the northern part of the continent

4. American (having copper-coloured skin, dark hair), which included all the inhabitants of the two Americas, except the Inuit

5. Malaysian (dark brown skin, curly hair, with a full nose and large chin), which included all the people living in the Pacific Islands

Noteworthily, Blumenbach prefers the term "variety". He softens the rigidity of the classification, underlining that it is impossible to draw a clear divider between skin colours and that there is no human variety characterized by a colour and other external physical traits so well defined that they cannot be significantly connected to other races. Other authors, instead, tried to prove that physical differences matched specific mental qualities [21].

The Ambiguity of the Term *Caucasian*

Later on, the term "Caucasian" was used to identify people with white skin. The word eventually became the medical term for generically defining the whites. However, we must be aware of the fact that there are Caucasian people who are not white at all – indeed, there is quite a distance between Ireland and the Panjab or the borders of Ethiopia to justify changes to skin colour among Caucasians. In 1799, Cuvier (1769–1832) had already brought up the topic of the *Falashas,* or Ethiopian Jews, and the debate has been on ever since [22]. As a matter of fact, all human "races" have populations whose skin is less or more pigmented. Dermatologists are so busy reminding everyone of the importance of skin phototypes that they miss the fact that the people who live in areas with intense ultraviolet radiation, like in the

Tibet Plateau or in South America, don't necessarily have their skin more pigmented. Conversely, someone living in the Punjab or in Balochistan may be Caucasian yet not necessarily have highly pigmented skin. Rather than race, we should therefore speak of human "clines". A "cline", as defined by the Oxford English Dictionary "is a gradual series of characters and differences that form within a species." Caucasians could be a "cline" of human beings who are genetically very close yet show different shades of pigmentation. Asians form another cline, Africans as well, and so on – scientists should have the task of working out how many clines can be identified.

When we use the term "Caucasian", we should be aware of the historical origin of this term, of the fact that it is a misnomer, of the time when it entered scientific literature and what we may understand it to mean (and what not) today [23, 24].

Colours and Migrations

Today, a number of scientists and, especially, the vast majority of the general public still consider skin colour as the most obvious evidence of the existence of human races. Even the colour and shape of the eyes and hair are seen as valid conditions that support the existence of a white race, a dark one, a yellow one, and so on. Many people still believe in the existence of races, despite the results of modern genetic, anthropology and molecular biology studies that confirm that under our skin we are biologically identical and that the concept of race is too unstable and indefinable to allow to build a scientific theory on it [25].

Geneticist Cavalli-Sforza underlined that the differences that impressed our ancestors and that continue to bother many people today include skin colour, eye shape, hair type, body and facial form – in short, the traits that often allow us to determine a person's origin in a single glance. Apparently, it is fairly easy to recognize a European, an African, an Asian. Many of these features are fairly homogeneous in a particular continent and can give us the impression that "pure" races exist and thus that the differences between races are pronounced. These traits are, at least partly, genetically determined. Skin colour and body size are less subject to genetic influence because they are also determined by sun exposure and diet. These differences form our beliefs to a major extent, because we can actually spot them out easily, and what you see is what you believe. Yet these differences are nearly all due to the great variety of environment and climates man has encountered while expanding throughout the entire world, starting from the world region we all originate from, Africa.

The expansion of the anatomically modern humans (AMH) from Africa to the other four continents led to the need to adapt to ecological conditions, especially climatic, which were very different from those of the original continent, except for Australia and other tropical regions. Adaptation, however, turned out to be both cultural and biological through the long period of time since then – about 50–60,000 years – and this led to the development of a truly genetic differentiation.

We can see clear traces of this differentiation exactly in the skin, eye and hair colour and in the size and shape of the nose and the body in general. Anthropologists have shown that differences among ethnic group have been genetically engineered under the influence of climate and diet [26].

Anthropology of Skin Colours

Today we know that race, which however we've shown earlier doesn't even exist, does not determine the colour of skin, just as skin colour does not define races. We can clearly state that there is no "Caucasian race", as there is no "dark race", and that the skin colour of an individual is given by the "interaction of several biological, genetic, environmental and cultural factors". One must also bear in mind that "dark skin" is not actually dark, that "white skin" is not really white and,

obviously enough, there is no such thing as "yellow skin". As a matter of fact, the different colours of skin are due to the variations in the red colour spectrum [27, 28].

Among all primates, only humans possess a skin that is almost completely hairless and that may take different hues. Today, many researchers agree that the different skin colours available in people around the world are not at all randomly determined but given by evolutionary processes of adaptation. In fact, people with darker skin tend to concentrate near the equator, while fair skin is found closer to the poles. It has long been believed that dark skin had evolved as such to protect against skin cancer, but recent observations offer a new interpretation of human pigmentation. Bio-anthropological and epidemiological data indicate that the worldwide distribution of human skin colour is due to natural selection acting to regulate the effects of ultraviolet radiation on certain nutrients essential for the reproductive process of human beings: *folates* and *vitamin D* [29]. Human pigmentation worldwide has evolved in a way that skin could be dark enough to prevent sunlight from destroying folates yet fair enough to trigger the production of vitamin D.

The evolution of skin pigmentation is connected to the progressive reduction of hair over skin. Humans have been evolving independently of apes for at least 7 million years, ever since our closest ancestors yielded from their closest relatives, chimpanzees, which instead over time have changed very little compared to man.

The skin of chimpanzees is clear and covered with thick hair. Younger individuals have pinkish face, hands and feet, which become darker over the years only due to prolonged sun exposure.

Also primitive humans almost certainly had fair skin covered by hair. Presumably, the loss of hair was an early event, whereas the colour of the skin changed only at a later stage.

But when did we actually lose most of the hair that covered our body for good, and how did it happen?

Lice: Best Friends with Skin

Studying lice has allowed us to understand why humans have lost their hair. In 2003, Mark Pagel, University of Reading, UK, and Walter Bodmer, of the John Radcliffe Hospital in Oxford [30], suggested that humans lost their protective covering to get rid of lice and other parasites that naturally thrive in mammalian fur; thus, the process of losing hair was triggered by the need to show we had healthy skin. According to the two scientists, this new theory explains why man is mostly hairless, unlike our closest relatives, apes. The hypothesis generally accepted so far stated that fur loss was an evolutionary process to allow man to control body temperature in hot weather. Instead, Pagel and Bodmer argue that man has lost his hair to get rid of insects and other parasites and, thereby, to increase their sexual attractiveness. Indeed, the body-heat-regulating theory has some issues related to situations where it is very hot or very cold. The two scientists point out that for a mammal to rid itself of its fur and its unwanted passengers, it must devise a better way of regulating body temperature. That, say the two scientists, is just what humans did when they harnessed fire and started wearing clothes, which, unlike fur, can be changed and laundered, making them far less parasite friendly. In an article published in the journal *Biology Letters*, Pagel and Bodmer say that their hypothesis better explains the differences between men and women. Loss of hair, in their opinion, allowed humans to more convincingly show their reduced susceptibility to parasite infections. The no-hair feature thus became a desirable trait in a mate, and women having less body hair than men could be due to the greater sexual selection that is conventionally exerted by men on women. It is therefore reasonable to expect that humans who evolved in regions with higher concentrations of disease-carrying parasites, such as tropical areas, have less body hair than people inhabiting other areas. Other research work has instead focused on body and head lice to figure out when our ancestors began to cover themselves with clothing. Although they feed on blood, body lice live in clothing. Consequently, their origin in time provides a decent estimate for when men started wearing clothes. Comparing the sequences of genes in organisms indeed allows to trace the origin of species. This research has shown that head lice have plagued humans since the beginning, while body lice evolved much later. The moment body lice appeared seems to suggest that human beings wandered around naked, though not entirely, for over a million years.

Multigenic Hypothesis for Human Pigmentation

The multigenic hypothesis for human pigmentation is confirmed by the evidence that the "dark" colour is not dominant in nature. The descendant of a mixed family often shows a significant change in skin colour, and pigmentation can also vary during the life of the individual due to the decrease in the number of active DOPA-positive melanocytes that accompany ageing.

Pigmentation in mammals is genetically determined, since genes act at different levels in the formation and distribution of the pigment granules.

The different populations around the planet show a broad variety of colours, from the dark skin in Western Africa and Southern India inhabitants to the olive-coloured skin of Pakistan people and the pale white of populations in the northern areas of the world [29].

Skin Colour Evolution

We ought to point out the fact that the "dark skin" is not dark, just as the "white skin" is not really white. In fact the different colours of the skin rather represent variations in the red spectrum. The colour of human skin is a subjective phenomenon influenced by the interaction of diverse factors such as the size, aggregation and diffusion of melanosomes; the dynamic state of cutaneous circulation which increases or decreases the amount of oxyhaemoglobin; the presence of biochemical substances or therapeutic agents such as haemosiderin or carotenoids; and certain pathological states of the epidermis or skin surface which alter skin colour.

Pigmentation in mammals is genetically defined, because genetic expression at different levels can lead to the formation and distribution of skin pigmentation.

A wide range of skin shades exists among different populations, from a deep dark in West Africa and Southern India to the olive colour in Pakistan to the pale white of northern people. In darks the pigment granules are large, and each one is surrounded by a membrane, while in Caucasians melanosomes are smaller and grouped in multiple units. The skin of Mongolians shows characteristics between the two extremes. Certain pathological states of the epidermis or skin surface can alter skin colour [31]. And so the question arises: are there differences between dark and white skin?

In the past, many authors were compelled to write texts on dermatology concerning the differences between skin diseases in white and dark patients. Some authors questioned whether these publications had any scientific basis. To account for dermatological problems in dark skin, one must investigate diseases which affect only dark skin and skin structures which differ from those in white skin. The study of scientific literature on this topic has revealed that there are few data which actually demonstrate peculiarities typical of dark skin.

Contrary to the past, when apparently ethnic-related illnesses were used to justify racist ideologies, today we can no longer do so. Other factors are more important than race in the incidence of certain diseases, including those affecting the skin, such as genetic, environmental, ecological, economic, social, nutritional, cultural and professional factors, especially the availability of adequate medical services and the possibility of receiving a correct diagnosis as well as appropriate and immediate treatment.

Taylor [29] noted that there is not a wealth of data on racial and ethnic differences in skin and hair structure, physiology and function. The studies that do exist involve small patient populations and often have methodologic flaws. Consequently, few definitive conclusions can be made.

All skin conditions seen in white skin are also found in darker skin; skin conditions exclusive to dark skin do not exist, so the treatment and diagnosis for both are essentially the same. However, it is evident that the doctor or medical worker must pay particular attention to how the same condition may look different in dark or white skin or how the same pathological process may provoke different reactions. In fact, many reactions in dark skin may be accentuated or else may not be so apparent, making diagnostic and therapeutic approaches necessarily different.

The structures of human populations are extremely complex and vary from region to region, from group to group; there are always shades of difference, due to continuous migration within and across the borders of all nations which make clear separations impossible.

The principal structures and functions of the skin are described in detail below, with the aim of detecting possible differences between dark and white skin.

Physiology of Skin Colour

The history of pigmentation biology requires the knowledge of the integration of evolution, genetics and developmental biology. The main factor affecting the skin colour primarily is the functions of melanocytes, the cells specialized in the synthesis and distribution of the melanin pigment. Melanocyte is connected through its dendrites with approximately 30~40 keratinocytes, establishing the so-called epidermal melanin unit. They are also connected to fibroblasts in the underlying dermis. Melanin synthesis occurs in specialized membrane-bound organelles of the melanocytes, termed melanosomes. Specific enzymatic apparatus, provided by tyrosinase and tyrosinase-related ones, directs the production of two melanins: dark-brown eumelanins, the major pigment found in dark skin and hair, and yellow/red pheomelanin, mainly observed in red hair and I/II skin phototypes. The number of melanocytes is very similar in skin of different colour, whereas this difference depends on the type (the relative quantity of pheo- and eumelanins) and the amount of melanin produced within melanosomes.

In light skin, melanosomes are smaller, mainly at an early stage of maturation (stages I and II), and transferred to keratinocytes as clusters. In dark skin, they are larger, at stage IV, and singly transferred to the surrounding cells. Their degradation appears also slower than that in the light skin. Finally, the pheomelanin-eumelanin ratio appears higher in dark versus light skins.

Thus the differences that can be observed among individuals are not racial but related to other factors, which we can list as follows:

1. Genetic factors
2. Adaptation to ecological conditions
3. Adaptation to climatic conditions
4. Access to education

As regards the genetic factors, a large number of novel loci have been recently discovered through several different large-scale genome-wide association studies. The polymorphisms within these pigmentation genes appear at different population frequencies and provide insight into the evolutionary selective forces that have acted to create this human diversity.

However, the genetics of pigmentation is complex: Melanocortin 1 receptor (Mc1R), a G protein-coupled receptor that regulates the quantity and quality of melanins, was the first gene identified in humans. Overall, "normal" pigmentation is regulated by 4250 genes (as per the latest count), and they function during the development, migration, survival, proliferation and differentiation of melanocytes and their precursors (melanoblasts). A relevant pigmentation pathway is that of the pro-opiomelanocortin (POMC)-derived peptides, mainly represented by melanocyte-stimulating hormone (MSH). Finally, melanocyte functionality and skin pigmentation are regulated by extracellular matrix (ECM) proteins and fibroblasts of the dermal compartment, which release many soluble factors able to modulate melanocyte activity, including stem cell factor (SCF) and hepatocyte growth factor (HGF) also released by keratinocytes.

A further pathway of pigmentation regulation is provided by the link between α-MSH and the peroxisome proliferator-activated receptor (PPAR)-γ in melanocytes [32, 33].

A dark skin colour protects those who live near the equator from ultraviolet radiation, which can cause skin cancer [26].

If we go beyond the analysis of the mere visible features, we comprehend how absurd it is to believe that there may be relatively "pure" races. In the past, we did not have the knowledge that to achieve "purity", that is genetic homogeneity (which in any case would never be to a full extent in higher animals), you should have very close relatives such as siblings or parents and their children mate over several generations (at least 20). This would obviously have very negative consequences on the fertility and health of the offspring, and this probably tells us why inbreeding has never occurred in human history, except for short periods and in very particular conditions like in some Egyptian or Persian dynasties. Hence, purity of race doesn't exist, is impossible to achieve and is totally undesirable [34].

Epidermis

There are conflicting data regarding ethnic differentials in stratum corneum structure. Taylor, in 2002, stressed that many of the studies reported in the literature have small patient populations and less-than-optimal study designs. Consequently, definitive conclusions cannot be made, and further researches are warranted [29].

Weigand et al. in 1974 [35] investigated the cell layers and density of the stratum corneum in dark- and light-skinned subjects, as measured by the number of tape strips necessary to completely remove the stratum corneum layer, microscopic observation and measurement of air density in the stratum corneum. In fair-skinned subjects, 6 to 15 tape strips (mean 10.3) were required to completely remove the stratum corneum compared with 8 to 25 strips (mean 16.6 strips) in dark subjects. The mean difference between the groups was significant. Microscopic visualization also demonstrated ethnic differences in the stratum corneum. Since the average stratum corneum thickness was found to be similar between the 2 ethnic groups, it was concluded that stratum corneum was more compact that the white one, possibly reflecting a greater intercellular cohesion.

Corcuff et al. [36] examined corneocyte surface area, mean surface area and spontaneous desquamation in African Americans, white Americans and Asian of Chinese extraction (18 to 25 subjects per group). There was no difference in corneocyte surface area between all three ethnic groups and no difference in spontaneous corneocyte desquamation between the Chinese and white groups. However, spontaneous desquamation was 2.5 times more significant in the dark group compared with the white and Asian groups. These data appear contradictory to Weigand's findings. More in-depth studies are required to explain this apparent contradiction between more frequent skin shedding and better cohesion. Some experimental studies suggest that the epidermis of darker subjects has a slightly higher epidermal lipid content, which could explain the better intracellular cohesion.

The melanocyte system, as above-mentioned, is responsible for skin pigmentation and hence for the colour it acquires. The main biological difference between dark and white skin is that the former has a particular capacity for producing and distributing melanin. There are no racial differences in the number of cells which produce melanin: in fact, all skin types have an equal number of melanocytes per square unit of surface area, but their structure is different [37, 38].

Melanin pigment in darks is constantly present in the upper part of the derma, while in whites it is rarely seen [39, 40]. Human skin colour is often modified according to sex. Women are generally slightly lighter coloured than men. Colorimetric and spectrophotometric studies show that this difference could lie in the different concentrations of haemoglobin and melanin. In whites, this is predominantly caused by a difference in haemoglobin levels. In Asians (Vietnamese and Chinese) both haemoglobin and melanin are involved, while in darks the difference resides only in melanin concentrations. The melanin concentration in the stratum corneum could also be responsible for the relatively dry appearance of dark skin, with a finer and more visible shedding process since the flakes are lighter than the background skin.

Melanin is an unstable molecule with numerous physical and chemical properties. Eumelanin also acts a scavenger of free radicals (superoxide anions, hydrogen peroxide) which are formed during photobiochemical processes [41].

Dark skin contains a larger quantity of melanin granules which are distributed by keratinocytes in the epidermis. Numerous melanosomes dispersed throughout the cells of the epidermis offer considerable protection against harmful ultraviolet radiation. Differences in the activities of melanocytes, in skin colour and the ability to resist excessive exposure to ultraviolet rays seem therefore to be under the control of genetics.

Dermis

Dark-skinned people are subject to massively disfiguring scarring, keloids and hypertrophic scarring. This phenomenon is even more common among groups from West Africa. It has also been observed that lichenification is more common in darker patients. It is surprising that recent research on collagen has not shown any differences in the role of fibroblasts in dark skin or in response to cytokines and the ability to produce collagen. It is probable that the ability of fibroblasts to replicate and produce collagen is genetically stimulated. The production of hypertrophic scarring and keloids is hereditary and not an ethnic or racial characteristic. We have observed numerous patients, both dark-skinned and white, who produce an abundance of collagen, with the formation of large keloids and hypertrophic scarring following episodes of nodulo-cystic acne, herpes zoster or even minimal surgical intervention. In dark subjects, in particular, skin biopsies should be performed with extreme care and avoiding, if possible, facial areas [42–44].

Eccrine Sweat Glands

The eccrine sweat glands are distributed all over the skin surface of humans, and the average person has two to three million of these. This significant variation in the number of glands seems to be due to environmental and individual adaptation rather than racial factors [45]. Kawahata and Sakamoto demonstrated that the total number of sweat glands per unit of skin surface for Japanese people born in Japan who subsequently migrated to tropical areas was the same as those who were born in Japan and remained there. However, parents and children born in the tropics have a significantly higher number of sweat glands [46].

This research implies that environmental factors such as climate, rather than racial background, are responsible for differences in numbers of eccrinal sweat glands. Some researchers have conjectured the existence of a relationship between skin pigmentation and higher levels of perspiration, due to the greater capacity of darker skin to absorb heat; however, there is no scientific evidence to confirm such a hypothesis. Other studies have suggested that there is no substantial difference between darks and whites. The quantity of perspiration produced at a given temperature is related to the level of acclimatization to heat, rather than anatomical or physiological characteristics related to race [47]. On the contrary, there are differences in perspiratory capacity between males and females [47, 48].

Apocrine Sweat Glands

The apocrine sweat glands are found over the entire body in all mammals with the exception of humans. They are absent or atrophied in humans everywhere except the armpits, inguinal, pubic, periumbilical, perianal and the external ear areas. There is observable variation between individuals in the distribution and size of apocrine glands, and these variations cannot be used to demonstrate racial superiority of any kind, as was attempted in the past.

In fact, some researchers observed that darks possess a higher number of apocrine glands, more diffusely distributed, than whites. These data were used to demonstrate that darks were more similar to other mammals than to whites.

The secretions of apocrine glands include iron, protein, glucides, ferric ions and ammonia ions. These substances, when subject to the action of gram-negative bacteria, are largely the cause of body odours, which people think are characteristic of different races, groups, genders and individuals. It is to be noted that they also play an important role in sexual attraction.

However, a person's body odour depends on eating, hygiene and cultural habits rather than racial and ethnic factors [49].

Sebaceous Glands

There are not many data on sebaceous gland secretion in darks, although some authors believe that their glands may be larger and more active than those of whites.

However, since gender and age can also influence sebaceous gland form and size, it is not possible to state whether true differences between whites and darks exist [49].

Hair and Nails

The difference between hair types for dark, white and Asian subjects lies in the cross section of the hair follicle. The cross section of white or Asian hair is round, and the hair strand is straight or rigid; in darks the cross section is elliptical or flattened, making the hair strand curly. The shape of the hair follicle determines the hair shape and cross section. The Negroid hair follicle, curved and helical, spiral shaped, explains the curliness of the hair. The Asian follicle is completely straight, while that of white people lies between the other two [50].

Curly hair is more fragile, breaks more easily and tends to spontaneously change. Structural analysis reveals weak cortical cell cohesion. The hairs on the rest of the body are weaker in darks, but baldness is rare. The chemical and physical properties of hair are exactly the same in darks and whites, confirming that the shape of hair is not related to a particular biochemical structure.

Four hair types exist: straight, wavy, helical and spiral (which appears as a flattened helix in cross section). In whites, hair type varies greatly, although hair is generally long, straight, wavy or curly.

In comparison to whites, dark subjects have less body hair per unit of surface area: the beard is quite sparse, and the thorax is less hirsute. Different hair types stem from genetic factors responsible for diversity in hair characteristics, particularly rate of growth.

The nails of darks and whites are identical, even though in the former linear pigmentation markings can be observed, which do not have any specific pathological meaning. However, significant differences can be found in nitrogen content, again without any apparent practical consequences [51].

Physiopathology of Pigmentation

It is important to be able to distinguish between what is physiological and pathological in dark skin.

Cutaneous Lines

Pigmentary demarcation lines are well-defined regions of sudden transition between contiguous areas, one of which is more deeply pigmented and the other less pigmented. The phenomenon was first described by Futcher who observed a colour demarcation on the flexor surface of the arm, whereas the medial area was lighter than the lateral surface [52]. However, Matsumoto was the first to describe this characteristic in detail. Other Japanese researchers reported this phenomenon, and Ito summarized this work and concluded that Futcher's line appeared in 4% of Japanese and was ten times more common in females than males [53].

Vollum observed this colour demarcation in 26% of Jamaican children between the ages of 1 and 11 years but, in contrast to the Japanese research, found no difference between males and females [54].

McDonald and Kelly observed that more than 50% of their patients exhibited this colour alteration bilaterally and less than 10% monolaterally. In monolateral cases they could find no correlation between this phenomenon and right- or left-handedness [55].

In our own experience, we have noted this line in about 30% of the adult darks we treated, while in children the frequency is 18%.

Forearm lines were observed in about 60% males and 70% females in McDonald and Kelly's cases, which often appeared to be continuations of Futcher's lines.

McDonald and Kelly observed thigh lines in about a quarter of their patients, about two-thirds of which were concurrent with Futcher's lines. These lines were generally located on the posteromedial surface of the thigh.

Cutaneous lines on the leg usually run from the popliteal region to halfway between the heel and the medial malleolus. In many cases they are an extension of lines on the thigh. All these lines are rarely seen in newborn, darks but many of them show similar lines corresponding to hair follicles. Also a remarkable linear colour modification can be observed between the darker lateral surface, which has downy hair, and the medial area which has no downy hair. A possible explanation for this observation is that hair follicles promote a darker skin colour, and this could be further confirmed by the clear demarcation between the darker pre-auricular area and the lighter surrounding area in newborns. Anatomically, Futcher's lines on the forearm, thigh and leg follow no particular nervous or venous path. As a result their nature and significance are still not understood.

Hyperpigmentation of Palmoplantar Areas

Hyperpigmented patches and marks on the palm can sometimes be observed in newborn darks but were present in 35% of the adults examined by McDonald and Kelly and in more than 60% of the subjects over the age of 65. Plantar hyperpigmentation seems to precede palmar hyperpigmentation by several years. Since neither is present at birth, repeated microtraumas, with successive post-inflammatory alterations, may be the cause of these phenomena.

Functional Features

Epidermic Hydration

The electrical resistance of skin in darks is about twice that of whites [56, 57]. Researchers claim that 80% of the skin's electrical resistance resides in the stratum corneum. Two hypotheses are suggested: the stratum corneum of darks is thicker, or the two different types of skin contain a different number of active eccrine sweat glands. Other researchers have put forward the possibility that it plays a role in skin hydration.

Greater skin hydration does of course mean greater skin conductivity and greater thickness of the stratum corneum. This would produce a mechanical blockage of pores and a decrease in perspiratory surface area in darks, who would thus have a less hydrated epidermis [58].

Thermoregulation

Adaptation is more essential for perspiration than either genetic or ethnic factors are [59, 60]. The amount of sweat produced at a given temperature is linked to acclimatization to heat rather than anatomical or physical factors of racial origin [61].

Experiments on the reaction of white and dark skin to a vasodilator yield essentially similar results, which could indicate either an identical percutaneous penetration of the substance and vasomobility or a difference in permeability compensated by different reactions [62]. Nevertheless, a different blood vessel reactivity seems to exist in darks. *Perspiratio insensibilis* increases in exactly the same way in both types of skin but is significantly higher in dark subjects over a range of temperatures [63].

Percutaneous Absorption

In general white skin is more permeable to certain chemical compounds than dark skin, but it is necessary to consider two hypotheses that may help explain this variation: a difference in the metabolism of the absorbed substance and a difference in the fixative capacity of the stratum corneum. In any case, the skin's effectiveness as a barrier is related to the compactness of the stratum corneum, and this is the reason why dark skin is less permeable [64].

The reasons for the variation in percutaneous absorption in white and dark skin are certainly more complex than had been thought of until recently [65].

Reaction to Irritants and Allergens

Traditionally, dark skin is thought to be more resistant to chemical irritation, and this has been confirmed by some studies [35]. In contrast to dark skin, white skin displays an erythematous reaction where exposed to lower concentrations of irritants, probably because dark skin is less absorbent. In fact, both types of skin have exactly the same reaction if the stratum corneum is absent [66].

A kind of irritation specific to dark skin is acne caused by creams: the acne, in this case, is a monomorphic acneiform eruption of comedones and microcysts on the forehead and temples which affects subjects who use greasy creams for prolonged periods. Its appearance is clinically and histologically the same as acne vulgaris, but inflamed papulopustular elements are rare.

In white subjects, on the other hand, prolonged use of comedogenic substances causes eruption and papulopustulosis with disturbance of hair follicles, and only secondarily do comedones appear. This experimental model clearly shows the different reactivity to irritants of the two types of skin: white skin becomes inflamed early on, cell walls rupture, and the contents of follicles pass into the dermis, while dark skin has a proliferative reaction with excess production and retention of corneous cells [67].

Sebaceous hair follicles in darks are more robust and hence more susceptible to a hyperkeratotic reaction; however, cutaneous reaction to irritants depends upon variation in permeability. Additional factors such as metabolic and inflammation mediators should not be underestimated [65].

Intradermic injection of histamine in nonatopic subjects, recorded by measuring the papule created, produces stronger reactions in darks than in whites [68].

Side effects such as lichenification and hyperpigmentation are also more significant in darks [69, 70]. The most common allergens involved both for white and dark skin are nickel and chrome.

Effects of Ultraviolet (UV) Light on Dark Skin

The photoprotective role of melanin is fundamental. The stratum corneum is a natural photoprotective barrier. Photo-induced epidermal hyperplasia is observed particularly in whites but is also found in dark-skinned subjects [75].

Protective elements in the stratum corneum have been identified as solar filters. The protective factor is calculated as a relationship between the lowest protected erythemal levels on skin and skin without protection [71]. The transmission of radiation is inversely proportional to the protective factor. The average transmission of UVB rays in the epidermis of dark subjects is 7.4%, against 24.9% in the epidermis of Caucasians. The transmission of UVB in the stratum corneum in dark individuals is 30.2%, while it is 47.6% in Caucasians. The protection degree of the epidermis of dark subjects is four times higher than that of whites for UVB, whereas the protective difference is less marked in the stratum corneum [71]. With regard to UVA, the average transmission level in the epidermis for darks is 17.5% and 55.5% for Caucasians.

The amount of melanin and the organization of melanosomes within keratinocytes vary in accordance with the type of pigmentation [72], implying that a difference in absorption of visible radiation exists in the skin [73]. The epidermis in whites is more translucent to ultraviolet, as well as visible light. At 300 nm the stimulation of melanocyte synthesis under repeated exposure to UVA produces a modest protection against the sun [71]: the lowest erythemogenic level increases by only two or three units. This process does not significantly increase the thickness of the stratum corneum and does not alter the thickness of melanosomes [74].

On the other hand, the stimulation of melanin by the administration of psoralens increases the lowest erythemogenic level by six units, making the distribution of melanosomes similar to the model for dark skin [75]. Even in dark subjects melanin is not only a photoprotective factor. According to various authors, the lowest erythemogenic amount in darks is between 10 and 30 times higher than that of whites. It is also difficult to measure erythema and determine the minimum erythemogenic dose [59, 71].

Dryness and skin flaking that appear a day after sun exposure are often the only indication of sunburn [45]. Photosensitivity is present in darks: it can be caused by medicines, contact and polymorphic lucites [59]. On the other hand, phototoxic reactions are infrequent in darks, as are pathologies caused by continuous exposure to UVA and UVB (actinic keratosis, keratoacanthoma, basal cell and spinocellular carcinoma, ageing of skin), all disorders due to prolonged absorption of high amounts of such radiations.

Effects of UV on the Immune System

UVB rays alter the function of Langerhans cells, causing temporary immunodepression [76]. Hollis and Scheibner observed a depletion of Langerhans cells after a single exposure to UVB rays, equally in both dark-skinned Australian aboriginals and light-skinned Australians of Celtic origin. The darker skin protects Langerhans cells more effectively than the light skin, but in neither case was photoprotection sufficient to prevent this reduction [77].

In white subjects, after being exposed to UV rays, Langerhans cells move from a median to a basal position in the epidermis, while in darks the opposite occurs. Melanocytes in darks respond more efficiently to solar stimulation and are more sensitive than those of whites. However, compared to the melanocytes in darks, they do not interfere with the activity of Langerhans cells nor protect them from depletion after multiple UV exposures [78].

Vitamin D Synthesis

Cutaneous synthesis of vitamin D is probably the only benefit of UV radiation in humans. Vitamin D is produced in the lowest area of the epidermis following exposure to UVB (290–320 nm) [79]. A large proportion of photons at this wavelength penetrate the epidermis in whites [80], but four times less photon penetration occurs in dark skin [71]. A lower amount of vitamin D is produced in the epidermis of darks, as was observed by Beadle [81]. The risk of vitamin D deficiency is therefore higher in darks. The capability of vitamin D production is identical in both whites and darks. However, the difficulty in vitamin D synthesis in darks resides in the extra melanin that acts as a barrier to UVB rays. Therefore, darks require a longer sun exposure than whites in order to achieve the same level of vitamin D production.

Melanogenesis

Melanocytes are the cells responsible for melanin synthesis. They are dendritic cells located in the basal layer of the epidermis and do not contain tonofilaments or desmosomes. Melanocytes are also present in hair follicles (external epithelial sheath, bulbus pili) and in mucous membranes. However, the melanocyte system is not limited only to the skin, pigmentation cells being also present in ocular structures (uvea, choroid, retina), internal ear and leptomeninges. The precursors of melanocytes are the melanoblasts, which are formed in the neural crest before moving towards the skin surface between the fourth and eighth week of the embryonic stage. It is at this point that melanoblasts become melanocytes and acquire the ability to produce melanosomes. Later, the melanocytes begin to colonize certain anatomical areas through mitotic division. The steps of melanogenesis can be outlined in the following scheme:

- Synthesis of melanosome components (enzymes, structural proteins)
- Formation of melanosomes
- Melanization of melanosomes
- Transfer of melanosomes to keratinocytes
- Degradation of melanosomes
- Elimination of melanin through the shedding of the stratum corneum, or at the dermal level, lymphatically [82]

Eumelanins are insoluble dark brown or dark pigments which contain carbon, hydrogen and nitrogen. Pheomelanin pigments are yellow, light brown or red and contain sulphur in addition to the above elements. Despite these differences, all melanic pigments have the same metabolic pathway. A sequence of oxidative reactions, some of which may be enzyme controlled, leads to the production of quinones that subsequently will enter in the composition of the terminal polymer. The addition of sulphur-containing substances (cysteine, glutathione) to the DOPA-quinone leads to biosynthesis of pheomelanins [83]. The synthesized molecules of cysteine-DOPA molecules polymerize. Various enzymatic systems regulate the intramelanocytic level of compounds containing sulphur. Most melanin pigments in mammals contain more or less the same proportion of sulphur compounds, independently of the colour of the pigment itself.

Skin pigmentation is genetically determined (see before). The genes which influence pigmentation act both directly on melanoblasts and/or melanocytes and indirectly through the environment surrounding these cells especially through keratinocyte activity.

There is also the effect of hormonal influence. The hypophysis produces various peptides which have a melanotrophic action. Within the steroid hormones, oestrogens have a stimulatory action. The effect of progesterone is more controversial, but oestrogen and progesterone work synergistically. Testosterone has a stimulatory effect on melanogenesis. The influence of thyroid hormones, although well known in amphibians, is still unclear in humans [84].

Dermatoses and Skin Colour

Sycosis cruris, a clinical condition which is observed in dark people in West Africa, is in part determined by ethnic and climatic characteristics and partly by the habit of applying certain oils to the skin. In other cases ethnic differences are well documented [85], for example, between Caucasians and Congoids, with particular reference to pigmentation, hair, hair follicles and the eccrine and apocrine sweat glands.

The terms "dark" and "white" have no relevance to geographical classification. They become inadequate as soon as attention is drawn to cultural categories rather than to an objective description of skin colour.

Pigmentation in darks is not uniform. Palmar and plantar regions and the periorbital area are not pigmented homogeneously, which can be problematic for elaborating a differential diagnosis. For example, multiple patches make a diagnosis of palmoplantar syphilis difficult.

Eczema may occur as hyperchromic or hypochromic. Pityriasis versicolor may occur in a hyperpigmented form with fine dark scales that give the skin a typical "crasseux" appearance. Hyperpigmentation with necrosis at the top of the bumps during toxidermia contrasts with the depigmentation of the skin below.

Hypopigmentation is found in about 40% of men and about 30% of women affecting the medio-sternal and lateral areas of the body. Pigmentation of areas exposed to the sun is often more intense than in areas that are usually covered. In chubby children pigmentation is less accentuated in skin folds [86].

Pigmentation of the mucous membranes is frequent, non-homogeneous and irregular and found in approximately 70% of subjects over the age of 50. Leuko-oedema, a greyish-white translucent film on the inside of the cheeks, is benign and found in about 50% of children. This leuko-oedema is due to an oedema of the Malpighian epithelium.

The gums are often pigmented, the colouration varying from blue to dark brown. In atypical forms, it is necessary to examine closely the pathological pigmentation of the mouth and check for exposure to mineral salts, synthetic antimalarial medicines, phenothiazine, Addison's disease, haematochromatosis and tattoos done with carbon. Tattooing of the gums sometimes provokes hyperpigmented gingival tumours.

In Europeans the erythematic macula, with little or no pigment, testifies to a previous inflammation, as it indicates vasodilatation of the skin. In subjects with slightly darker skin, erythema assumes a brownish colour. In even darker skin, erythema appears as a slate blue colour. In very dark patients like the Senegalese, the colour is a dark blue skin and may not be noticeable at all. The skin temperature and oedema when palpated are the best indicators to evaluate the degree of inflammation in dark skin [87].

Dark-skinned African children never show roseola. Early oculonasal catarrh and late furfuraceous flaking are the only symptoms of the illness. Simple lesions in dark subjects are sometimes observed in unusual forms and dimensions with respect to those found in whites. The initial markings of Gibert's pityriasis rosea are sometimes two to three times larger than those seen in whites. These large-sized lesions quickly become covered with numerous scales [88]. Lesions which last for long periods of time can become sites of lichenification. According to some authors, this is provoked by personal hygiene habits. The use of vegetable or cocoa fibre sponges for personal hygiene (similar to a horsehair glove) gives normal skin a shiny or satin finish but is severely harmful for people with dermatoses. Vigorous buffing by the patient aggravates and prolongs symptoms, provoking a generalized Koebner phenomenon.

Mobile Human Population

The world's mobile human population, people who temporarily or permanently cross borders for reasons of employment, politics or tourism, comprised 1.4 billion people in 2019. In particular, 258 million people travelled in search of employment. This demonstrates increasing desperation in the world: in the 1980s the number was 70 million. Mobility has always been a necessity for humanity and has constantly been mixing human geography and state of health. Travelling always includes danger and the risk of illness; the word itself possesses a relationship to illness. The profoundly rooted idea that travelling is an experience that builds character and tests the health of the traveller is seen clearly in the German adjective bewandert that today means "shrewd" or "expert" but in the fifteenth century simply meant "well-travelled". The English verbs to fare and to fear have the same etymological root and have the experiential terrain in common, within the idea of travelling.

Ethnomedicine

Another feature of recent history, paralleling the phenomenon of immigration, is the growing interest in ethnomedicine in the West countries. This discipline protects and reclaims the medicinal culture of developing countries. The forms and qualities of natural or traditional therapies used by people in tropical or "distant" countries continually stimulate anthropological and medical curiosity and interest in Europe. The remedies used are often perceived as a mix between medicine and magic, where it is difficult to separate one from the other. We have no difficulty in admitting that certain plants have unanimously recognized therapeutic qualities, but we view the rites, celebrations and attitudes of appeasement that often accompany therapeutic events or are themselves viewed as therapeutic events, with healthy scepticism. But more than anthropological interest, the clinical and scientific interest that

"other" cultures have raised in Europe and the United States has resulted in millions of patients using remedies and therapies defined "complementary" or "natural". Furthermore, these disciplines are taught in many universities, and many hospitals have created or are planning to open wards that incorporate and study these new/ancient medicines.

In contrast to the past, researchers now rarely go to distant countries to study other habits and medicines. The phenomenon of immigration means that patients, with their different cultures, rites and habits, "bring" the concrete use of "other" medicines to Italy and Europe.

In today's multi-ethnic societies, ethnomedicine can be a useful aid for Western physicians and healthcare personnel in understanding immigrant illness.

In fact, whether in an intercultural or intracultural context, patients present themselves with the totality of their experiences and their knowledge and are examined by people who are likely to have a completely different perspective. Misunderstanding is often an obstacle to effective treatment. Knowing what is being talked about and how to discuss it together, and knowing in what overall scheme the patients' comments are contextualized, leads to a better understanding of how to treat their suffering and improves the effectiveness of treatment.

We have seen a return of scientific attention to natural treatments, remedies derived from ancient medical practices such as Ayurveda, centuries-old Indian medicine, based on an extraordinary body of work or the long tradition of Chinese medicine and particularly acupuncture in recent years. There are many forms of complementary medicine, and international debate between the proponents and detractors of these practices is lively. In this article, we will limit ourselves to describing certain skin conditions most frequently observed as side effects of alternative medical practices, putting aside for the moment the debate on the usefulness of complementary or alternative medicine, as dealt with by Witkowski and Parish in 2002 [89].

Ethnodermatology

Our service has an extremely varied patient group, coming from different and distant geographical and cultural situations. In our outpatient clinic we see more and more frequently people of different-coloured skin, with skin lesions that are difficult to identify. It is very important to understand the country of origin and related cultural behaviours, which often have an effect on skin and venereal clinical pictures. It is thus possible, after taking an accurate case history and doing a careful medical examination, to reveal particular and varying behaviours that may lead to the appearance of certain skin lesions. Some of these conditions derive from peculiar cosmetic practices, such as acquired ochronosis, alopecia and follicular-occlusive disturbances. Others are linked to traditional medical practices such as cupping, coining, scraping, moxibustion or to anthropological and ritual reasons, such as female genital mutilation and keloids resulting from perforation. At the Centre for Preventive Medicine for Migration, Tourism and Tropical Dermatology of the San Gallicano Institute, numerous dermatological disturbances related to various common cultural practices in use in the country of origin have been observed. The difficulty of diagnosing and doing a differential diagnosis and follow-up due to the particular "mobility" of this population is critical.

These cultural behaviours can be subdivided into:

1. Cosmetic habits
2. Traditional medical practices
3. Anthropological and ritual motives
4. Psychocultural motives
1. Among traditional cosmetic practices that produce dermopathologies, we find the use of:
   - Depigmentation substances
   - Hair products
   - Greasy creams

The use of depigmentation products containing hydroquinone can have the opposite effect from that intended and lead to ochronotic-type hyperpigmentation of dark skin. The pathogenic mechanism lies in the inhibition of oxidase of homogentisic acid in the skin, with a consequent local accumulation of the acid in the skin and successive polymerization and production of ochronotic fibre. The characteristic xerosis of dark skin and particularly of the skin of immigrants from the Indian subcontinent induces them to use continually greasy substances, with a consequent development of follicular-occlusive phenomena. The clinical picture is often that of so-called pomade acne, made up of usually comedogenic lesions, with few inflammatory elements, but which may leave pigmentary results for a long time.

2. The principal traditional medical practices leading to lesions are:
   - Cupping
   - Coining
   - Moxibustion
   - Piercing

Lesions resulting from traditional medicine must often be looked at using differential diagnosis with sexual abuse, in particular in infancy.

Cupping consists in the application of hot glass cups or suction cups in which a vacuum has been created. In dry cupping the interior of a round glass cup is covered with alcohol. The alcohol is then burned and the cup applied to the skin. In the wet method an incision is made on the skin, and the cup is applied in such a way as to encourage bleeding. The vacuum created by the combustion of air creates suction on the skin within the cup, with consequent local hyperaemia. There are many hypotheses for the use of cupping, from biophysical mechanisms to magic-ritual practices. The most common are:

- Driving evil spirits out (medicine men in primitive cultures)
- Draining of "humours" from diseased internal organs (ancient Greece)
- Theory of "counterirritation"
- Nerve and hormone theories
- Psychosomatic theories
- Chinese theory of energy

In the humoural theory, cupping drains "humours" from the area below the skin, therefore eliminating pathologies from internal organs damaged by an excess of humour. The theory of counterirritation states that irritation of the skin, in producing local hyperaemia with an increase in blood flow to the surface, eliminates congestion in diseased internal organs. The nerve and hormone theories state that irritation of the skin causes a nervous or hormonal reflex reaction that produces favourable circulatory or trophic effects on the organs below.

Coining consists in vigorously rubbing a coin over the chest or back after applying hot oil or Tiger Balm, to the point of creating ecchymosis and linear petechiae. The idea is to "liberate the breath" and has a therapeutic goal in curing a myriad of adult disturbances but particularly fever in children. Superficial observation often causes coining lesions (cao-gio in Cambodian) to be mistaken for child abuse.

Moxibustion uses heated sticks, incense or herbal sticks such as *Artemisia vulgaris*. The material used takes the name of moxa. The *Artemisia* is placed inside burning cones, or moxa cigars are used, which may cause burns, generally in the abdominal, neck or heel regions. It is often used as a last resort when other methods have not been effective or for chronic respiratory illness.

Piercing (perforation of the skin) is traditionally used to distinguish the roles of members within a tribe. It regulates the relations between individuals, both day to day and during ceremonies, establishing with a single glance the position of the individual in relation to the group. Nowadays it is very fashionable among young people in the West. It often causes dermatitis due to contact with nickel sulphate.

3. Among anthropological-ritual dermopathologies found are:
   - Female genital mutilation (FGM)
   - Scarification (scraping, branding, cutting)
   - Tattoos
   - Perforation (lip plates, ear plates)

Female genital mutilation (FGM) is a condition that, while originating in distant countries and regions, is frequently observable in our country due to the continuous flow of people from the African continent, particularly Egypt, the Horn of Africa and sub-Saharan Africa. While being frequently practiced by people of the Islamic religion, it is also observed among Christian populations, animists and Jews (Ethiopian Falashas).

In this connection, for a clear definition of FGM, it would be appropriate to report here the joint statement issued in April 1997 by the World Health Organization (WHO), by the United Nations International Children's Emergency Fund (UNICEF) and by the United Nations Population Fund (UNFPA): "Female genital mutilation comprises all procedures involving partial or total removal of the external female genitalia or other injury to the female genital organs whether for cultural or other non-therapeutic reasons". The three agencies also classified the different types of FGM as follows:

- Type 1. Excision of the prepuce, with removal of all or part of the clitoris.
- Type 2. Excision of the clitoris, with removal of all or part of the labia minora.
- Type 3. Excision of all or part of the external genitalia and narrowing of the vaginal opening (infibulation).
- Type 4. Unclassified: includes perforation, penetration or incision of the clitoris and/or labia; stretching of the clitoris and/or labia; cauterization by burning the clitoris and surrounding tissue; scraping of the tissue surrounding the vaginal opening (angurya cuts) or incision of the vagina (gishira cuts); introduction of corrosive substances or herbs into the vagina to cause bleeding in order to close or tighten it; and any other procedure falling under the definition of FGM.

The complications observed are serious, both physical (haemorrhagic shock, vaginal fistulae, keloids, dermoid cysts) and psychosexual. A specially created law prohibits the practice being carried out in Italy [90–92].

Scarification is the creation, through whatever technique, of one or more permanent scars in any area of the skin. It is used in African societies for decoration of the face or for medical reasons.

Branding is a particular form of scarification using heated metal instruments.

Cutting is carried out by incision of the skin, repeated in the same spot over time, with the goal of obtaining a clear and visible mark. In other cases, the wounds are temporarily kept open in order to create a pronounced scar like a keloid.

Cutaneous perforations are common in ethnic groups from Central Africa. One of these is the lip disk. The women of the Mursi tribes in Ethiopia use a rounded disk made of clay, and the perforated lip is continually manipulated to make it more elastic and capacious. Sometimes the lower incisors are removed to create more stability. In Sudan, Suma women use a rectangular plate made of light balsa wood. The lower incisors are removed for greater stability. If the lip, freed from its plate, reaches up to the top of the woman's head, she will be especially prized and her dowry extremely large.

4. Among psychocultural motivations found are:
   • Dhat syndrome

The term "Dhat syndrome" was coined by Wig in 1960 and describes a culture-bound syndrome common in the Indian subcontinent, related to a Hindu theory according to which seminal fluid is rich in a particular vital force and losing it impoverishes the physical and psychic energy of the individual.

This disorder is characterized by profound anxiety over the loss of seminal fluid through ejaculation and wet dreams. The term "culture-bound" means a psychopathological entity of defined geographic prevalence determined by the beliefs and paradigms of a specific cultural area. Clinical symptomatology often mimics prostatitis, aspecific urethritis or epididymitis, with consistent negative results of microbiological exams. Patients complain of anxiety, feeling unwell, burning sensations, weakness, psychic distur-

bance and trembling. Most clinical studies have investigated the phenomenon of "Dhat syndrome" in the resident population in the country of origin. In Italy, an increasing number of cases can be seen in immigrants. A multidisciplinary approach is very important, with the presence of anthropologists, ethno-psychologists and the help of linguistic-cultural mediators.

Conclusions

In every era and in every human population, a particular vision of the world and perception of health and illness is constructed through culture and knowledge. People interpret their own situation in forms and ways based on their culture's knowledge, which is transmitted and used in everyday life, through different rites and rituals.

From this knowledge, each group focuses on and develops whatever appears most useful for their well-being and turns it into tradition. Representations of good and evil, wisdom and foolishness, physiology and pathology are articulated through a variety of cultural models. Differing classifications are made according to different knowledge, and the meeting of complementary and conventional medicine produces complex and fluid situations. Today we have the fascinating task of reading and developing these, for our own future and the future of our children. Dermatology is the medical-scientific discipline that, more than any other, may help all of us in this historical challenge.

References

1. Nadel SF. The Nuba. Oxford: Oxford University Press; 1947.
2. Barth JF. Ethnic groups and boundaries. The social organization of culture difference. Bergen-Oslo: Universitets Forleget; 1969.
3. Amselle JL, M'Bokolo E, editors. Au Coeur de l'ethnie. Ethnies, tribalisme et ètat en Afrique. Paris: La Découverte; 1985.
4. Fabietti U. L'identità etnica. Storia e critica di un concetto equivoco. Carocci: Roma; 1995.
5. Gallissot R, Kilani M, Rivera A. L'imbroglio etnico, in quattordici parole-chiave. Dedalo: Bari; 1997.

6. Levi- Strauss C. Razza e storia e altri studi di antropologia. Torino: Einaudi; 1967.

7. Marazzi A. Lo sguardo antropologico. Processi educative e multiculturalismo. Carocci: Roma; 2006.

8. Tullio-Altan C. Ethnos e civiltà. Identità etniche e valori democratici. Feltrinelli: Milano; 1995.

9. Morrone A. Racism and medicine. In: Bolaffi G, Bracalenti R, Braham P, Gindro S, editors. Dictionary of race, ethnicity and culture. London: Sage; 2003.

10. Fabietti U, Remotti F, editors. Etnicità, in Dizionario di Antropologia. Bologna: Zanichelli; 2001. p. 271.

11. Balandier G. Le società comunicanti. Laterza: Bari; 1971.

12. Fabietti U. Elementi di antropologia culturale. Milano: Mondadori Università; 2004.

13. Van Der Berghe PL. Race and racism. A comparative perspective. New York: Wiley; 1967.

14. Smith AD. Le origini etniche della nazione. Il Mulino: Bologna; 1992.

15. Renan E. Che cos'è una nazione? Donzelli: Roma; 1993.

16. Amselle JL. Ethnie. In: Encyclopaedie Universalis, corpus VIII. Paris: E.U. Edit à Paris. p. 971–3.

17. Redcliff-Brown AR, Forde D, editors. African systems of kinship and marriage. Oxford: Oxford University Press; 1950.

18. Fortes M, Evans-Pritchard E, editors. African political systems. Oxford: Oxford University Press; 1940.

19. Darwin C. The descent of man and selection in relation to sex. London: John Murray; 1871. p. 11.

20. Linneus C. Systema Naturae per Regna Tria Naturae, secundum classes, ordines, genera, species, cum characteribus, differentiis, synonymis, locis. Holmiae: Imprensis Laurentii Salvii, 1758. 2 volumi.

21. Blumenbach JF. Ueber die natürlichen Verschiedenheiten im Menschengeschlechte. Breitkopf und Härtel, Leipzig; 1798.

22. Cuvier G. Tableau élementaire de l'histoire naturelle des animaux. Paris: Baudoin. p. 1799.

23. Chardin J. Voyage de Paris a Ispahan. In: Voyages en Perse et autres lieux etc. Vo1. I, Edité par Amsterdam aux Depens de la Compagne; 1735.

24. Holubar K. What is a caucasian? J Invest Dermatol. 1996;106(4):800. https://doi.org/10.1111/1523-1747. ep12346434.

25. Morrone A. Health system and skin diseases: the case of Ethiopia. Roma: Di punto in bianco Ed; 2007.

26. Bastonini E, Kovacs D, Picardo M. Skin pigmentation and pigmentary disorders: focus on epidermal/dermal cross-talk. Ann Dermatol. 2016;28(3):279–89. https:// doi.org/10.5021/ad.2016.28.3.279.

27. Mahe YF, Michelet JF, Billoni N, et al. Androgenetic alopecia and microinflammation. Int J Dermatol. 2000;39(8):576–84.

28. Mahé A, Ly F, Aymard G, Dangou JM. Skin diseases associated with the cosmetic use of bleaching products in women from Dakar, Senegal. Br J Dermatol. 2003;148:493–500.

29. Jablonski NG, Chaplin G. The evolution of human skin coloration. J Hum Evol. 2000;39(1):57–106. https://doi.org/10.1006/jhev.2000.0403.

30. Taylor SC, Cook-Bolden F. Defining skin of color. Cutis. 2002;69(6):435–7.

31. Langton AK, Alessi S, Hann M, et al. Aging in skin of color: disruption to elastic Fiber organization is detrimental to skin's biomechanical function. J Invest Dermatol. 2019;139(4):779–88. https://doi.org/10.1016/j.jid.2018.10.026.

32. Morrone A. Atlas of dermatological diseases on dark skin, medical communications Srl Ed. Torino. 2007.

33. Hearing VJ. Milestones in melanocytes/melanogenesis. J Invest Dermatol. 2011;131(E1):E1. https://doi.org/10.1038/skinbio.2011.1.

34. Cavalli-Sforza LL. Genes, peoples, and languages. Proc Natl Acad Sci U S A. 1997;94(15):7719–24. https://doi.org/10.1073/pnas.94.15.7719.

35. Weigand DA, Haygood C, Gaylor JR. Cell layers and density of Negro and Caucasian stratum corneum. J Invest Dermatol. 1974;62(6):563–8. https://doi.org/10.1111/1523-1747.ep12679412.

36. Corcuff P, Chaussepied C, Madry G, Hadjur C. Skin optics revisited by in vivo confocal microscopy: melanin and sun exposure. J Cosmet Sci. 2001;52(2):91–102.

37. Fellner MJ, Chen AS, Mont M, McCabe J, Baden M. Patterns and intensity of autofluorescence and its relation to melanin in human epidermis and hair. Int J Dermatol. 1979;18(9):722–30. https://doi.org/10.1111/j.1365-4362.1979.tb05009.x.

38. Bang J, Zippin JH. Cyclic adenosine monophosphate (cAMP) signaling in melanocyte pigmentation and melanomagenesis [published online ahead of print, 2020 Aug 10]. Pigment Cell Melanoma Res. 2020; https://doi.org/10.1111/pcmr.12920.

39. Novales RR. On the role of cyclic AMP in the function of skin melanophores. Ann N Y Acad Sci. 1971;185:494–506. https://doi.org/10.1111/j.1749-6632.1971.tb45276.x.

40. Vasilevskiĭ VK, Zherebtsov LD, Spichak AD, Feoktistov SM. Tsvet i morfologicheskie osobennosti kozhnogo pokrova u liudeĭ razlichnykh rasovykh grupp [color and morphological characteristics of the skin in people of different racial groups]. Biull Eksp Biol Med. 1988;106(10):495–8.

41. Zhong G, Yang X, Jiang X, et al. Dopamine-melanin nanoparticles scavenge reactive oxygen and nitrogen species and activate autophagy for osteoarthritis therapy [published correction appears in Nanoscale. 2019 Dec 28;11(48):23504–23505]. Nanoscale. 2019;11(24):11605–16. https://doi.org/10.1039/c9nr03060c.

42. Yousef H, Alhajj M, Sharma S. Anatomy, skin (integument), epidermis. In: StatPearls. Treasure Island (FL): StatPearls publishing; July 27, 2020.

43. Kapoor R, Dhatwalia SK, Kumar R, Rani S, Parsad D. Emerging role of dermal compartment in skin pigmentation: comprehensive review [published online ahead of print, 2020 Apr 3]. J Eur Acad Dermatol Venereol. 2020; https://doi.org/10.1111/jdv.16404.

44. Kiprono SK, Chaula BM, Masenga JE, Muchunu JW, Mavura DR, Moehrle M. Epidemiology of keloids

in normally pigmented Africans and African people with albinism: population-based cross-sectional survey. Br J Dermatol. 2015;173(3):852–4. https://doi.org/10.1111/bjd.13826.

45. Garcia RI, Mitchell RE, Bloom J, Szabo G. Number of epidermal melanocytes, hair follicles, and sweat ducts in skin of Solomon islanders. Am J Phys Anthropol. 1977;47(3):427–33. https://doi.org/10.1002/ajpa.1330470314.

46. Kawahata A, Sakamoto H. Some observations on sweating of the Aino. Jpn J Physiol. 1951;2(2):166–9. https://doi.org/10.2170/jjphysiol.2.166.

47. Mujahid N, Liang Y, Murakami R, et al. A UV-independent topical small-molecule approach for melanin production in human skin. Cell Rep. 2017;19(11):2177–84.   https://doi.org/10.1016/j.celrep.2017.05.042.

48. Sonnenschein RR, Kobrin H, Janowitz HD, Grossman MI. Stimulation and inhibition of human sweat glands by intradermal sympathomimetic agents. J Appl Physiol. 1951;3(10):573–81. https://doi.org/10.1152/jappl.1951.3.10.573.

49. Hodge BD, Brodell RT. Anatomy, skin sweat glands. In: StatPearls. Treasure Island (FL): StatPearls Publishing; August 16, 2020.

50. Cavallini C, Vitiello G, Adinolfi B, et al. Melanin and Melanin-like hybrid materials in regenerative medicine. Nanomaterials (Basel). 2020;10(8):E1518. Published 2020 Aug 3. https://doi.org/10.3390/nano10081518.

51. Hein K, Cohen MI, McNamara H. Racial differences in nitrogen content of nails among adolescents. Am J Clin Nutr. 1977;30(4):496–8. https://doi.org/10.1093/ajcn/30.4.496.

52. Zieleniewski Ł, Schwartz RA, Goldberg DJ, Handler MZ. Voigt-Futcher pigmentary demarcation lines. J Cosmet Dermatol. 2019;18(3):700–2. https://doi.org/10.1111/jocd.12884.

53. Belzile E, McCuaig C, Le Meur JB, et al. Patterned cutaneous hypopigmentation phenotype characterization: a retrospective study in 106 children. Pediatr Dermatol. 2019;36(6):869–75. https://doi.org/10.1111/pde.13913.

54. Vollum DI. Skin markings in negro children from the West Indies. Br J Dermatol. 1972;86(3):260–3.   https://doi.org/10.1111/j.1365-2133.1972.tb02226.x.

55. McDonald CJ. Polyamines in psoriasis. J Invest Dermatol. 1983;81(5):385–7. https://doi.org/10.1111/1523-1747.ep12521665.

56. Davies DJ, Heylings JR, Gayes H, McCarthy TJ, Mack MC. Further development of an in vitro model for studying the penetration of chemicals through compromised skin. Toxicol In Vitro. 2017;38:101–7. https://doi.org/10.1016/j.tiv.2016.10.004.

57. Berardesca E, de Rigal J, Leveque JL, Maibach HI. In vivo biophysical characterization of skin physiological differences in races. Dermatologica. 1991;182(2):89–93. https://doi.org/10.1159/000247752.

58. Fowles DC, Rosenberry R. Effects of epidermal hydration on skin potential responses and levels.

Psychophysiology. 1973;10(6):601–11. https://doi.org/10.1111/j.1469-8986.1973.tb00810.x.

59. Plikus MV, Van Spyk EN, Pham K, et al. The circadian clock in skin: implications for adult stem cells, tissue regeneration, cancer, aging, and immunity. J Biol Rhythm. 2015;30(3):163–82. https://doi.org/10.1177/0748730414563537.

60. Yousef H, Ramezanpour Ahangar E, Varacallo M. Physiology, thermal regulation. In: StatPearls. Treasure Island (FL): StatPearls Publishing; June 19, 2020.

61. McDonald CJ. Some thoughts on differences in dark and white skin. Int J Dermatol. 1976;15(6):427–30. https://doi.org/10.1111/j.1365-4362.1976.tb00229.x.

62. Tur E, Maibach HI, Guy RH. Spatial variability of vasodilatation in human forearm skin. Br J Dermatol. 1985;113(2):197–203. https://doi.org/10.1111/j.1365-2133.1985.tb02065.x.

63. Forslind B, Engström S, Engblom J, Norlén L. A novel approach to the understanding of human skin barrier function. J Dermatol Sci. 1997;14(2):115–25. https://doi.org/10.1016/s0923-1811(96)00559-2.

64. Roberts MS. Solute-vehicle-skin interactions in percutaneous absorption: the principles and the people. Skin Pharmacol Physiol. 2013;26(4–6):356–70. https://doi.org/10.1159/000353647.

65. Larouche D, Lavoie A, Paquet C, Simard-Bisson C, Germain L. Identification of epithelial stem cells in vivo and in vitro using keratin 19 and BrdU. Methods Mol Biol. 2010;585:383–400. https://doi.org/10.1007/978-1-60761-380-0_27.

66. Callender VD. Acne in ethnic skin: special considerations for therapy. Dermatol Ther. 2004;17(2):184–95. https://doi.org/10.1111/j.1396-0296.2004.04019.x.

67. Modena DAO, Miranda ACG, Grecco C, Liebano RE, Cordeiro RCT, Guidi RM. Efficacy, safety, and guidelines of application of the fractional ablative laser erbium YAG 2940 nm and non-ablative laser erbium glass in rejuvenation, skin spots, and acne in different skin phototypes: a systematic review [published online ahead of print, 2020 May 29]. Lasers Med Sci. 2020; https://doi.org/10.1007/s10103-020-03046-7.

68. Van Niekerk CH, Prinsloo AE. Effect of skin pigmentation on the response to intradermal histamine. Int Arch Allergy Appl Immunol. 1985;76(1):73–5. https://doi.org/10.1159/000233664.

69. Fisher AA. Contact dermatitis in dark patients. Cutis. 1977;20(3)

70. Fairhurst DA, Shah M. Comparison of patch test results among white Europeans and patients from the Indian subcontinent living within the same community. J Eur Acad Dermatol Venereol. 2008;22(10):1227–31. https://doi.org/10.1111/j.1468-3083.2008.02787.x.

71. Kaidbey KH, Agin PP, Sayre RM, Kligman AM. Photoprotection by melanin–a comparison of dark and Caucasian skin. J Am Acad Dermatol. 1979;1(3):249–60.   https://doi.org/10.1016/s0190-9622(79)70018-1.

72. Quevedo WC, Szabó G, Virks J. Influence of age and UV on the populations of dopa-positive melanocytes in human skin. J Invest Dermatol. 1969;52(3):287–90.

73. Willis I. Photosensitivity reactions in dark skin. Dermatol Clin. 1988;6(3):369–75.

74. Parrish JA, Anderson RR, Ying CY, Pathak MA. Cutaneous effects of pulsed nitrogen gas laser irradiation. J Invest Dermatol. 1976;67(5):603–8. https://doi.org/10.1111/1523-1747.ep12541699.

75. Danno K, Toda K, Ikai K, Horio T, Imamura S. Ultraviolet radiation suppresses mouse-ear edema induced by topical application of arachidonic acid. Arch Dermatol Res. 1990;282(1):42–6. https://doi.org/10.1007/BF00505644.

76. Yan B, Liu N, Li J, et al. The role of Langerhans cells in epidermal homeostasis and pathogenesis of psoriasis [published online ahead of print, 2020 Sep 11]. J Cell Mol Med. 2020; https://doi.org/10.1111/jcmm.15834.

77. Hollis DE, Scheibner A. Ultrastructural changes in epidermal Langerhans cells and melanocytes in response to ultraviolet irradiation, in Australians of Aboriginal and Celtic descent. Br J Dermatol. 1988;119(1):21–31. https://doi.org/10.1111/j.1365-2133.1988.tb07097.x.

78. Morison WL. Effects of ultraviolet radiation on the immune system in humans. Photochem Photobiol. 1989;50(4):515–24. https://doi.org/10.1111/j.1751-1097.1989.tb05557.x.

79. Holick MF, Smith E, Pincus S. Skin as the site of vitamin D synthesis and target tissue for 1,25-dihydroxyvitamin D3. Use of calcitriol (1,25-dihydroxyvitamin D3) for treatment of psoriasis. Arch Dermatol. 1987;123(12):1677–1683a.

80. Holick MF, McNeill SC, MacLaughlin JA, Holick SA, Clark MB, Potts JT Jr. Physiologic implications of the formation of previtamin D3 in skin. Trans Assoc Am Phys. 1979;92:54–63.

81. Beadle PC. The epidermal biosynthesis of cholecalciferol (vitamin D3). Photochem Photobiol. 1977;25(6):519–27. https://doi.org/10.1111/j.1751-1097.1977.tb09122.x.

82. Hida T, Kamiya T, Kawakami A, et al. Elucidation of melanogenesis cascade for identifying pathophysiology and therapeutic approach of pigmentary disorders and melanoma. Int J Mol Sci. 2020;21(17):E6129. Published 2020 Aug 25. https://doi.org/10.3390/ijms21176129.

83. Schlessinger DI, Anoruo M, Schlessinger J. Biochemistry, melanin. In: StatPearls. Treasure Island (FL): StatPearls publishing; July 10, 2020.

84. Bertolesi GE, McFarlane S. Melanin-concentrating hormone like (MCHL) and somatolactin. A teleost specific hypothalamic-hypophyseal axis system linking physiological and morphological pigmentation [published online ahead of print, 2020 Sep 8]. Pigment Cell Melanoma Res. 2020; https://doi.org/10.1111/pcmr.12924.

85. Ting HC. Dermatitis cruris pustulosa et atrophicans: case reports. Med J Malaysia. 1984;39(1):82–4.

86. Bach MA, Chatenoud L, Wallach D, Phan Dinh Tuy F, Cottenot F. Studies on T cell subsets and functions in leprosy. Clin Exp Immunol. 1981;44(3):491–500.

87. Kohli I, Braunberger TL, Nahhas AF, et al. Long-wavelength ultraviolet A1 and visible light Photoprotection: a multimodality assessment of dose and response. Photochem Photobiol. 2020;96(1):208–14. https://doi.org/10.1111/php.13157.

88. Takaki Y, Miyazaki H. Cytolytic degeneration of keratinocytes adjacent to Langerhans cells in pityriasis rosea (Gibert). Acta Derm Venereol. 1976;56(2):99–103.

89. Knapowski J, Wieczorowska-Tobis K, Witowski J. Pathophysiology of ageing. J Physiol Pharmacol. 2002;53(2):135–46.

90. Morrone A, Hercogova' J, Lotti T, Dermatology of Human Populations, Bologna: MNL; 2004.

91. Dave AJ, Sethi A, Morrone A. Female genital mutilation: what every American dermatologist needs to know. Dermatol Clin. 2011;29(1):103–9. https://doi.org/10.1016/j.det.2010.09.002. PMID: 21095534.

92. Morrone A, Female genital mutilation. In: Morrone A, Hay R, Naafs B editors. Skin disorders in migrants. Cham: Springer Nature Switzerland; 2020. pp 191–207.

Index

© Springer Nature Switzerland AG 2021
B. S. Li, H. I. Maibach (eds.), *Ethnic Skin and Hair and Other Cultural Considerations*, Updates in
Clinical Dermatology, https://doi.org/10.1007/978-3-030-64830-5

Printed in the United States
by Baker & Taylor Publisher Services